# ARTICULATION AND PHONOLOGY RESOURCE GUIDE FOR SCHOOL-AGE CHILDREN AND ADULTS

# SINGULAR RESOURCE GUIDE SERIES

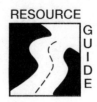

## EDITOR

**Ken Bleile, Ph.D.**
Department of Communicative Disorders
University of Northern Iowa
Cedar Falls, Iowa

## ASSOCIATE EDITORS

**Brian Goldstein, Ph.D.**
Communication Sciences
Temple University
Philadelphia, Pennsylvania

**Sharron Glennen, Ph.D.**
Department of Communication Sciences and Disorders
Towson University
Towson, Maryland

**Carole Roth, Ph.D.**
Department of Speech Pathology
Hennepin County Medical Center
Minneapolis, Minnesota

**Amy Weiss, Ph.D.**
Department of Speech Pathology and Audiology
University of Iowa
Iowa City, Iowa

**Tricia Zebrowski, Ph.D.**
Department of Speech Pathology and Audiology
University of Iowa
Iowa City, Iowa

# ARTICULATION AND PHONOLOGY RESOURCE GUIDE FOR SCHOOL-AGE CHILDREN AND ADULTS

## Ann Bosma Smit, Ph. D.
Communication Sciences and Disorders
School of Family Studies and Human Services
Kansas State University
Manhattan, Kansas

THOMSON

DELMAR LEARNING

Australia  Canada  Mexico  Singapore  Spain  United Kingdom  United States

MW

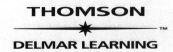

# THOMSON
## DELMAR LEARNING

Articulation and Phonology Resource Guide for School-Age Children and Adults
by Ann Bosma Smit

**Vice President,**
**Health Care Business Unit:**
William Brottmiller

**Editorial Director:**
Cathy L. Esperti

**Developmental Editor:**
Marjorie A. Bruce

**Marketing Director:**
Jennifer McAvey

**Channel Manager:**
Lisa Osgood

**Marketing Coordinator:**
Jill Osterhout

**Editorial Assistant:**
Chris Manion

**Art/Design Coordinator:**
Connie Lundberg-Watkins

**Project Editor:**
Bryan Viggiani

**Production Coordinator:**
Jessica Peterson

Library of Congress Cataloging-in-
Publication Data

Smit, Ann Bosma.
   Articulation and phonology resource
guide for school-age children and adults /
Ann Bosma Smit.
       p. cm. — (Singular resource guide
series)
Includes bibliographical references and
index.
   ISBN 0-7693-0075-8
 1. Articulation disorders. 2. Articulation
disorders in children. 3. Speech therapy
4. English language—Phonology. I. Title.
II. Series.
   RC424.7.S637 2003
   616.85'5—dc22

                                2003055605

### International Divisions List

**Asia (including India):**
Thomson Learning
60 Albert Street, #15-01
Albert Complex
Singapore 189969
Tel 65 336-6411
Fax 65 336-7411

**Australia/New Zealand:**
Nelson
102 Dodds Street
South Melbourne
Victoria 3205
Australia
Tel 61 (0)3 9685-4111
Fax 61 (0)3 9685-4199

**Latin America:**
Thomson Learning
Seneca 53
Colonia Polanco
11560 Mexico, D.F. Mexico
Tel (525) 281-2906
Fax (525) 281-2656

**Canada:**
Nelson
1120 Birchmount Road
Toronto, Ontario
Canada M1K 5G4
Tel (416) 752-9100
Fax (416) 752-8102

**UK/Europe/Middle East/Africa:**
Thomson Learning
Berkshire House
1680-173 High Holborn
London WC1V 7AA
United Kingdom
Tel 44 (0)20 497-1422
Fax 44 (0)20 497-1426

**Spain (includes Portugal):**
Paraninfo
Calle Magallanes 25
28015 Madrid
España
Tel 34 (0)91 446-3350
Fax 34 (0)91 445-6218

## NOTICE TO THE READER

5/29/04

# CONTENTS

## SECTION 1: CORE KNOWLEDGE                                                          1

## SECTION 2: EFFECTIVE ASSESSMENT OF SPEECH SOUND DISORDERS          35

## SECTION 3: ASSESSMENT: THE EARLY SCHOOL-AGE CHILD WITH POOR
##                   INTELLIGIBILITY                                                  57

## SECTION 4: ASSESSMENT OF SCHOOL-AGE CHILDREN AND ADULTS WHO HAVE
##                   RESIDUAL ERRORS                                                  75

## APPENDIX A: EVALUATING SUCCESS     215

## APPENDIX B: MATERIALS USEFUL FOR OLDER SCHOOL-AGE CLIENTS AND FOR ADULTS WHO SPEAK ENGLISH AS A SECOND LANGUAGE     233

## GLOSSARY     253

## REFERENCES     263

## INDEX     273

# LIST OF TABLES

## SECTION 6: INTERVENTION FOR EARLY SCHOOL-AGE CHILDREN WITH PHONOLOGICAL DISORDERS

## SECTION 8: APPLICATIONS TO PARTICULAR POPULATIONS: DEVELOPMENTAL VERBAL DYSPRAXIA, ENGLISH AS A SECOND LANGUAGE, AND DEVELOPMENTAL DELAY

The emblem for this series is a stylized road ending in an arrow. This symbol is intended to represent the goal of the series: to create books that serve as road maps to the care of communicative disorders. Like good road maps, each book gives the clinician an honest depiction of the territory, shows the various routes, and allows you the traveler to select the route best suited for your particular type of journey. Each book author is someone who knows the territory about which he or she is writing, both as a clinician and a researcher. The editorial board that advises the editors and authors is composed of some of the most respected persons in our profession. The hope of all involved in the series is that you will find the books useful and readable. Good traveling!

Ken Bliele, Ph.D.<br>
Series Editor

# PREFACE

In writing this book, my goal is to encourage practicing speech-language pathologists to make use of current information about articulation and phonology as they affect school-age children and adults who are learning English. This area of practice can be both exciting and rewarding. The exciting part comes when the speech-language pathologist discovers ways to help an individual to make progress. The rewarding part is that people in the client's environment typically let you know when they hear the client start to make changes.

Difficulties with speech sound formation are also quite important in the client's life. Children may be teased about their immature speech, and parents may be concerned to the point that affect their interactions with a child. Adults who speak English as a second language may be passed over for academic or job placements because their English is not readily intelligible.

Unfortunately, in visiting with many speech-language pathologists, I have sensed that treating persons who have articulatory or phonological deviations is merely a bread-and-butter part of their professional lives. They may work with a lot of cases, but there is not much excitement about them, nor is there much in the way of challenge. Consequently, one of the goals of this book is to share some of the passion that I have about working with children and adults with speech sound differences and show the way to improved clinical practice. For me, every new case is a challenge to see how quickly I can help the client achieve acceptable or intelligible speech so that she does not carry the inevitable stigma for any longer than necessary.

In order to improve our work with articulation and phonology, we as speech-language pathologists need to have some understanding of how sound systems might be organized in the human mind, especially the child mind. Casting light on sound system organization is the role of theory and research. Since the "phonological revolution" started about 30 years ago, the way that we view preschoolers and their speech sound difficulties has changed remarkably. We now view the preschool child's difficulties as primarily cognitive and linguistic in nature, rather than motoric. It is worth noting that, at this point, there are certainly many different theoretical orientations in child phonology. Fortunately, all of them shed new light on various areas within child phonology.

There has been no comparable revolution with respect to speech sound problems in older children or adults. However, during this same period, a great deal of work on motor learning has taken place. This new information can help us plan our intervention to be more efficient and in line with current knowledge when we work with this population.

With my personal emphasis on eliciting the greatest amount of change in the shortest period of time, I run up against many phenomena that make me question what we do in practice. For example:

- Why do we wait until a child is out of the period of greatest speech sound learning before we treat the late-developing sounds that are in error?

- Why is a "terminal" /r/ (or /s/) so difficult to correct? Is it because we start too late? Or because we use ineffective methods?

- Would it be possible to do short-term interventions to stimulate future sound production with children who are not stimulable, thereby preventing later long-term treatment? (This question applies to both preschoolers and school-age children.)

- Can auditory bombardment increase "readiness-to-become-stimulable" for preschoolers and young school-age children with speech sound errors and thereby shorten intervention times?

- What is the nature of stored phonological forms in children who have speech sound errors? How do these forms relate to perceptual performance? To motor performance? Do we need to change them? If so, how?

- What is the nature of the interaction between motor capabilities and cognitive/linguistic abilities in Developmental Verbal Dyspraxia in young children? How can we promote change in all relevant domains?

- In developmentally disabled children, what are the components of effective interventions for speech sound disorders? Do we need to devise particular strategies to get around particular cognitive impediments in this population?

- With English as a Second Language speakers, why do we focus almost exclusively on output? Would the use of auditory bombardment improve outcomes for this population?

Although I touch on all of these questions in this book, I do not have the answers—like everyone else, I sometimes have to work with clients without knowing everything that there is to know. As work progresses in this area, it will be exciting to me to discover answers to some of these questions.

My approach to intervention can best be characterized as more client-dependent than theory-dependent. No child comes prepackaged as a specimen that exemplifies one theory or another. Human beings are notoriously "messy" as subjects—in fact, statistics were developed to deal with the data provided by humans and other messy systems. As a result of this inherent "noise" in the system, we are compelled to pay attention to what the child can show us about his or her speech sound deviations. In particular, the child can show us at what point change in the system can take place so that we can take advantage of it in planning intervention.

In my experience, the large majority of children *do* provide evidence about where the next changes are likely to occur, but we have to go looking for it. Of course, we can make educated guesses (based on theory and existing research) about where to look. For example, if a child uses no fricatives, we might probe first in final position for a fricative that can be elicited. The reason is that acquisition data show that children often learn a fricative first in final position.

If that educated guess is not confirmed by the child's responses, then we can try other word positions or even /s/-clusters.

Adult clients, especially those learning English as a second language, can also show us where and how to make changes. Some of these clients already know what specific aspects of English phonology they need to learn. Others may not know so precisely what they need, but they are willing to attempt a wide variety of tasks because of their high level of motivation.

Finally, when I work with clients, I am always aware that speech involves a motor system in the service of a cognitive and linguistic system. Of course, people have other such systems—think of transferring the musical symbols on a page into the motor movements need to play that composition on the piano. However, speech is by far the most complex motor activity that children and adults will ever undertake.

I hope that practicing speech-language pathologists will find this book helpful to their understanding of speech sound disorders and their work with school-age and adult clients.

Ann Bosma Smit, Ph.D.<br>
Kansas State University<br>
Manhattan, Kansas

*Delmar Learning grants users permission to reproduce forms in Appendix A for class and clinical use*

# ACKNOWLEDGMENTS

This book could not have been written without the ongoing encouragement of Ken Bleile and Brian Goldstein, the Editor and Associate Editor, respectively, of the Resource Guide series. They have been helpful at every juncture. The editorial staff at Singular, and later Delmar, persisted with this project despite the length of time it took, and I am grateful to them, especially to Marge Bruce who brought it to completion.

Because of my interest in maintaining readability, this book is not studded with references. Nevertheless, the book builds on the work of many researchers, whether referenced or not. I hope that I have been fair to their work and ideas when summarizing and explaining the research in the area, even as I owe them a debt of gratitude for their achievements. Particular thanks go to persons who permitted me to reproduce some aspect of their work: Lawrence D. Shriberg, Joan Kwaitkowski, Linda Hand, Joseph Freilinger, Ann Bird, Barbara Bernhardt, John Bernthal, and J.P. Stemberger.

Finally, this book also owes its existence to the many child and adult clients who have taught me about their difficulties in speaking and who have shown me how to help them help themselves.

## DEDICATION

This book is dedicated to the memory of my father, James F. Bosma, M.D.,
who showed me the road to the study of speaking and swallowing
and the disorders that affect them.

# SECTION

# CORE KNOWLEDGE

• • • • • • • • • • • • • • • • • • • • • • • • • • • • • • • • • • • • • • • •

The ability to produce and perceive the sounds of speech is the stuff of human interaction. The quality of speech is so important that the general public can readily identify those whose speech is poorly intelligible or otherwise deviant. In particular, parents of young children are often very aware that their child is not understood by others. The older child who has a very prominent distortion of, say, fricatives, may be acutely embarrassed, even to the point of avoiding communication because his speech calls attention to itself. Adults who cannot clearly produce the sounds of English may find their vocational options limited.

The focus of this book is on assessing and changing speech sound production. For the most part, the clients with whom we work to improve speech sounds have developmental disorders affecting speech sound production. The aspect of developmental speech sound disorders that complicates the picture is that speech sounds are acquired over time and at different rates in typically developing children. Thus, the child who exhibits a speech sound disorder often differs only in degree from his or her peers.

Speech sound disorders are also present in other categories of communication disorder, such as dysarthria, apraxia, cleft palate speech, and hearing loss. In clients who have grown up with these problems, there may be a complex interaction between typical patterns of phonological development and the direct effects that the underlying disorder may have on the production of speech sounds.

Finally, we may serve bilingual children who are having difficulties with speech sounds in both languages. We may even serve young adults who speak English as a second language who elect to improve their intelligibility by improving their speech sound production. The techniques used to bring about change in speech sound production in monolingual clients with disorders are useful for these clients as well.

1

## DEFINITIONS RELATING TO SPEECH SOUND PRODUCTION

In this book, the term **speech sounds** covers all types of oral production of sounds intended for communication. The word **articulation** will be used to refer to the motoric and phonetic aspects of production. The word **phonology** will be used whenever the issue is how a sound system works. The following are some examples of the usage of these terms:

| | |
|---|---|
| Speech sounds | "While this infant clearly does not yet produce speech sounds, she does engage in vocal experimentation that results in speech-like sounds." |
| Articulation | "This man has difficulty with the articulation of /r/. He does not pull the tongue far enough back in the mouth, nor does he distinguish between acceptable and unacceptable /r/ when he listens to them." |
| Phonology | "This child's phonology includes no final consonants and no clusters in any word position." |

## DEMOGRAPHICS

The **prevalence** of developmental speech sound disorders is the proportion affected in the population at any one point of time. There is little information about the prevalence of speech sound disorders as separate from other speech disorders. However, we know that they are very common. For example, data from the 2000 ASHA Omnibus Survey showed that 97% of school-based **speech-language pathologists (SLPs)** served children with articulation or phonological disorders (ASHA Leader, 2000). About one-third of disorders served by SLPs are related to "articulation" (Slater, 1992). Another 50% of the caseload are children with childhood language disorders, many of whom undoubtedly have concomitant speech sound disorders. That is, in the preschool and school age years, speech sound disorders and other types of language difficulties tend to co-occur, with estimates of the proportion of children exhibiting both disorders ranging from 50-80% (Paul & Shriberg, 1982; Shriberg & Kwiatkowski, 1988, 1994; Tyler & Watterson, 1991). At the same time, about 30% of the caseloads of school speech-language pathologists is comprised of preschoolers, most of them in the 3- to 5-year-old range (Peters-Johnson, 1992) and it is likely that many, if not most, of these children have phonological problems.

Linguistic diversity has no doubt had an increasing effect on caseloads, because the United States is becoming increasingly diverse (Goldstein, 2000). There is no reason to think that the proportion of children learning English as a second language who have speech sound disorders is any different from the proportion of children learning a different first language who also have speech sound disorders. In fact, the diagnostic process involved in assessment of second language learners is complicated by the dual influences of development and second language acquisition (Yavas & Goldstein, 1998).

Adults who speak English as a second language constitute still another group of diverse speakers. Very often, these adults are in the United States on a short-term basis for educational reasons. Many of them have good reading and writing knowledge of English, but they lack exposure to spoken English. The large majority of these clients do not have speech sound disorders *per se*. In most of these cases, the SLP is working on what is sometimes called "accent reduction," but is probably more accurately labeled "intelligibility improvement."

## THE TOOLS OF THE SLP TRADE

The speech-language pathologist needs to have certain proficiencies in order to work effectively with speech sound disorders. Perhaps the most important of these is the ability to describe the client's speech. Without an accurate transcription of the client's speech, the analysis of error patterns and the subsequent recommendations with respect to treatment will very likely be faulty.

In order to do good transcriptions, the SLP also needs the capacity to make good recordings, whether audio or video. Inexpensive little cassette recorders will not suffice for the level of transcription that we typically require. However, we do not need the most expensive equipment either, if we pay attention to the conditions under which we record and play back our recordings.

## Transcription Tools

Transcription of speech is almost always an educated guess about what the client did with the articulators in the process of producing that speech. However, with practice, a clinician can become quite reliable about those educated guesses. That is, she may agree with her own previous transcriptions a high percentage of the time, and she may agree with other transcribers a high percentage of the time. This type of reliability can give confidence that others are describing the same phenomenon and ascribing it to the same set of articulatory gestures. Nevertheless, the fact remains that we will usually not know exactly what the client did unless we employ invasive techniques.

The first job of the transcriber is to **gloss** the speech sample, that is, write down the words that he understands the speaker to say. This step is very important because most subsequent transcription and analysis uses the intended word as its reference. In the case of poorly intelligible speakers, trying to understand what the client said can be a difficult task, requiring that the transcriber listen again and again to the sample.

Transcription is typically done at one of two levels, **broad** or **systematic transcription**, and **narrow** or **phonetic transcription.** Broad transcription uses the traditional consonant and vowel symbols to indicate the phoneme class and identity of the speech sound that was produced. Narrow transcription captures additional details about the way the sound was produced. Both kinds of transcription are needed to do an adequate analysis of children's speech sound errors. Broad transcription is useful to indicate intended phonemes and entirely correct productions, while narrow transcription is needed to pinpoint the nature of errors.

## English Syllable and Word Shapes

When denoting **syllable shapes** and **word shapes**, we customarily use the symbol **C** to represent a consonant and the symbol **V** to represent a vowel. English has a wide range of syllable shapes, as is indicated by this partial list:

| | | |
|---|---|---|
| Open Syllables | V | a, eye |
| | CV | see, chew |
| | CCV | ski, slow |
| | CCCV | screw, spray |
| Closed Syllables | VC | eat, ace |
| | CVC | pot, judge |
| | CVCC | cast, pump |
| | CVCCC | casts, pants |

As this list of single-syllable examples demonstrates, English has very complex syllable structures, including two- and three-element **consonant clusters** or sequences. In addition,

English has a relatively large consonant inventory and an extremely large vowel inventory compared to other languages in the world. These facts mean that English speakers can create an enormous number of different single-syllable words, some of them very complex, for example, *squints* (CCCVCCC). Of course, multisyllabic words can be even more complex, and English has plenty of those as well.

The point of this discussion is that English syllable structure can be difficult for children who are having trouble acquiring English phonology. They face complexities that few of the world's children have to deal with, because very few languages of the world allow this level of complexity at the syllable level. For example, at the opposite extreme, Hawaiian has eight consonants and five vowels, and allows only CV syllables (Goldstein, 2000). As we might expect, Hawaiian words tend to consist of strings of CV syllables, exemplified in Hawaiian names (Honolulu, Kamehameha). If speakers of Hawaiian want to come up with a new word, it probably means that they have to add a CV syllable to an existing word.

This is not to say that in an overall sense, English is more difficult to learn than other languages. After all, Mandarin has primarily CV syllable structure, but babies learning Mandarin have to acquire the tonal contrasts on Mandarin vowels. Hawaiian itself may present difficulties because of the length of strings of CV syllables that the child must remember.

## Broad Transcription of Consonants

The symbols used in broad transcription of consonants are shown in Table 1-1. This is actually a three-dimensional chart organized by place, manner, and voicing of the consonant. This chart shows the consonant **singletons**, that is, consonants that are not in clusters. Ordinarily we use **slashes** / / to indicate phonemes, which are actually abstractions, and **brackets** [ ] to indicate the way a sound was actually said. On the consonant chart, one of the symbols shown is the glottal stop [ʔ], which is not a phoneme. Rather, [ʔ] serves as a variant (allophone) of some of the other consonants.

**TABLE 1–1**  Consonants of American English arranged by place of articulation, manner of articulation, and voicing (where relevant).

| Manner Voicing | Place | | | | | | |
|---|---|---|---|---|---|---|---|
| | Labial | Labiodental | Interdental | Alveolar | Palatal | Velar | Glottal |
| Nasals | m | | | n | | ŋ | |
| Stops | | | | | | | |
| Voiceless | p | | | t | | k | ʔ* |
| Voiced | b | | | d | | g | |
| Fricatives | | | | | | | |
| Voiceless | | f | θ | s | ʃ | | h** |
| Voiced | | v | ð | z | ʒ | | |
| Affricates | | | | | | | |
| Voiceless | | | | | tʃ | | |
| Voiced | | | | | dʒ | | |

| Manner Voicing | Place | | | | | | |
|---|---|---|---|---|---|---|---|
| | Labial | Labiodental | Interdental | Alveolar | Palatal | Velar | Glottal |
| Glides | w | | | | j | | |
| Liquids | | | | | | | |
| Retroflexed | | | | | r | | |
| Lateral | | | | l | | | |

*The glottal stop is used as an allophone, not as a phoneme in its own right.

**The /h/ is considered to be a glide by many phoneticians.

The consonants of English are often grouped into classes of sounds for purposes of analysis because they are often affected in the same way by certain phenomena. This grouping is often based on distinctive features. A **distinctive feature** is the smallest characteristic that can make a difference between two phonemes. There are a number of distinctive feature systems, some more abstract than others. Table 1-2 shows a distinctive feature system based on work by Chomsky and Halle (1968).

Some of the classes of sounds are quite familiar. For example, the phonemes in the class of nasals all share the feature [+nasal], and the class of fricatives includes all sounds made with continuous air forced past an obstruction ([-sonorant] and [+continuant]). In other words, these classes are a kind of shorthand. Some of the classes of sounds that are mentioned frequently in the literature are these:

**Glides**: /w j/ (and /h/ in some systems)

**Nasals**: /m n ŋ/

**Stops**: /p t k b d g /

**Fricatives**: /f θ s ʃ v ð z ʒ/

**Affricates**: Single phonemes composed of a stop-like portion followed by a fricative-like portion, as occurs in /ʧ ʤ/ ([+delayed release])

**Obstruents**: All sounds made with increased oral pressure, including the stops, fricatives, and affricates

**Stridents**: All fricatives except /θ ð/

**Liquids**: /l r/

**Approximants**: Glides (except /h/) and liquids

**Alveolars**: /t d n s z/

**Palatals**: /ʃ ʒ ʧ ʤ/

**Velars**: /k g ŋ/

**Glottals**: /h/ and [ʔ]

Position in the word or syllable can influence consonant production in English. The meaning of terms like **word-initial** and **syllable-final** are self-evident. The term **intervocalic** refers to a consonant occurring between two vowels, for example, the /z/ in the word *easy*. Although some SLPs may use the term **medial**, meaning anywhere between the beginning and the ending of a word, that term has not proved helpful in understanding phonological structures.

**TABLE 1–2**  Distinctive feature specifications for the consonantal phonemes of English. *After Chomsky and Halle (1968).*

|  | p | b | t | d | k | g | f | v | θ | ð | s | z |
|---|---|---|---|---|---|---|---|---|---|---|---|---|
| Consonantal | + | + | + | + | + | + | + | + | + | + | + | + |
| Vocalic | − | − | − | − | − | − | − | − | − | − | − | − |
| Sonorant | − | − | − | − | − | − | − | − | − | − | − | − |
| Continuant | − | − | − | − | − | − | + | + | + | + | + | + |
| Strident | − | − | − | − | − | − | + | + | − | − | + | + |
| Delayed Rel. | − | − | − | − | − | − | − | − | − | − | − | − |
| Voiced | − | + | − | + | − | + | − | + | − | + | − | + |
| Coronal | − | − | + | + | − | − | − | − | + | + | + | + |
| Anterior | + | + | + | + | − | − | + | + | + | + | + | + |
| Nasal | − | − | − | − | − | − | − | − | − | − | − | − |
| Lateral | − | − | − | − | − | − | − | − | − | − | − | − |
| High | − | − | − | − | + | + | − | − | − | − | − | − |
| Low | − | − | − | − | − | − | − | − | − | − | − | − |
| Back | − | − | − | − | + | + | − | − | − | − | − | − |
| Round | − | − | − | − | − | − | − | − | − | − | − | − |

|  | ʃ | ʒ | tʃ | dʒ | m | n | ŋ | r | l | w | j | h |
|---|---|---|---|---|---|---|---|---|---|---|---|---|
| Consonantal | + | + | + | + | + | + | + | + | + | − | − | − |
| Vocalic | − | − | − | − | − | − | − | + | + | − | − | − |
| Sonorant | − | − | − | − | + | + | + | + | + | + | + | + |
| Continuant | + | + | − | − | − | − | − | + | + | + | + | + |
| Strident | + | + | + | + | − | − | − | − | − | − | − | − |
| Delayed Rel. | − | − | + | + | − | − | − | − | − | − | − | − |
| Voiced | − | + | − | + | + | + | + | + | + | + | + | − |
| Coronal | + | + | + | + | − | + | − | + | + | − | − | − |
| Anterior | − | − | − | − | + | + | − | − | + | − | − | − |
| Nasal | − | − | − | − | + | + | + | − | − | − | − | − |
| Lateral | − | − | − | − | − | − | − | − | + | − | − | − |
| High | + | + | + | + | − | − | + | − | − | + | + | − |
| Low | − | − | − | − | − | − | − | − | − | − | − | + |
| Back | − | − | − | − | − | − | + | − | − | + | − | − |
| Round | − | − | − | − | − | − | − | − | − | + | − | − |

An alternative way to talk about syllable shapes is more common in linguistics than in speech-language pathology. The concepts are the onset and the rime of a syllable, with the rime including a nucleus and possibly a coda. The **onset** of a syllable includes all the consonants at the beginning of the syllable, which in English can range from zero to three. The **rime** is the rest of the syllable, and it consists of a **nucleus** (usually a vowel or a syllabic consonant) and a coda. The **coda** includes all the consonants at the end of the syllable, which in English can range from zero to four.

Most English consonants can occur in all positions, but some cannot. The glides can occur only in syllable-initial (onset) and intervocalic positions, and the nasal /ŋ/ can occur only in intervocalic and syllable-final (coda) positions. In addition, some consonants can occur in clusters in syllable-initial or syllable-final positions, while others cannot. The English syllable-initial clusters are shown in Table 1-3.

**TABLE 1–3** English word-initial consonant clusters.

| /w/-clusters | tw | twin | /j/-clusters (rare; some consider /ju/ a diphthong) | pj | pure |
| --- | --- | --- | --- | --- | --- |
| | kw | queen | | bj | beauty |
| | | | | mj | music |
| | | | | kj | cube |
| /s/-clusters | sp | spoon | /l/-clusters | pl | play |
| | st | stick | | bl | blue |
| | sk | ski | | kl | climb |
| | sw | swim | | gl | glue |
| | sl | slide | | fl | fly |
| | sf | sphere (rare) | | | |
| /r/-clusters | pr | prize | Three-element clusters | skw | square |
| | br | bread | | spl | splash |
| | tr | tree | | spr | spray |
| | dr | drop | | str | straw |
| | kr | cry | | skr | scream |
| | gr | grow | | | |
| | fr | free | | | |
| | θr | throw | | | |

Syllable-final clusters are far more numerous and varied than syllable-initial clusters. In fact, English morphology routinely results in consonant clusters at the end of words, for example,

| | | | | | |
| --- | --- | --- | --- | --- | --- |
| *run* | *runs* (/nz/) | *Jim* | *Jim's* (/mz/) | *face* | *faced* (/st/) |
| *punt* | *punts* (/nts/) | *ask* | *asked* (/skt/) | *hand* | *hands* (/ndz/) |

## Broad Transcription of Vowels

English vowels are usually described in terms of their location on the vowel quadrilateral, shown in Figure 1-1. In this figure the vertical dimension of the quadrilateral represents the vowel height in terms of location of the bunching of the tongue, and the horizontal dimension represents "frontness" or "backness" of the bunching of the tongue. In fact, the two-dimensional figure is an abstract representation of the oral cavity. Another dimension of the vowel space is represented in the arrangement of the vowels along the edges of Figure 1-1, with **tense vowels** arranged on the outside and **lax vowels** on the inside, except that /ɝ/ is also a tense vowel. The vowels shown on the quadrilateral are considered to be phonemic monophthongs even though the tense vowels are often diphthongized. Monophthongs are phonemically considered to be single vowels.

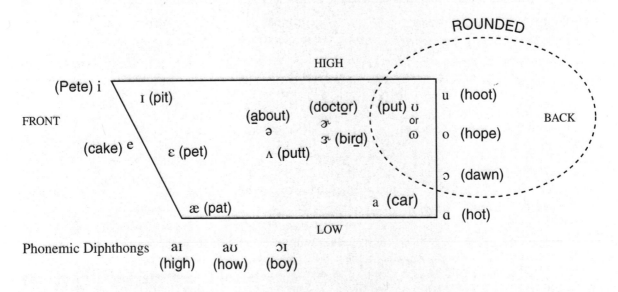

**Figure 1–1**   *Vowels of American English shown on the vowel quadrilateral.*
The dimensions of the quadrilateral represent vowel height and tongue bunching anterior to posterior. The dotted line encloses the rounded vowels. Phonemic diphthongs are shown at the bottom. Each symbol is accompanied by a representative word.

Tense vowels are produced with more tension than lax vowels and are usually longer in duration. However, the defining feature of tense vowels is that they can occur in **open syllables** (CV syllables), while lax vowels cannot. The existence of words like *pea, pay, Pooh, Poe, paw, Pa,* and *purr* demonstrates that the vowels /i e u o ɑ ɝ/ are tense vowels. Phonetically speaking, English tense vowels are typically diphthongized. That is, they are produced with an off-glide: [biɪ] for /bi/ (*bee*), [peɪ] for /pe/ (*pay*), [kuʊ] for /ku/ (*coo*), and [boʊt] for /bot/ (*boat*). Incidentally, English is one of the few languages to make a distinction between tense and lax vowels at similar locations on the vowel quadrilateral. For example, many languages do not distinguish between the two high front vowels /i/ and /ɪ/.

Some English vowels have still other features that are not represented in this diagram. For example, the /æ/ is the most open English vowel in the sense that the jaw is opened the farthest for this vowel. Some of the back vowels have lip rounding, indicated in a dotted line on the vowel chart. For the two sets of vowels in the middle of the space, the symbol used depends on whether the vowel occurs in a stressed or an unstressed syllable. Thus /ʌ/ and /ɝ/ (an /r/-colored vowel) are used in stressed syllables, for example, *duck* /dʌk/ and *dirt*

/dʒɚt/, and the /ə/ and /ɚ/ symbols are used in unstressed syllables, for example, *away* /əwe/ and *baker* /bekɚ/.

English also has three phonemic diphthongs that are shown at the bottom of the chart. **Diphthongs** involve the successive articulation of two different vowels, and they make a difference in meaning, but they are considered to represent one phoneme. English has both phonemic and non-phonemic diphthongs, depending on whether the diphthong makes the minimal difference between two words or not. The three generally accepted phonemic diphthongs in English are /aɪ aʊ ɔɪ /, and some consider /ju/ also to be a phonemic diphthong. The non-phonemic diphthongs are usually diphthongized tense vowels.

As is the case for the consonants, it is possible to label groups of vowels in a kind of shorthand. In addition to tense vowels and lax vowels, some of the common categories are these:

High front vowels: /i ɪ e ɛ/

High back vowels: /u ʊ/

Low back vowels: /ɔ ɑ/

Rounded vowels: /u ʊ o ɔ /

/r/-colored vowels: /ɚ/ as in *doct<u>or</u>*, /ɜ/ as in *purr*, /ɪr / as in *peer*, /ɛr/ as in *pair*, /ʊr/ as in p*oor*, /ɔr/ as in *pore*, and /ar/ as in *par*

Point vowels: the vowels at the corners of the quadrilateral. English has four point vowels (/i u ɑ æ/), but most languages have only three (/i u ɑ/).

We should note that most of the dialects of American English differ primarily in their vowel structure, including /r/-colored vowels (Small, 1999). For example, most Midwesterners do not use the vowel /ɔ/. Instead, they use /ɑ/ in more words than East Coasters do. In New Jersey, the names *Don* and *Dawn* are typically pronounced as /dɑn/ and /dɔn/, respectively, but in Kansas, both names are produced as /dɑn/. Another example is the Southern dialects' treatment of diphthongs as elongated monophthongs. In Seattle, the word *fine* would be said as [faɪn], but in Alabama, it is said as [fa:n], where the [:] represents lengthening.

## Narrow Transcription

**Narrow transcription** is focused on capturing phonetic details about speech production. For example, although both a typical [s] production and a lateralized [s] production are phonemically /s/, there is a marked difference in the actual production, and it is this type of difference that narrow transcription can help to record.

In most narrow transcription systems, there is a large set of **diacritics**, that is, symbols that can be placed adjacent to the phoneme symbol to represent a particular feature (e.g., Kent & Shriberg, 1995). Systems of diacritics represent a mapping of symbols to labels (e.g., a dentalized [n] is transcribed as [n̪]). The use of diacritics can be daunting if they are not used frequently. Furthermore, if a clinician does not use diacritics frequently, then using diacritics probably increases errors because of the heavy memory load involved in storing and searching a system of diacritics at the time of transcription.

It is far more important that the clinician be able to give a name to the features of the production that he wants to note. These labels can be written near the phoneme symbol without the clinician engaging in a tedious memory search process to find the right diacritic. This way, no information is lost, and in fact, the relevant information may be more accessible than if it were recorded solely in diacritics. The interested reader may wish to examine the narrow transcription system used in the *Smit-Hand Articulation and Phonology Assessment* (*SHAPE*, Smit & Hand, 1997). This test uses a checklist of phoneme symbols and labels of possible phonetic events. The choices that are provided for each phoneme target are arranged in order of frequency of their appearance in a large sample of children, that is, in order of probability of occurrence.

The speech-language pathologist who was not trained to use a system of narrow transcription may wish to choose a system and then start listening for the events that system covers. Some of the important phenomena affecting classes of sounds are these:

1. Glides can be lengthened, shortened, or nasalized.

2. Nasals can be lengthened, shortened, or denasalized.

3. Stops in initial position can be aspirated or deaspirated, while stops in final position can also be unreleased.

4. Stops can be frictionalized.

5. Alveolar and palatal fricatives can be produced with a number of distorting elements such as lateralization, dentalization, post-alveolar distortions, and affrications (addition of a stop, e.g., [tsun] for *sun*).

6. The liquid /r/ can be labialized, or derhotacized, or both, and it can also be velarized.

7. The liquids /l r/ can be substituted by vowels when they are syllable-final.

8. The nasals and the liquids can be syllabic, that is, they can themselves function as syllables.

An excellent way to learn how to apply these concepts is for the clinician to record and transcribe the English of non-native speakers. There is one caveat: In this author's experience in teaching narrow transcription to hundreds of practicing clinicians, many clinicians tend to credit the client with too much. This means that the clinician tends to miss omissions, possibly because there is a very strong expectancy that the phoneme will be present. Some clinicians also give children too much credit for /r l/ productions, for example by recording the child's [tw] in *train* as [tr] or the child's [o] for syllabic /l/ in *candle* as acceptable.

There are at least four computerized narrow transcription systems available, including the *Logical International Phonetic Programs* (*LIPP*—Oller & Delgado, 2000), *Programs to Examine Phonetic and Phonologic Evaluation Records* (*PEPPER*—Shriberg, 1986), *Computerized Profiling* (Long, Fey, & Channell, 2000), and the *Macintosh Interactive System for Phonological Analysis* (*MASPA*—Masterson & Pagan, 1994). These systems do not relieve the clinician of the need to label the child's production; rather they provide for computerized storage of the diacritics that the SLP chooses to represent the production. The SLP who does a lot of work with phonology may benefit from learning one of these systems to make the transcription process go faster. Masterson, Long, and Buder (1998) have reviewed a number of the computerized transcription programs, and the interested clinician may wish to consult that work.

## Making Good Audio and Video Recordings

Good recordings of speech samples are very important to the speech-language pathologist and are indispensable for those doing narrow transcription. The most important principle in making good recordings is to put the microphone as close as possible to the speaker's mouth in order to get an optimum signal-to-noise ratio. One way to do this is to use a tie-tack microphone along with a cassette recorder that has a remote microphone input. Or, if recording a child who will be moving about the room, one can use an FM (wireless) system with the microphone and transmitter attached to the child's clothing and the receiver providing line input to the recording system.

Video recordings can be beneficial if they have a good audio track and if the client's face is in view most of the time. Some of the current systems provide excellent sound quality as well as good video representation. With some models, it is possible to lead the signal from a remote microphone into the video camera. Again, it is best to have the microphone and camera as close to the speaker's face as is feasible.

In making both kinds of recordings, there are some ways to maximize the quality of the audio signal. These include the following:

- Record at the highest level possible without overdriving the signal, that is, without "going into the red" (indicator on the VU meter).

- Do your recording in the quietest place possible to eliminate/reduce extraneous noise.

- Use a windscreen on the microphone to reduce popping sounds from certain types of sounds, such as aspirated stops. Windscreens are routinely included with new microphones.

- Use a heavy cloth table covering if you have the client seated at a table looking at pictures or playing with toys. This will reduce environmental noises on the recording.

- If the client is a child who moves a lot and tends to kick table legs and chair legs, pad the furniture legs with foam sheets.

- Use a new cassette tape or videotape.

- To the extent possible, choose toys that are relatively quiet and cannot be banged loudly.

The device that is used for playback, whether cassette player or video player, should have a heavy duty transport system that makes it easy to listen over and over to a particular short sample. Generally, systems sold as "portable" have less sturdy drive mechanisms than tabletop models. In fact, it is possible to record the client using a relatively inexpensive portable system that permits microphone input, but then do the playback and transcription on a sturdier machine.

## CONCEPTS FROM PHONOLOGY

The term phonology has two related meanings. On the one hand, the **phonology of a language** is the speech sound system of that language. On the other hand, **phonology** denotes the study of speech sound systems to determine common principles. The field of speech-language pathology has borrowed extensively from linguistics in using concepts of phonology, and there are several different approaches to phonology in the linguistics literature.

**Natural phonology** is oriented toward discovering the common features of languages and especially the common aspects shown by children acquiring speech sound systems, no matter what language they are learning. Research into child speech acquisition has shown that English-speaking children tend to be highly predictable in the types of sound patterns that they use in their early phonology, although the details may vary from child to child. Several different investigations of children's early words (Davis & MacNeilage, 1990; Dyson, 1988; Locke, 1983; Robb & Bleile, 1994; Stoel-Gammon, 1985) have reported on the following:

- The early words of children tend to have the syllable shapes V, CV, CVCV, and sometimes CVC.

- The early vowels have received relatively little attention; however, the early vowels in words tend to be mid to low, and front to central. A majority may be used incorrectly.

- The early developing consonants tend to be glides, nasals, and stops, with a fricative [f] or [s] showing up a bit later

Phonologists who have studied the progression of speech acquisition have also made the case that the first 50 words or so tend to be learned as wholes, or "smears" of speech, whereas after the **50-word point**, children start to behave as if their words have phoneme-sized parts. That is, if they change the /d/ in *dog*, then they change the /d/ in *dumb* the same way, suggesting that they understand that these two sounds are in some sense the same.

The concept of phonological processes also came from the study of word use in the first two to three years of life. **Phonological processes** are statements about regularities in a child's phonology as compared to adult forms. For example, the phonological process called **final consonant deletion** describes the phenomenon of the child who leaves off syllable-final consonants that are present in the adult version of the word. There are a number of phonological processes that appear in the literature. Some of them are so common among young children that they are considered to be **natural processes**, that is, phonological processes that appear to be part of every child's biological predisposition.

**Syllable structure processes** affect syllable and word shapes. Most syllable structure processes result in CV syllables. Consequently, they may reflect a human preference for CV forms (Pickett, 1999). They include:

- **Final consonant deletion**—Use of open syllables (i.e., lack of syllable-final C)
- **Cluster reduction**—Deletion of one or more elements of a consonant cluster
- **Weak syllable deletion**—Deletion of a weak (unstressed) syllable
- **Reduplication**—Production of a CVCV form. In full reduplication, the two CVs are the same (e.g., [baba] for *blanket*), while in partial reduplication either the two Cs or the two Vs may differ (e.g., [babo] for *bottle*).
- **Metathesis**—The shifting of a phoneme-sized unit from one position to another (e.g., [nupɪs] for *Snoopy*)
- **Epenthesis**—The addition of elements not present in the adult form (e.g., [bəlu] for *blue*.

**Substitution processes** involve the substitution of one phoneme-sized unit for another. They include:

- **Stopping**—Substitution of a stop for a fricative or an affricate (e.g., [du] for *zoo*)
- **Fronting**—Substitution of an alveolar for a velar consonant (e.g., [tʌm] for *come*)
- **Depalatalization**—Substitution of an alveolar for a palatal consonant (e.g., [tsɪp] for *chip*)
- **Gliding**—Substitution of a glide for a liquid in initial or intervocalic position (e.g., [waɪt] for *light*)
- **Vocalization**—Substitution of a vowel for a liquid in final position (e.g., [wio] for *wheel*)
- **Backing**—Substitution of a velar for an alveolar (e.g., [gɪr] for *deer*)

**Assimilation processes** describe the change of a consonant to make it similar to a consonant elsewhere in the word. There are many possible assimilation processes, but only a few are commonly used. Although these processes may initially look like substitution processes, in fact the "substitutions" are conditioned by other consonants in the word. They include:

- **Velar assimilation**—An alveolar consonant early in the word changes to a velar, matching the place of articulation of a consonant later in the word (e.g., [gagɪ] for *doggie*)
- **Alveolar assimilation**—A velar consonant early in the word changes to an alveolar, matching the place of articulation of a consonant later in the word (e.g., [dot] for *goat*)

**Idiosyncratic processes** are processes that are very uncommon in child phonology. They may be peculiar to a particular child and so are definitely not considered to be "natural." A number of processes have been reported in the literature, for example:

- **Glottal replacement**—Some or all consonants are replaced with glottal stops (e.g., [ʔɪʔ] for *fish*).
- **Favorite sound**—The child chooses to say words with this sound, and also uses this sound to substitute for other consonants (e.g., [t], as in [ti] for *see*, [tɪp] for *ship*, [tin] for *green*, and [bɛt] for *best*).
- **Word recipes**—Words of a given type are produced in a similar way (e.g., *bunny* said as [bʌji], *tummy* said as [tʌji], *monkey* said as [mʌji], and *baby* said as [beji]).

## Phonological Idioms and Frozen Forms

Occasionally the SLP will encounter a child who says certain words in a surprisingly advanced form compared to the rest of the child's phonology. These forms are called **phonological idioms** (Moskowitz, 1973). For example, the child may say *orange juice* in adult-like fashion at a time when /r/ is usually substituted by [w] and /ʤ/ is substituted by [d]. These advanced forms tend to show regression later when they are recast in terms of the child's then-current phonology.

A child may also use **frozen forms**. These are versions of words that the child used at a much younger age but has kept in the same form despite advances in his phonological system. The most common example of this phenomenon is the word *yellow* said as [lɛlo] at a time when the child says *you*, *yes*, and *yell* with correct [j]. The use of [lɛlo] also represents an assimilation of the type that children usually use in the second year and perhaps the third year of life.

## Importance of Phonological Processes

Although most of the phonological processes mentioned previously were based on studies of typically developing children, they are very important for children with speech sound disorders as well. That is, these children tend to use many of the common phonological processes well past the age when typically developing children would have stopped using them. Children with severe speech sound disorders may use idiosyncratic processes as well, a fact that would contribute greatly to poor intelligibility.

One further point is that most children vary somewhat in their use of processes. For this reason, we need a criterion to determine when a child uses a particular process productively and not just occasionally. Consequently, Hodson and Paden (1991) have suggested the **40% rule**: A child uses a process productively if she uses it in 40% or more of the opportunities to use the process.

McReynolds and Elbert (1981) considered the issue of the number of exemplars needed to declare that the child uses a process productively. An **exemplar** is a single word or phoneme that can be affected by a process, that is, a word in which there is an opportunity for a process to occur. For example, the words *can*, *face*, *suit*, *cloud*, and *witch* could all be exemplars of final consonant deletion because they all have final consonants. McReynolds and Elbert recommended that clinicians use a **4-exemplar rule**: A child cannot be said to use a process unless there are at least four exemplars in the speech sample.

## Analyses of Phonology

Stoel-Gammon and Dunn (1985) have provided an important framework for the assessment of phonology in children with speech sound disorders. They view the child's phonology as both a self-contained system (independent) and a system that is related to the adult system (relational). Consequently, a complete assessment of the child's system would include both independent analyses and relational analyses.

**Independent analyses** treat the child's system as self-contained, that is, not compared to the adult system. The two parts of an independent analysis include a phonetic inventory and a syllable and word shape inventory. The **phonetic inventory** is an organized list of the types of speech sounds the child produces, whether correct or not. The **syllable and word shape inventory** is a listing of the types of syllables and words the child uses, using C and V notation. Both of these inventories are used to determine what structures the child is lacking, compared to typical performance of children at the child's current age. A statement of **sequential constraints** is an indication of what kinds of sounds can follow each other (e.g., the child lacks clusters). Forms to assist in these analyses are found in Section 9.

**Relational analyses** compare the child's performance to the adult standard. One kind of relational analysis is familiar to all SLPs, that is, the listing of results of a typical test of articulation, where the adult target phoneme is listed and the child's version is written next to that target. Another kind of relational analysis is the **segmental inventory**, to be used when the clinician must work from a connected speech sample or other sample for which a scoring sheet is not available. (Following the usage of Shriberg and Kwiatkowski, 1982a, the term *segmental* rather than *phonemic* is used to describe this inventory). The third part of a relational analysis is a **list of phonological processes** used by the child, together with the percent of use of each. The clinician can then apply the 40%-or-more rule and the minimum-of-four-exemplars rule to determine which processes the child uses productively.

## The Contribution of Generative Phonology

**Generative phonology** has a focus on the nature of the child's knowledge about the word forms that are affected by phonological processes. This knowledge takes the form of the child's **underlying representation (UR)**, a kind of stored form that serves as an internal reference. When we talk about phonological processes, we make the stored adult form our reference. However, one cannot assume that the child's underlying representation is in fact adult-like. The question of what the child's UR might look like is difficult to resolve, although Elbert and Gierut (1986) have devised some clever procedures to discover what phonological structures are represented in the UR. These procedures result in **knowledge hierarchies** that are used to plan intervention.

## The Contribution of Cognitive Phonology

**Cognitive theories** of phonology (e.g., Macken & Ferguson, 1983) focus on the child as an active processor of phonological information. The child brings to the acquisition of a sound system a tendency to hypothesize about patterns in the sound system and a tendency to try out new structures. Evidence supporting this theory includes the existence of patterns unique to individual children, the existence of phonological idioms that later are fitted into the current pattern (regression), and children's selectivity about what words they choose to say. Perhaps the most important evidence is the child's ability to generalize on the basis of imperfect exemplars, an ability without which the child would face failure in phonological treatment.

## The Contribution of Nonlinear Phonology

Most theories of phonology have viewed speech as a string of phoneme-sized units that are independent of each other. **Nonlinear phonology** (e.g., Bernhardt & Stoel-Gammon, 1994) emphasizes the hierarchical relationships that exist within words and phrases. By way of example, consider that in traditional child phonology approaches, phenomena such as assimilation (e.g., [lɛlo] for *yellow*) and vowel harmony (e.g., [bibi] for *baby*), both of which leap over segments, cannot be explained. Nonlinear phonology posits different levels of formal representation of the word and allows elements at each level to interact with each other. Clinically, the biggest contribution of nonlinear phonology has been its attention to multisyllabic words and to the way therapy is organized.

## The Contribution of Frame-and-Content Ideas

MacNeilage and Davis (1990) developed the metaphor of **frame and content** to describe the child's differentiation of consonants and vowels. They view the basic mechanism of speech to be the opening and closing of the jaw, which the infant acquires almost from birth. The tongue at first is not differentiated from the jaw in any functional way; rather, it "goes along for the ride." This basic movement pattern constitutes the "frame." However, eventually independent movement of tongue and other articulators is apparent, and MacNeilage and Davis consider this change to represent the "content," as in their statement "First frame, then content."

Frame-and-content theory was developed explicitly to understand phenomena in the first year or so of life. However, as a metaphor, this idea can sometimes apply to children with speech sound disorders, especially those who use idiosyncratic processes. For example, the child who has a favorite sound appears to have a frame consisting of favorite sound and any adjacent vowels. Similarly, the child who has "word recipes" clearly has a frame for words of a certain length and type into which she fits those words. In these cases, the clinician must help the child achieve long overdue differentiation, that is, change the content that goes into the frame.

## SPEECH ARTICULATION

For many years, before phonological theories began to influence speech-language pathology, speech sound disorders were called *articulation disorders*. The assumed cause of articulation disorders was a difficulty in learning the motor actions needed to produce particular phonemes. Several authorities attributed the difficulties in learning motor patterns to difficulties in perceiving the phonemes in error. While phonological approaches did not eliminate consideration of motor difficulties, motor problems have taken a back seat to abstract phonological systems. This is unfortunate. Whatever else it may be, speech is a complex series of motor activities involving several motor systems and a linguistic system. We should not be surprised if some children have difficulty acquiring the sounds of their language in part because of a balky speech mechanism.

In order to provide effective treatment, the SLP should be aware of certain phenomena in speech production. First of all, the physical realization of a phoneme is different depending on where in the utterance it occurs. By way of example, consider the three different versions of /k/ in this sentence: <u>K</u>ick the ball ba<u>ck</u>! (/kɪkðəbɔlbæk/)

> First [k]: There are no acoustic transitions into this [k], but there are transitions away from it into the vowel, which is a high front vowel. These transitions result from movements of the articulators. This [k] is aspirated, as are all English voiceless stops in word-initial position.

> Second [k]: There are transitions from the preceding high front vowel into this [k] and also transitions away from it. In fact, this [k] may not even have an audible release, because the release can occur as part of the next consonant production, [ð].

Third [k]: Production of this [k] is affected by transitions from the preceding low front vowel [æ]. There are no transitions away from this [k] because it is at the end of the utterance. However, there is a choice for the speaker to make, because English stops at the end of an utterance can be released, aspirated, or unreleased.

It is clear from this example that each version of the phoneme /k/ has different motor constraints on it, with the second [k] having perhaps the most complex interactions with surrounding phonemes. The speech-language pathologist who keeps these complexities in mind will probably wish to schedule production first in initial or final word position, and only later in intervocalic or medial position.

A second point about articulation is that despite its complexity, speech occurs at fast rates. Adult speaking rates as fast as 19 phones per second have been reported (Tiffany, 1980). Studies of motor control systems (Schmidt & Lee, 1999) suggest that accurate motor activity does not occur at fast rates until it is highly practiced, that is, the person doing the movement has become skilled and accurate at performing the movement. One implication of this information is that if we want the client to use a new articulatory structure in speech that is produced at a typical rate, we will need to use procedures that result in overlearning.

## Influences of the Speech Mechanism on Production in Children

The speaking mechanisms of children are growing and changing during the period when they are acquiring their phonology. For example, there are substantial changes in the angle between the oral and pharyngeal cavities. Whereas early on, the angle is obtuse, by the time the child is about 12 months old, the angle is close to 90 degrees, as it is in adults (Kent & Murray, 1982). This change means not only that the child learns to move the articulators over increasingly long distances, but also that the directions of movements change. There are still further changes after the first year, as the child acquires teeth (and a dental arch) and loses the sucking pads in the cheeks.

Another shift that occurs during the entire period of childhood is a change in speaking rate. Children on average have longer segment durations (and therefore slower speech) than adults (Kent & Forner, 1980). Of course, during this period some acceleration is to be expected because children eventually will achieve adult rates of speech. Table 1-4 shows some of the changes in speaking rate as children mature.

**TABLE 1–4**   Speaking rates of preschool and school-age children and adults, in syllables per minute.

*Sources: Pindzola, Jenkins, and Loken (1989); Guitar (1998); Andrews and Ingham (1971).*

| Preschool children (conversational speech) | |
| --- | --- |
| Age | Syllables per minute |
| 3 | 116-163 |
| 4-5 | 109-183 |
| School-age children (conversational speech) | |
| Age | Syllables per minute |
| 6 | 140-175 |
| 8 | 150-180 |
| 10-12 | 165-220 |

Adults (conversational speech)

Syllables per minute

162-230

## Speech Universals

Despite the very large differences among languages of the world, the speech mechanism imposes certain common characteristics on all human beings, and these characteristics affect children also. For example, **utterance-final lengthening** means that the last word in an utterance is almost always longer than the same word would be if it were embedded in the utterance (Kent & Read, 1992). This phenomenon is true of most speakers most of the time, no matter what their first language, and it is also true for children. This fact may be used in planning treatment sequences. For example, the SLP can plan to teach a new structure in an utterance-final word first and then teach the structure embedded in the utterance.

Many languages demonstrate **context-related shortening of a segment** such as a phoneme or syllable. For example, an [s] produced in isolation is usually longer than the "same" sound produced in a syllable. Even more shortening of the [s] is seen when the [s] occurs in a cluster. At the level of the syllable, using the sequence *speed*, *speedy*, *speedily*, if we measure the length of the *speed* syllable, we see that it shortens as the suffixes are tacked onto it, and the greater the number of suffixes, the shorter the duration of *speed* (Kent & Read, 1992). The SLP can manipulate context so as to increase or decrease the demand for rapid production of a new sound.

Another constraint imposed by the speech mechanism on all speakers is the breath group. A **breath group** refers to the syllables that are produced on one breath. The number of syllables can vary quite a bit, but the boundaries of the breath group typically occur at major syntactic boundaries. A related constraint on the mechanism is **final declination** in breath groups, that is, the decrease in both intensity and pitch that occurs at the end of a breath group. The final declination is attributed to falling subglottal pressure (Cruttenden, 1986). Virtually all breath groups show this declination except those in which the speaker over-rides the tendency to reduce pressure, for example, in English when there is an upward pitch inflection to indicate a question. The SLP sometimes needs to make sure that the client does not use inappropriate breath groups when trying to produce new sounds in the stream of speech.

**Coarticulation** is the overlapping of articulatory gestures for adjacent speech sounds. Coarticulation, which is also a universal phenomenon, has both mechanical and acoustic consequences. The example of the phrase presented earlier, "Kick the ball back," suggests some of the influences that coarticulation can have on production of a particular phoneme. For example, the stop closure for the second [k], spoken after the high front vowel [ɪ], is made in a more anterior position on the palate than is the stop closure for the third [k], spoken after the low front vowel [æ]. The acoustic consequence is that the most prominent energy in the [k]-release is higher in frequency following the high front vowel than when it follows the low front vowel.

Coarticulatory effects are the basis for many of the "tricks" that SLPs use to elicit correct productions. (See Bernthal and Bankson, Appendix—Procedures for Teaching Sounds, 1998, for some of these "tricks.") A good example is the recommendation that the child use the /t/-position to segue to [s], which is also an alveolar consonant. Another example is the frequent recommendation that the SLP elicit /r/ in a clustered context, specifically clustered with a velar consonant as in the words *green* or *bark*.

## Prosody

**Prosody** refers to the rhythm, intonation contours, loudness contours, rate, and perceived stress in an utterance. All of these variables are considered to be **suprasegmentals** because they transcend the segments (phonemes) in the stream of speech. Although speech-language pathologists who work primarily with children most often focus on segments, suprasegmentals can have a large influence on intelligibility. A case in point is the person who speaks English as a second language (ESL) and is difficult to understand: There is general agreement that when an ESL speaker is poorly intelligible, prosody is often a major contributor. The prosodic difficulties tend to manifest themselves as misplaced syllable stress and non-English intonation contours.

### Word-level Stress

There are several aspects to prosody, including word-level stress patterns and utterance-level stress patterns. An example of **word-level stress** is the word *amaze*: We know that the "-maze" syllable is stressed because it is usually louder, longer in duration, and spoken at a higher pitch level than the "a-" syllable. Word-level stress is an important concern in children because children with severe phonological disorders tend to have difficulty with it.

There are a number of systems to transcribe word-level stress, with some systems having as many as five levels. For clinical purposes, however, three levels of word-level stress are generally sufficient, with a rating of "1" given to the syllable with the most stress, "3" given to the syllable with the least stress, and "2" given to syllables with intermediate stress. Examples of this system follow:

| 1  2 | 3   1 | 1  3 | 3  1  2 | 1 3  2 |
|------|-------|------|---------|--------|
| Haldol | between | center | connection | argument |

| 3  1  3  2 | 2 3  1  3 2 |
|------------|-------------|
| establishment | alphabetical |

Suprasegmentals are conditioned by the nature of the language the child is learning. English is a **stress-timed language**, meaning that the basic unit of rhythm is the **foot**, that is, one stressed syllable with one or two adjacent unstressed syllables (Lehiste, 1970). On the whole, English tends to have alternating stress. In fact, the alternating stress in English is readily apparent in this bit of doggerel that is a mnemonic for the names of the cranial nerves:

3   1   3   1   3    1    3    1
On old Olympus' towering tops

3  1   3   1   3    1   3   1
a Finn and German sat at hops.

The early two-syllable words of children are usually **trochees** (with stress on the first syllable, as in *doggie*), and occasionally **iambs** (with stress on the second syllable, as in *away*).

Many other languages are not stress-timed but **syllable-timed**, meaning that the basic rhythmic unit is the syllable. Syllables tend to be equally stressed in syllable-timed languages like French and Spanish. Probably more world languages are syllable-timed than are stress-timed, and sometimes speakers of those languages have a difficult time learning English stress patterns.

Stress timing in English has several implications for the SLP. First of all, without unstressed syllables, there would be none of the **vowel reduction** for which English is known. Vowel reduction is the use of a more central vowel for a vowel that is less central. In terms of the vowel quadrilateral (see Figure 1-1), the actual vowel produced would be closer to the center of the figure than is the target vowel. For example, the first vowel in *mistake* is /ɪ/ (in the upper left-hand corner of the vowel quadrilateral), and we would use an /ɪ/ in careful speech. However, most of the time in connected speech we substitute [ə], which is in the center of the quadrilateral.

In other words, reduction of non-central vowels toward more central vowels occurs only in unstressed syllables. For example, consider the second vowel in the words *resign* and *resignation*. In *resign*, the second vowel is in a stressed syllable and is said as /aɪ/, but in *resignation*, that same vowel is now located in an unstressed syllable and is reduced to [ɪ] or to the most central vowel, [ə].

A second important aspect to stress timing is that there are several populations seen in clinics that have particular difficulty with alternating stress (and with vowel reduction). These include some ESL speakers, some dysarthrics (particularly those with monopitch and monoloudness), telegraphic aphasics (who delete function words, which are unstressed), and finally, children with severe speech sound disorders. In the child population, the process of syllable reduction occurs only on unstressed syllables. Children who reduce syllables are also likely to leave out function words, which are unstressed (Smit & Bernthal, 1983). The result is that the child's speech sounds somewhat jerky because stressed syllables are all that is left.

**Sentence-level stress** refers to the location of emphasized words in an utterance, and this location is dependent on the speaker's intent. For example, in this simple sentence, the implied meaning changes depending on the location of the emphasis:

Algernon (and not Edward) loves Penelope.

Algernon loves (not merely likes) Penelope.

Algernon loves Penelope (and not Sybil).

In English, emphasis on a word in an utterance is usually signaled by an increase in vocal pitch, increase in loudness, and increase in duration of that word. In some other languages, emphasis is signaled by adding a syllable to the emphasized word. Obviously, ESL clients whose first language works this way will have particular difficulty with sentence-level stress.

**Durations of speech sounds** play as important a role as spectral frequency in the production and perception of speech. Coordination of articulatory movements must happen within certain timing constraints or the clarity of the utterance will be muddied. Moreover, we have already mentioned that there is a developmental course to most durational aspects of speech.

**Intonation contours** and **loudness contours** describe characteristics of the whole utterance by indicating perceived changes in pitch (intonation) or loudness over the course of an utterance. This can be noted by drawing a contour over the printed utterance, for example:

Pitch contour          Algernon loves Penelope.

Loudness contour          Algernon loves Penelope.

There are also computerized programs to extract the fundamental frequency—the physical correlate of pitch, and the amplitude—the physical correlate of loudness. These programs produce contours that can be printed out and annotated. Some of them also permit the clinician to model a production, and then have the client imitate and compare the two productions with respect to these contours.

## Characteristics of Speaking Situations

The situational context in which a person speaks an utterance can greatly influence the motor and phonological aspects of that utterance. The most frequent effects appear to be on segment durations and on carefulness of articulation.

**Citation forms** are single words spoken as single words in an isolated utterance. When we model a word for a child to imitate, we produce that word as a citation form. Citation forms are typically longer in duration, that is, spoken at a slower rate, than the same word embedded in an utterance. Citation forms also tend to be spoken with attention to all the phonemes in the word. For example, most people, when they say the word *government* in a conversation, never say the /n/ in the second syllable. In fact, in some parts of the United States, the word is said as "gummint." However, if a clinician is trying to teach a client the word *government*, she will be careful to produce that /n/. **Clear speech** is the connected-speech equivalent of citation speech. That is, clear speech is relatively slow, and it has emphasis on acoustic differences (Kent & Read, 1992).

**Conversational** or **colloquial speech** is the everyday, ordinary version of speech. It is informal, slangy, and characterized by elisions (deletions and contractions) and extreme vowel reductions (Kent & Read, 1992). Colloquial speech is also spoken at relatively fast rates. Perhaps the best-known example of the phonology of colloquial English is the utterance [ʤiʔʤɛʔ], meaning "Did you eat yet?" This production is a great example of **syllable coalescence**, in which two or more syllables are said as one syllable, but aspects of the two original syllables are preserved. In [ʤiʔʤɛʔ], it is clear that the four syllables are coalesced into two syllables. The [ʤiʔ] syllable preserves the stops of *did* (albeit in affricate form), the palatal place of articulation of the /j/ in *you*, and the central vowel of the more meaningful word, *eat*. The second resulting syllable, [ʤɛʔ], preserves the approximate place of articulation of the final stop in *eat*, the palatal nature of the /j/ in *yet*, and the center vowel [ɛ] in *yet*. Another aspect of this much shortened production is the fact that assimilation is going on: There is no /ʤ/ in the full version of this question. However, the alveolar obstruents /d/ and /t/ and the palatal glide /j/ have combined to form the palatal obstruent /ʤ/ in the colloquial form.

**Formal speech** is the type of speech that people tend to use when making presentations, speaking to a person deemed worthy of respect, engaging in professional interactions, and giving a sermon. Compared to colloquial speech, formal speech tends to show fewer elisions and fewer instances of syllable coalescence, and to use less extreme vowel reduction. In formal speech, the question "Did you eat yet?" is produced [dɪdjuiʔjɛʔ]. Formal speech is probably the closest to the printed versions of words, in that there is a closer mapping between the graphemes and the phonemes produced.

**Exaggerated speech** is a form of speech used to emphasize words in a dramatic way. Exaggerated speech is also used to differentiate two or more words that can fit into the same frame, for example, "I said <u>Mary</u>, not Susan." Exaggeration is accomplished through lengthening in duration and through atypically large variations in pitch and loudness.

In speech-language pathology, we most often encounter exaggerated speech when presenting members of minimal pairs (e.g., "ba<u>t</u>," "ba<u>d</u>"). In spoken minimal pairs, the segments that differentiate the two words may have characteristics that are maximally different. This is also called **contrastive speech**. For example, in "bat" the /æ/ may be very short and the /t/

may be aspirated, while in "bad" the vowel may be much longer in duration and there may be voicing for a relatively long time during the /d/.

## ASSESSMENT CONCEPTS

Accurate assessment is crucial to providing effective services to change speech sound production. Accurate assessment includes not only describing the client's speech pattern, but also generates information about the best approach to this client's difficulties. For example, we may serve two school-age children who have similar speech patterns, but for one, we may have a strong home program as a component, and for the other, we may work more intensively in the school setting. The information that might lead to this differentiation could be that the parent of one child expresses this interest and appears to have the skills to undertake a home program, while the parent of the other child may be either too anxious or too stressed to do a good job.

A recent focus in speech-language pathology has been that of dynamic assessment. **Dynamic assessment** refers to ideas that originated with Vygotsky (1978; 1986), who argued that a child's cognitive development occurs <u>in</u> a social environment and occurs <u>because</u> of the social environment. In particular, he claimed that knowledgeable adults in the child's environment guide her participation in the social and cultural context. Applied to speech and language disorders, dynamic assessment refers to the clinician's search for ways that help the child change toward social and cultural expectations with respect to speech and language (Bain, 1994; Olswang, Bain, & Johnson, 1992). Dynamic assessment also implies that (a) the ways in which we can best assist the child are likely to change over time, and (b) assessment needs to occur relative to the child's social interactions. Dynamic assessment plays a role in an initial assessment to help answer the question of whether the client can benefit from intervention at this time. However, the larger role for dynamic assessment is during the course of treatment, when the clinician needs to remain alert for signs of impending change and for new behaviors toward which he can guide the client.

### Normative Information

Virtually all forms of assessment in speech-language pathology and audiology depend on normative information for their interpretation. **Norms** represent the typical behavior of persons at specific chronological ages in the population sampled. In other words, in much of our assessment, a developmental model is used. Sometimes, however, a norm represents a kind of physiological normalcy, for example, the zero dB HL level on audiograms. Speech-language pathologists working with speech sound disorders typically use three kinds of norms: standardized test norms, ages of acquisition of phonemes, and ages of "suppression" of phonological processes.

### *Standardized Tests*

The majority of **standardized tests** for articulation and phonology provide an inventory of the client's production of most or all of the phonemes in English as well as a sampling of consonant clusters. Most of these tests are normed on a large number of children who represent the demographics of the population of the United States. Some examples include the *Goldman-Fristoe Test of Articulation-2* (Goldman & Fristoe, 2000), the *Bankson-Bernthal Test of Phonology* (*BBTOP*—Bankson & Bernthal, 1990), and the *Smit-Hand Articulation and Phonology Evaluation* (*SHAPE*—Smit & Hand, 1997). Other tests are not normed themselves but "borrow" norms from other work. Typically, the test user consults the test manual for the mean score for children at the age of the client, the confidence interval, and the cutpoints to determine if the child's performance is outside normal limits.

Standardized tests must meet certain statistical standards in order to be considered valid tests of what they purport to test. The statistical terms that are most often used in describing test data are these:

- The **mean** (the average score of the group in question)
- The **standard deviation** (a mathematically defined measure of variation about the mean)
- The **confidence interval** (a range about the score in which the clinician can be relatively sure that the true score would fall)
- The **cutoff for the lowest 10%** (a point that is often used in defining clinical populations)
- The **cutpoint at two standard deviations below the mean** (another point that is used in defining clinical populations)
- **Percentile ranks** (how high or low the child's score is in the distribution of scores for children of the same age)

In addition, many tests make provision for **standard scores**, which represent a transformation of the basic test statistics. The transformation is usually to a scale with a mean of 50 or 100 and a standard deviation of 10.

The standard deviation and other measures of variability are important because typical behavior for a given age cannot be reduced to a single point (the mean); rather, typical behavior represents a range of abilities. At the same time, we often need to know how far away from the mean a child must be in order to be considered "not normal." For this purpose, the two cutpoints (two standard deviations below the mean and the lowest 10 percent) can be very helpful.

Speech-language pathologists may also use **special-purpose tests**. These are tests that do not claim to be normed but rather are descriptive in nature. For example, to describe a child's use of phonological processes, the clinician might administer the *Assessment of Phonological Processes—Revised* (*APP*—Hodson, 1986). In order to examine the degree to which the client varies in production of a target phoneme when the phoneme is produced in a variety of phonetic contexts, the SLP could use the *McDonald Deep Test* (McDonald, 1964a).

### *Ages of Acquisition for Phonemes*

Some of the earliest studies of speech development were done in order to determine by what age a child should have mastered each phoneme. These investigators typically studied groups of children at succeeding ages in whole- or half-year intervals, gave them single-word inventory tests, and determined the number (and percentage) of children at each age level who had mastered a particular phoneme. The **age of acquisition** of a phoneme was defined as the age level at which at least 75% (or sometimes 90%) of children used the phoneme correctly in all word positions tested. These ages of acquisition have been used extensively in standards set by each state for providing speech-language pathology services to children in public schools. School-age children (and adults) who continue to make errors on individual phonemes past the age of acquisition for that phoneme are said to have **residual errors** (Shriberg, 1994).

Table 1-5 shows the recommended ages of acquisition that resulted from the most recent study of this type (Smit, Hand, Freilinger, Bernthal, & Bird, 1990). This table is based on 90% levels of acquisition for phonemes tested in word-initial and word-final positions. In some cases, such as /f/, there was such a large disparity between initial and final positions that the word positions are reported separately. In addition, in this table males and females are reported separately, at least for the preschool years, because their performance differed somewhat. Finally, in Table 1-5, a range is given for /s z/ and any cluster containing /s/ because of the nature of the errors. That is, some errors on /s z/ are considered to be developmental and others are not. The only error for these sounds that is considered to be developmental is dentalization (either dentalized [s̪ z̪] or *theta* and *eth* substitutions).

**TABLE 1–5**  Ages of consonant acquisition, adapted with permission from the Iowa-Nebraska Norms Project. The ages indicated are based on 90% levels of acquisition. *Smit, Hand, Freilinger, Bernthal, and Bird (1990).*

| | Recommended Ages of Acquisition (years:months) | |
|---|---|---|
| **Phoneme** | **Females** | **Males** |
| /m/ | 3:0 | 3:0 |
| /n/ | 3:6 | 3:0 |
| /-ŋ/ | 7:0-9:0 | 7:0-9:0 |
| /h/ | 3:0 | 3:0 |
| /w-/ | 3:0 | 3:0 |
| /j/ | 4:0 | 5:0 |
| /p/ | 3:0 | 3:0 |
| /b/ | 3:0 | 3:0 |
| /t/ | 4:0 | 3:6 |
| /d/ | 3:0 | 3:6 |
| /k/ | 3:6 | 3:6 |
| /g/ | 3:6 | 4:0 |
| /f/ /f-/ | 3:6 | 3:6 |
| /-f/ | 5:6 | 5:6 |
| /v/ | 5:6 | 5:6 |
| /θ/ | 6:0 | 8:0 |
| /ð/ | 4:6 | 7:0 |
| /s/ | 7:0-9:0* | 7:0-9:0* |
| /z/ | 7:0-9:0* | 7:0-9:0* |
| /ʃ/ | 6:0 | 7:0 |
| /tʃ/ | 6:0 | 7:0 |
| /dʒ/ | 6:0 | 7:0 |
| /l/ /l-/ | 5:0 | 6:0 |
| /-l/ | 6:0 | 7:0 |
| /r/ /r-/ | 8:0 | 8:0 |
| /-ɚ/ | 8:0 | 8:0 |

*(continues)*

**TABLE 1–5**    Continued

| Recommended Ages of Acquisition (years:months) | | |
|---|---|---|
| **Word-Initial Clusters** | **Females** | **Males** |
| /tw kw/ | 4:0 | 5:6 |
| /sp st sk/ | 7:0-9:0 | 7:0-9:0 |
| /sm sn/ | 7:0-9:0 | 7:0-9:0 |
| /sw/ | 7:0-9:0 | 7:0-9:0 |
| /sl/ | 7:0-9:0 | 7:0-9:0 |
| /pl bl kl gl fl/ | 5:6 | 6:0 |
| /pr br tr dr kr gr fr/ | 8:0 | 8:0 |
| /θr/ | 9:0 | 9:0 |
| /skw/ | 7:0-9:0 | 7:0-9:0 |
| /spl/ | 7:0-9:0 | 7:0-9:0 |
| /spr str skr/ | 7:0-9:0 | 7:0-9:0 |

*Assess and remediate non-developmental errors before age 7:0. Errors not considered to be developmental include lateralizations and other post-alveolar distortions.

## Ages of "Suppression" of Phonological Processes

Because most of the errors of preschool children can be described under the rubric of phonological processes, the age at which children no longer use them is important for assessment. The term *suppression* has been criticized on the grounds that it suggests that children actually know the correct form but actively change it because of production constraints. This criticism has merit, because it is entirely possible that the child does not know the adult form. However, there do not appear to be other shorthand ways to describe the concept of a criterion age when children no longer use a particular process.

There are two or three sources of information about the age of suppression of processes. Each source is likely to list somewhat different ages of suppression from the others because of variations in how the data were collected. The most recent data are shown in Table 1-6, which is taken from the *SHAPE* (Smit & Hand, 1997). This table shows the ages of suppression for processes in the type of single-word sample elicited in the process of norming this test. The age of suppression is the age at which 90% or fewer of children in the norming population continued to use a process productively, that is, used the process in 40% or more of the opportunities to use it.

**TABLE 1–6**    Ages at which children suppress common phonological processes (i.e., no longer use them productively). Data are taken from the *SHAPE*.

*Smit and Hand (1997).*

| **Process** | **Age of "Suppression"*** |
|---|---|
| Voicing of initial voiceless obstruents | <3:0 |
| Assimilations | <3:0 |
| Final consonant deletion | 3:0 |

| Process | Age of "Suppression"* |
|---|---|
| Stopping of initial fricative and affricate singles | 3:6 |
| Fronting of initial velar singles | 4:0 |
| Cluster reduction—clusters without /s/ | 4:0 |
| Depalatalization of final singles | 4:6 |
| Depalatalization of initial singles | 5:0 |
| Weak syllable deletion | 5:0 |
| Cluster reduction—/s/-clusters | 5:0 |
| Gliding of initial liquids | 7:0 |
| Vocalization of postvocalic liquids | 7:0 |

*Age at which 10% or fewer use the process productively. Productive use is defined as use of the process in 40% or more of exemplars.

Table 1-6 deals with the very common processes. However, the *SHAPE* manual also provides information about how to determine if a child uses any of the many possible unusual or idiosyncratic processes. Other tests of phonological processes include similar tables showing the age at which particular processes are no longer used.

## Global Assessment of Speech

In assessment of speech production it is important to characterize the overall effect or contribution that the speech has to a child's communication difficulty. Three very important areas are the intelligibility of the speech, the severity of the speech disorder, and the effects of the speech on the child's communication function. Clearly, global assessment is consistent with the focus on social use of speech that characterizes dynamic assessment practices.

**Intelligibility** is a measure of how understandable the child's conversational speech is to others. The clinician can quantify intelligibility through the use of rating scales that have equal-appearing intervals, such as this one:

| | | | | | |
|---|---|---|---|---|---|
| 1 | 2 | 3 | 4 | 5 | 6 |

Most intelligible          Least intelligible

Another way to quantify intelligibility is to listen to a recorded sample and to count up the number of glossable words as well as the total number of words. **Glossable words** are the words that a listener understands well enough to **gloss** or write down. The percent of glossable words is then used as an estimate of intelligibility (Shriberg & Kwiatkowski, 1982b). It is important to keep in mind that intelligibility can be influenced by factors such as familiarity of the listener with the child's speech patterns, the nature of the interaction (which may result in short choppy sentences or long complex sentences), whether or not the listener knows the context, and the quality of the recording and recording conditions. For this reason, it is good to collect speech samples under uniform conditions and to gloss them in a uniform way.

Another assessment instrument that has been developed recently is the *Preschool Speech Intelligibility Measure* (Wilcox & Morris, 1999). This instrument is based on single words imitated by the child. The listener has a multiple-choice response form to use in recording what the child said. The authors developed this instrument primarily as a means to track intelligibility changes over time.

**Severity** is a measure of how disordered or deviant the child's speech is in terms of its deviation from some internalized standard. In order to measure severity, the SLP can use a scale similar to that shown earlier for intelligibility, but with "severity" substituted for "intelligibility." However, there is another measure of severity that is widely used, namely the Percent of Consonants Correct (PCC—Shriberg & Kwiatkowski, 1982b). Details of this measure will be given in Section 2.

**Distinctiveness/bizarreness** is the degree to which the client's error pattern draws attention to itself and away from the content of her speech. In the early days of the profession of speech-language pathology, this concept was routinely used in evaluations to determine if intervention services were required. This criterion is still used extensively in the area of fluency disorders, and it is still relevant to some cases of articulation and phonology disorders. For example, if a young girl has lateral productions of /s z ʃ ʒ tʃ dʒ/, the listener is likely to be distracted by the unusual acoustic and visual patterns of her speech. In fact, the distraction may be so great that the listener does not receive the content of the utterance.

**Functionality** is a measure of how ecologically useful the child's speech is. For example, if a child has poor intelligibility and her speech is severely disordered, but she can communicate effectively with the people in her environment, that child is better off than another child whose few errors are developmental but who cannot use speech effectively during the early language learning period. Functionality is difficult to quantify, because it has to be based on reports from significant others. These must all be clinician-constructed tools, because as yet, there are no standardized or commercial tools to assess functional communication in children. These tools will most likely be questionnaires with questions such as these:

How do you communicate with your child?

Does your child ever show signs of frustration or anger when he or she is not understood?

Does your child sometimes just walk away when misunderstood?

How do you try to help your child?

How often do you or others have to "interpret" for your child?

## Related Areas

In our assessment of articulation and phonology disorders, we may assess many other areas of function in order to determine what impact they may have on the child's difficulties or on our findings. Positive findings in these areas will need to be interpreted as part of the clinical picture. Some of these areas include the child's dialect or second-language status, the client's social and medical history, the adequacy of the oral and respiratory structures and their functions, hearing status, linguistic status (comprehension and production), cognitive status, metaphonological status, and social-familial interactions.

Shriberg and Kwiatkowski (1982a) have discussed some of these areas in terms of what they call "causal-correlates." **Causal-correlates** are variables that have been identified in the past as related to the presence of a speech sound disorder or that are plausible on the basis of phonological and other types of theories. These variables in general are potentially causative either by themselves or in combination with other variables, but the mechanisms of causation have not been elucidated. Causal-correlates are conceptualized in three areas: those that relate to the mechanism, those that reflect cognitive-linguistic function, and those that are considered to be psychosocial. These are useful classifications for the clinician to use in conceptualizing diagnostic information.

The areas encompassed under causal-correlates include all of the areas that the SLP typically assesses. To examine variables related to the physical mechanism, we consider the child's health and developmental history, we assess hearing status, and we evaluate the speaking mechanism (articulators, respiration, phonation, and resonance) in terms of both structure and function. Causal-correlates related to language and cognition include receptive and expressive language measures, pragmatics, and sometimes, estimates of cognitive functioning, and these also are typically assessed. The psychosocial causal-correlates include variables related to inputs, for example, parental behaviors, and the existence of friends of an appropriate age. The psychosocial causal-correlates also include outputs, for example, aggression, dependency, and responsiveness on the part of the child, as well as the child's interest in communicating.

## Dialect and/or Second-Language Status

Our primary concern with respect to dialect is whether a child's speech sound patterns might be due to the child's dialect. **Dialects** are distinctive but mutually intelligible varieties of a language that are spoken by large groups of people. Many dialects are regional in nature, for example,"Bostonian" or "Southern," but some appear to be based on ethnicity or social class, such as "African American Vernacular English" or the variety of British English known as "Cockney." Within dialects there is often a great deal of "optionality," meaning that the speaker is free to use or not use particular features of the dialect.

Most American dialects differ from each other primarily with respect to vowels and diphthongs, but there are also some consonant differences, most of which affect post-vocalic /r/ (Small, 1999). The issue with respect to dialects and assessment is that many test norms and most published sets of normative data are based on children who speak a dialect close to General American. If we are evaluating a child growing up in Boston who does not always use post-vocalic /r/, she should not be penalized for lack of /r/ because that is a characteristic of her dialect.

The issues related to English being learned as a second language can be quite complex. If the first language is very different from English, there may be interference in learning English. For example, if a Japanese-speaking child of age 7 starts to learn English at that age, we can expect that at first the child will not produce English clusters or final consonants because Japanese has few, if any, of these structures.

The biggest issue for assessment is whether the child is making adequate progress in the second language, including its phonology. Some of the variables that can have an impact on this issue include the length of time the child has been exposed to English, whether that exposure comes only at school or from peers, how many hours per week he is exposed to English, whether reading instruction is underway, whether the child is having difficulty acquiring the first language, and so forth. Goldstein (2000) has an excellent chapter on these issues. One important point he makes, quoting Cummins (1984), is that children who go to school in English should be able to converse with peers within two years, but it may take five to seven years before the child develops academic skills in English.

## Metaphonology and Phonological Awareness

**Metaphonology** is the ability to think about and evaluate one's own phonological productions. Self-evaluation of production is an important part of many intervention approaches, particularly for children older than about 6 years of age. Younger children may not have this ability, at least for the acoustic results of oral movements, but they may be able to assess or report on their own physical movements of the articulators before that age.

**Phonological awareness** is the capacity to think about phonemes, syllables, and words and also to manipulate these segments (e.g., by rhyming words). Phonological awareness is related to learning to read and becoming a fluent reader (Kamhi & Catts, 1991). Some of the skills that seem to be critical for learning to read include encoding of phonological information, retrieval of phonological information, and using phonological codes in working memory. Children with phonological difficulties are considered to be at risk for later reading problems and also have been shown to have more difficulties with phonological awareness than children without phonological disorders.

## Prognosis and Prognostic Indicators

We can think of a **prognosis** as an educated guess or forecast about the client's future with respect to the speech sound disorder. Prognosis is one of the least researched areas in the study of speech sound disorders. However, with respect to speech sound disorders, there is some research to go on concerning stimulability and inconsistency or variability. **Stimulability** is the ability to imitate correctly an errored sound under specified conditions. Stimulability is generally tested informally.

**Inconsistency** or **variability** refers to a client's tendency to vary or not to vary in production of a given phoneme or phonological structure. In general, variability is considered to be positive because the client has not settled on a "final" version of the structure and the system is considered to be malleable. If the variable productions include one or more that are closer to the target than the others, variability is an even more positive prognostic indicator.

It is probably safe to say that typically developing children are quite variable in their productions of specific sounds in the period before the sound is firmly entrenched in the phonology. In fact, in the motor control literature, reduction in variability is considered to be an indicator of skill. On the other hand, children with severe speech sound disorders may have relatively stable systems. For example, the existence of idiosyncratic processes over a period of time (favorite sound, word recipes, and glottal substitutions) suggests that the child has a default setting that is relatively stable. In this case we may prefer to think of the child as "stuck" rather than as "skilled." Clearly the goal of treatment for this child is to introduce variability.

## *Environmental and Status Variables*

Many variables can influence a prognosis. Some of them are related to the child's environment, and others are related to the child's status in specified areas (e.g., cognitive delay). Clinical Note 1-1 suggests that prognosis may vary in ways that are related to environmental and status variables. The reader should be warned, however, that the evidence for these statements is scant because there is little research in this area.

---

CLINICAL NOTE 1-1:  Possible Tendencies in Prognosis

- "Uncomplicated" speech sound disorders probably have a better prognosis than disorders complicated by such variables as a significant medical history, behavioral disorders, and so on.

- Younger children may have a better prognosis than do older children.

- Mild speech sound disorders may have a better prognosis than more severe disorders.

- Speech sound disorders that are largely developmental may have a better prognosis than speech sound disorders that have bizarre or idiosyncratic components.

*(continues)*

*(continued)*

- If the client is old enough for motivation to be assessed, the motivated client may have a better prognosis than the unmotivated client.
- The child who has a speech sound disorder may have a better prognosis if she is growing up in an accepting environment than in a punitive, rejecting, or critical environment.

## Diagnostic Groups

It makes sense to talk about diagnostic groups within the spectrum of speech sound disorders, so long as these divisions are useful for differential treatment and for determining prognosis. Certain groups have been delineated for many years, and these are based on **etiology**, that is, on the presumed cause of the speech sound disorder. So, for example, the speech of the severely to profoundly hearing impaired can be distinguished from the speech of those with cleft palate. Children with cerebral palsy are often considered to be dysarthric, and children with severe developmental delay are often considered to form a unique group. Treatment for these diagnostic subgroups tends to differ from group to group.

It should be mentioned, however, that children with some of the organically based disorders are just as likely to use phonological processes as other language-learning children. In other words, during the period of phonological acquisition, not all of the child's speech sound errors can be attributed to the effects of an underlying organic disorder. What is more likely is that the characteristics associated with the organic deficit interact with the basic biologically driven tendencies of the language-learning child.

Among children with speech sound difficulties who do not have an obvious etiology, there has been relatively little research into other meaningful subgroups (see Shriberg, 1994, for a review of this literature). Ideally, if a group can be defined functionally, on the basis of assessment and history, then there should be either a more appropriate type of treatment, or a distinct prognosis for the members of the subgroup compared to members of other subgroups. In this respect, we might consider the prognostic portraits presented in Clinical Note 1-2.

The distinction made between phonological and motor-based approaches in Clinical Note 1-2 reflects the idea that the child with phonological disorders (abstract, linguistic) is functionally different from children with motor-based or residual errors. Consequently, the type of treatment is different. In addition, two of the portraits in the Clinical Note (4 and 7) would most likely be considered to demonstrate **Developmental Verbal Dyspraxia (DVD),** sometimes called **Developmental Apraxia of Speech (DAS),** both of which refer to a presumed difficulty in the sequencing of speech movements. Those who use this terminology make reference to adult neurogenic apraxia of speech, which is thought to be a disorder of motor sequencing. In this view, DVD is also a motor sequencing disorder but with a developmental cast. Then there are those who say that DVD does not exist as a unique disorder in children, and that children who are said to show DVD really have just a very severe phonological disorder.

It is the position of this author that DVD does exist as unique symptomatology and unique history embedded within a phonological disorder, a group that Shriberg (1994) calls "Speech Delay plus DAS." In my view, the unique symptoms include groping behaviors of the articulators, a very slow rate of speech, markedly restricted phonetic and phonemic inventories, presence of both natural phonological and idiosyncratic processes, and often prosodic changes. The unique history may include a relatively long history of treatment with relatively little improvement, a history of **sensory aversions** (e.g., extreme dislike of certain textures) in the limbs, face, and mouth during the early years; a history of reluctance to imitate; and possibly feeding difficulties in early life.

CLINICAL NOTE 1-2: Prognostic Portraits

1. Preschool or early school-aged child; intelligibility mild-moderate; many phonological processes; no idiosyncratic processes; no complicating issues.

   Prognosis: Positive for normalization within one to two years, but only if phonological process approaches are used.

2. Preschool or early school-aged child; intelligibility moderate-severe; many phonological processes; one or two idiosyncratic processes; expressive language delayed, receptive language normal; no other complications.

   Prognosis: Positive for normalization within two to three years, if a combination of phonological processes and motor articulation approaches is used.

3. Preschool or early school-aged child; intelligibility moderate-severe; many phonological processes; one or two idiosyncratic processes; expressive and receptive language delayed; no other complications.

   Prognosis: Fair for significant improvement within two to three years, assuming that language and phonology are treated simultaneously and that a phonological process approach is used.

4. Preschool or early school-aged child; intelligibility severely-profoundly impaired; many phonological processes, and many idiosyncratic processes; receptive language normal to low-normal; expressive output extremely limited; child appears to have difficulty with volitional oral-nonverbal movements.

   Prognosis: Guarded for significant improvement within two to three years, assuming specialized treatment.

5. School-aged child; intelligibility fair to good; residual errors; stimulable for all errors; motivated; language and cognition within normal limits; no previous treatment or treatment only many years previously.

   Prognosis: Excellent, assuming that motor-based approaches are used.

6. School-age child; intelligibility moderate to fair; residual errors; stimulable for only some errors; long history of treatment; motivation questionable; language and cognition in low-normal range.

   Prognosis: Guarded, assuming that motor-based approaches are used.

7. School-aged child; intelligibility poor; many errors, not all residual; stimulable for some errors with difficulty; long history of treatment; language and cognition in low normal range, with language output very limited; difficulties with volitional oral-nonverbal movements.

   Prognosis: Guarded, even with appropriate approaches; may need to supplement with AAC device.

## REMEDIATION CONCEPTS

The continuum of treatment is a concept discussed by Bernthal and Bankson (1998) in their classic text on disorders of articulation and phonology. The **continuum of treatment** is a way to conceptualize the sequence of treatment from an initial establishment phase through a phase of facilitation of generalization and finally to maintenance of the newly acquired skills. Different goals and procedures are required at each stage.

During the **establishment phase**, the client learns to produce the target phoneme or structure voluntarily and repeatedly. At the end of this phase, the target should be stable (90% accurate) in at least one linguistic or phonetic context, no matter how restricted. During the next phase, the **generalization phase**, the client learns to use the target in a greater variety of contexts and a greater number of speaking situations. For example, if the elicitation phase ended with stable production of /s/ in the syllable /is/, then generalization to other nonsense syllables will likely occur first, and later generalization to words, phrases, and sentences. If the establishment phase ended with stable production of an /s/-plus-stop cluster in the word *spit*, then generalization proceeds to words such as *spoon*, *stick*, and *ski*. During the **maintenance phase**, the clinician gradually transfers responsibility for carryover to other speaking situations and contexts to the client.

## The Technology of Behavioral Methodology

The most important technology in the speech-language pathology tool kit is the methods borrowed from behavioral modification and motor learning. These techniques are powerful in their ability to change behavior. They have generally been associated only with motoric approaches to remediation, but this is a wrong-headed view. That is, behavioral techniques are useful under any approach, including those intended to stimulate cognitive processing, and the informed use of these tools makes treatment more efficient and effective than if they are not used.

Bernthal and Bankson (1998) divide behavioral strategies into those that are concerned with **antecedent events** (occurring before the response), **response definition** (the criteria for an acceptable response), and **consequent events** (occurring after the response). The antecedent events include models and cues provided by the clinician, while the consequent events include reinforcement and other forms of feedback to the client.

### *Technology of Antecedent Events: Models and Cues*

The models and cues provided to the child immediately prior to his attempt to produce the target are critical to his success. Models are the clinician's production of the target, said as a citation form (at least for syllable and word targets). Cues are added instructions, visual stimuli, or phonetic placement reminders (e.g., iconic hand gestures). Effective use of models and cues increases the probability that the child will respond correctly. In the early stages at a particular level, models and cues may be needed, but then they are faded as the client progresses.

### *Technology of Response Definition*

The **response definition** is the statement of criteria for considering a production acceptable. In most cases, the response definition is not something we even consider, since the accepted default is "correct production" of the target, whatever that may be. However, there are times when response definition becomes critical. Consider the case of the client whose error on the alveolar and palatal fricatives is a unilateral fricative with a definite jaw slide toward the side from which air exits. This error is both acoustically and visually deviant. If the client corrects the acoustic product without correcting the jaw slide, his speech will still call attention to itself. In this case, the clinician decides to reinforce only acoustically acceptable productions that have no jaw slide. In other words, the response definition has two criteria, both of which must be met.

## *Technology of Consequent Events: Contingencies/Reinforcement*

The speech-language pathologist can manipulate consequent events as well as antecedent events. When used appropriately, consequent events provide important feedback to the child about the correctness of his response. The clinician may provide **positive reinforcement** if the response met the response criteria, or the clinician may say "No" followed by a statement of how to improve the production. For example, in the case mentioned above with a prominent jaw slide:

Clinician: [s:]

Client: [s:] (acoustically correct, but with jaw slide)

Clinician: No. Make sure your jaw only moves up and down.

Most often SLPs use verbal/social reinforcement ("Good," said with a smile). Sometimes a token economy is used with a client who appears to need motivation. A **token economy** is a system of tangible rewards (tokens) that the client can accumulate and exchange later for a desired object. Tokens can be poker chips, beads, paper clips, or M&Ms, and they are usually accompanied by verbal/social reinforcement.

Besides the nature of the reinforcement, the **schedule of positive reinforcement** is an important variable. Here are some sample schedules of reinforcement, arranged from the most responsive (top) to the least responsive (bottom).

Based on Counts

100% : reinforce every correct response

50%: reinforce every other correct response

50% variable: on average, reinforce half of the correct responses

10%: reinforce every tenth correct response

10% variable: on average, reinforce every tenth response

Based on Intervals

Reinforce at the end of each specified interval (e.g., one minute)

Reinforce on a schedule that that averages out to once per minute

Intensive reinforcement schedules are used when quick attainment of a goal is needed. However, behaviors acquired with a 100% schedule tend to extinguish (be lost) easily. Therefore, as soon as the behavior is stable, the clinician reduces the reinforcement schedule. Sparse reinforcement schedules tend to make a behavior resistant to extinction.

## Approaches to Treatment

Although a great many therapy programs have been published, most can be classified into two major categories. These two categories are nicely summarized by Elbert and Gierut (1986) as "training deep" and "training broad." **Training deep** implies an emphasis on remediating one or just a few sounds, taking them from the establishment phase through the maintenance phase. The emphasis is on the motor patterns and the resulting acoustic products. Traditional Van Riper-type treatment is a good example of "training deep." **Training broad** is used to refer to phonological treatments that target several exemplars of one phonological process and/or several processes all at once. These programs solicit involvement of the cognitive/linguistic capacities of the child. The explicit goal of "training broad" approaches is rapid generalization to spontaneous speech.

There are, of course, certain treatment regimes that do not appear to fit into either category. Examples might be the motor-kinesthetic treatments such as PROMPT (Chumpelik, 1984) and McDonald's Sensory-Motor Approach (1964b), both of which will be discussed in Section 8. Such treatments appear to focus on the establishment phase by enhancing motor and sensory precursors considered necessary to produce the target sound.

## SUMMARY

This chapter has given the areas that are basic to the practice of speech-language pathology in the areas of speech sound disorders and intelligibility improvement. I hope that practicing SLPs are generally familiar with most of these concepts. Knowledgeable use of this information can benefit our clients in ways that are clear-cut and noticeable to the client and to the people important to her. This is, therefore, one of the very rewarding areas of practice in our profession.

# SECTION

## 2

# EFFECTIVE ASSESSMENT OF SPEECH SOUND DISORDERS

• • • • • • • • • • • • • • • • • • • • • • • • • • • • • • • • • • • • • •

**W**hen we see a client for the first time, it is usually in the context of beginning a diagnostic evaluation with that client. Our plan for this evaluation depends on several pieces of information, most important of which is a statement about the problem made by the client or the client's parent, or by someone else who knows the client. Sometimes these statements are very general ("We have trouble understanding her"), but quite often they indicate what the respondent thinks the problem might be ("She does not make the 'r' sound right"). Based on this information, we determine what procedures and assessments to follow.

As part of the planning process, we work under several constraints. One of these is the general standard for evaluations that guides all professionals in communication disorders. Another is the accepted practice for communication disorders of the type that this client may have. In school settings, there are additional standards relating to the need for multiple types of assessment in the relevant areas. And still another constraint is the preferences of the speech-language pathologist.

# PROFESSIONAL STANDARDS FOR DIAGNOSTIC EVALUATIONS

There is no generally accepted statement of professional standards for diagnostic evaluations. However, virtually all speech-language pathologists understand that a diagnostic evaluation should be conducted according to this rule: "Assess in all areas relevant to communication." The assessment may need to be only a screening, but the speech-language pathologist must at least comment on each of the relevant areas. These include:

- Case history, both developmental and recent
- Speech sound production
- Language
- Hearing
- Voice and resonance
- Fluency
- Prosody and speaking rate
- The oral mechanism

Clearly, if you are evaluating a child, you will want to document language performance across several domains: receptive, expressive, content, form, and use (pragmatics). If you are assessing a older teenager with a distorted /s/, then it may be sufficient to note that the client's linguistic abilities are most likely adequate since the client has progressed annually from grade to grade and is on the honor roll at school.

Another professional standard, this one external to speech-language pathology, has been adopted in public laws relating to education. This standard is that the SLP must assess an area in at least two distinctly different ways before deciding that the child has a deficiency in that area. So, for example, if speech sound production appears to be an area of difficulty for the child, it could be assessed using a standardized test and an analysis of connected speech. The important idea is that one test or one screening should never be the sole basis on which the child receives intervention. This principle is a good one for all settings.

The profession of speech-language pathology changes as we learn more about communication and related areas. For example, we now know that information about feeding and swallowing is important when you are assessing preschoolers, school-age children with severe impairments, and adults with neurogenic or craniofacial disorders. For such clients, the SLP needs to make sure to assess in these domains. Another example is of phonological awareness and its relationship to reading and reading problems. Many clinicians now routinely assess phonological awareness when evaluating preschool and early school-age children.

There are a number of excellent resources available for the speech-language pathologist that deal with the general topic of assessment (e.g., Tomblin, Morris, & Spriestersbach, 2000). The present chapter will deal with issues that are specific to speech sound disorders within the context of assessment. In addition, Reproducible Form 1 in Appendix A provides a checklist of areas typically covered in a diagnostic evaluation.

# THE CASE HISTORY

Most often, a partial case history can be obtained in writing from the client or from a person who is close to the client. This information is usually supplemented through the use of interview questions posed to the informant. Most published case history questionnaires include questions about developmental history, medical history, and current status (communicative, social, behavioral). Examples can be found in Haynes and Pindzola (1998) and Shipley and McAfee (1998).

It is difficult to overestimate the importance of the case history for helping the clinician to think about the whole person and to interpret the rest of the assessment data. Appropriate interpretation is the goal of every evaluation because the course of intervention will be based on that interpretation. Some examples of possible interpretations may be seen in the next few pages.

## *THE CASE HISTORY*

### Background

**WHO?**      All clients with suspected communication difficulties.

**WHAT?**     The typical case history includes the following:

- Statement of the concerns of the client, parents, or caregiver

- Perinatal and developmental history, including achievement of milestones

- Medical history, including feeding (if considered relevant), sensory defensiveness or aversions (if considered relevant), ear infections, hospitalizations, diagnoses, and medications

- Social history, including family constellation and child's general behavior

- Communication history, including ages of first word and word combinations, how the child uses communication, and any history of intervention

- Current communication status, including how the child talks at present, any use of gestures, and the client's reaction to his/her own speech

- Nature of communication interactions, including an estimate of how much of the time familiar and unfamiliar listeners understand the client, and what listeners do to help the child

**WHY?**      The information obtained in the case history influences both the interpretations and the outcomes of the evaluation. For example, if there are potential delays due to slow overall development and or repeated bouts with illness, then any delays in communication may need to be interpreted in that light. The information about social and communication function helps the SLP determine the magnitude and severity of the child's communication difficulties. The case history information may also support the need for referral to other specialists.

**WHEN?**     The case history is obtained as part of every initial evaluation and may be supplemented as information becomes available.

**SUPPORT:**  Use of case history information has been part of the practice of speech-language pathology since its inception.

# THE CASE HISTORY

## *Procedures and Interpretation*

The case history information may be obtained using questionnaires and interviews. Most agencies offering speech-language pathology services have adopted a standard case history form that they use. In some cases the form may be sent out and returned before the evaluation is scheduled. In other cases the client may be asked to fill out the form on-site.

Interviews are usually based on the case history questionnaire, and they offer the SLP an opportunity to follow up on information obtained from it. The best information is obtained using open-ended questions, for example, "You mentioned that your child's teacher is concerned about communication. What are those concerns?"

The information obtained from the case history feeds into interpretation in various ways. Some examples follow.

- The child with delayed overall development may have speech sound development that is commensurate with mental age but not chronological age. In such cases, the SLP may recommend a wait-and-see stance if the child is young, but she may recommend treatment with a functional communication approach if the client is an adolescent or adult.

- The child who is showing signs of frustration with communication is a prime candidate for treatment.

- At least one adult in the child's immediate environment should understand most of what the child says. The child who is not understood readily by anyone in the immediate environment is a candidate for immediate intervention.

- If the child is in a situation where failures in communication are constantly brought to her attention, she is a candidate for immediate intervention.

- The child who does not respond readily to speech directed at him or her and who also does not communicate effectively should be evaluated by an audiologist and possibly also by a psychologist and a pediatric neurologist.

- Children with a history of feeding problems and/or sensory defensiveness may be at risk for Developmental Verbal Dyspraxia (see Section 8).

- Teenage or adult clients may express the concern that their speech will hold them back in their vocational choices. The SLP will want to weigh this concern and provide counseling on this issue, whether or not there is a problem.

---

# ASSESSING SPEECH SOUND PRODUCTION

Perhaps in no area of practice is interpretation of test results as critical for intervention as in the area of speech sound disorders. As was mentioned in Section 1, there are two major constellations of difficulty, the one that characterizes school-age children and adults, and the other that characterizes preschoolers. Typically, the older group shows "residual errors" or "phonetic errors," which are thought to have a motor learning basis, and the younger group shows "phonological processes," which have a linguistic basis.

The difference between these two constellations is critical to successful treatment. In particular, approaches based exclusively on motor drills are ineffective with phonological disorders and generally should not be used with such cases. Similarly, phonological approaches are likely to be useless with residual errors. We should note, however, that the picture becomes much more complicated when there are elements of Developmental Verbal Dyspraxia.

With respect to tools for assessing segmental (phoneme-level) production, there is an old adage to the effect that "If all you have is a hammer, then everything looks like a nail." With respect to speech sound disorders, if you use a standard test of articulation, you will be led to diagnose a problem with a motoric basis, even if the underlying problem is linguistic. Consequently, it is very important to decide beforehand if a phonological assessment is needed or not. Clinical Note 2-1 indicates some guidelines that the SLP can use.

---

**CLINICAL NOTE 2-1: Guidelines for Choosing an Assessment Approach**

- If the client is younger than 3 years of age, and likely to be within normal limits cognitively (based on the case history), your tentative assumption is that the difficulties are phonological/linguistic. In this case, "informal" phonological assessment instruments are appropriate, including the phonetic and segmental inventories.

- If the child is a preschooler or early school age, and likely to be within normal limits cognitively, a reasonable working assumption is that the difficulties are phonological, especially if the case history suggests that intelligibility is seriously impaired. Phonological test instruments are appropriate if the child's mental age is 3 or older. With children who use few segments, the procedures used with the 0–3 population may be more appropriate.

- If the client is age 7–8 or older, and within normal limits cognitively, it is highly likely that the difficulties consist of residual errors and are motor-based. In such cases, traditional assessment of articulation is appropriate.

- If the client is developmentally delayed, the child's approximate mental age should be your guide.

---

## NON-STANDARDIZED LINGUISTIC ANALYSES

Particularly with infants and toddlers, the SLP may need to use various linguistic analyses to understand the child's phonology. Among these are the determination of the child's phonetic inventory, the syllable and word-shape inventory, and perhaps the segmental inventory. Section 3, which is devoted to assessment of the preschool and early school-age child whose speech is poorly intelligible, describes these types of analyses.

It should be noted that none of these analyses is standardized across large numbers of children. However, in each case, there is information on typical performance of young children on such measures, and the data obtained about your client can often be compared to the published data.

## STANDARDIZED TEST INSTRUMENTS

Standardized tests are those for which the psychometric characteristics are known. For example, the test manual will typically provide a mean or average score for a particular age group, as well as information related to variation about that mean. These tests are frequently used in school situations because of the need to justify inclusion of a child on the caseload. Typically, justification is achieved by demonstrating that the child's speech performance is outside of normal limits.

There is a variety of standardized test instruments available to the SLP. Some of these are tests that are oriented toward phonological processes and yet are standardized. In general, these instruments are appropriate for preschoolers who are 3 years old or older and for some children in kindergarten and first grade. Again, Section 3 describes these tests in greater detail.

Numerous standardized tests are available that are appropriate for school-age and older persons likely to have residual errors. Section 4 discusses assessment in these populations, and it includes information about these tests, as well. We should note that very few of these tests are useful for the population of teenagers and older adults who speak English as a second language. The reason is that most of these instruments are based on the naming of pictures that are likely to be known by young children. As a result, it is somewhat demeaning to an adult to respond to a test of this nature.

## MEASURES BASED ON CONNECTED SPEECH

The standardized test instruments that are commercially available are used widely, in part because of their appearance of objectivity. However, most of them lack face validity because they are based on the naming of pictured objects. As we SLPs know all too well, everyday speech is spoken in the give-and-take of conversation, is connected, and is composed of more than nouns. As a result, measures of speech sound production that are based on conversational speech are absolutely essential to every diagnostic evaluation. Such measures also help us toward our goal of dynamic assessment of the child's function in typical situations. For example, if we find that the child uses most final consonants in single-word treatment tasks, but uses almost none in conversation, we need to find a way to assist the child in using final consonants in more interactive contexts.

Connected speech measures can contribute enormously to our understanding of a client's difficulties. For example, we can measure intelligibility both directly (Percent of Intelligible Words) or indirectly (estimated percent of time that the client is understood by family members and by others). We can measure severity directly or indirectly. We can determine the percent of time that a particular phonological form is used correctly and incorrectly. We can compare the client's production of words spoken in citation form with her production of the same words in connected speech. And finally, we can observe suprasegmentals such as the appropriateness of the pitch and loudness contours over an utterance relative to the content of the utterance.

## MEASURING INTELLIGIBILITY

Intelligibility is the capacity to communicate with others in a way that they can understand. In many ways, intelligibility is what makes us human. When people lose this capacity, for example, through stroke, they sometimes report feeling less than human because they cannot make wants, needs, and feelings known to others.

Intelligibility is also one of the constructs that connects speech, language, and hearing professionals with the general public. Family members are concerned when they do not understand a child, and that is often the presenting complaint even when subsequent evaluation shows that far more than speech sound performance is involved. Older adults who have a hearing loss are concerned that they are missing important information. Coworkers may become concerned if they repeatedly misunderstand a fellow employee. In other words, the general public understands that intelligibility is important.

Finally, intelligibility can have implications for other areas of communication. A graduate student at Kansas State University, Marcia Hurt, studied the interactions of several parent-child dyads in play (1991). At the outset of her study, the children had poor intelligibility. As the child benefited from intervention and became more intelligible, the nature of parental input to the child changed. Early in the study, some parents spent a lot of their talk time repeating what they thought their child said, as if for confirmation. Other parents simply held the floor and did not give the child much opportunity to bring up new topics or even to comment on current topics. However, both of these tendencies decreased as the child became more intelligible. That is, parents made more substantive contributions to the conversation, and so did their children. In short, the conversations (and the nature of the linguistic input to the child) became more typical.

Besides the speaker's speech sound production, a number of factors can influence intelligibility. For example, people who are familiar with the client usually understand more of her speech than people who are not familiar. For another example, if the conversational partner knows the context of what the client is talking about, he will usually understand more than if he does not know the context.

Given these potential complications to assessing intelligibility, it is not surprising that normative data on child intelligibility have not been published in a refereed journal. Consequently, it is in this area of assessment that clinical judgment becomes critical. If the child is rarely understood, if the parents are anxious about the child's difficulties, or if the child is frustrated, all of these situations warrant a decision to recommend intervention.

There are several ways to measure the intelligibility of a client's connected speech. One of them is relatively straightforward: We count up the total number of words spoken in a recorded conversational sample and determine what percentage of the total another listener is able to gloss (Shriberg & Kwiatkowski, 1982a).

Another extremely important measure of intelligibility is determined by asking significant persons in the child's environment to describe how intelligible the child is. These indirect measures of intelligibility could be relatively informal measures such as asking teachers what percentage of a student's speech they typically understand. Alternatively, we can use rating scales with defined intervals and endpoints, or we can use categories. Finally, there is a single-word measure of intelligibility that the SLP can use. These measures are delineated in the next few pages.

---

## MEASURING INTELLIGIBILITY

### Background

| | |
|---|---|
| **WHO?** | Virtually all clients with speech-sound disorders. |
| **WHAT?** | Intelligibility refers to how well the client is understood. This quality can be measured directly or indirectly. |
| **WHY?** | The ability to make oneself understood by others is basic to our function as human beings. |
| **WHEN?** | We assess intelligibility at the initial evaluation and intermittently thereafter. |
| **SUPPORT:** | Measures of intelligibility have been used in speech-language pathology since its inception as a profession. |

# MEASURING INTELLIGIBILITY

## *Procedures*

A. Measures Based on Connected Speech

**Direct Measures** (Based on a word-by-word gloss of a recording of the client's speech)

- **Percentage of Intelligible Words (Shriberg & Kwiatkowsky, 1982):** While making the recording of the child's speech, the SLP repeats what he understood the client to say immediately after the client's utterance. This recording is then played for another person who writes down what the client said before hearing the clinician's gloss. The listener has only one opportunity to hear the tape. The SLP then calculates the percent of words that the listener glossed correctly and using the glosses made on-line as the standard, determines what percentage of the total words the listener understood.

- **Comment:** This measure is appropriate for all clients. Presentation to two or more listeners who are not familiar with the client would improve reliability. This technique has considerable face validity. However, it is not standardized. As a measure of change over time, this measure is likely to be relatively insensitive to small changes, a difficulty made more salient by the fact that content of conversation cannot be controlled from administration to administration. Additionally, the SLP who is eliciting the sample must be extraordinarily skilled at deciphering poorly intelligible speech on-line.

**Indirect Measures** (Estimates are obtained from significant others, and sometimes from the SLP)

- **Percentages:** What percent of the time do you understand this client:

    If you know the topic? _____%

    If you do not know the topic? _____%

- **Defined Scale:** Please rate how well you understand this client on the following scale. You should assume that the intervals are equal, and that "1" represents normal speech and "6" represents speech that is impossible to understand. Please circle one number.

    | If you know the topic: | 1 | 2 | 3 | 4 | 5 | 6 |
    |---|---|---|---|---|---|---|
    | If you do not know the topic: | 1 | 2 | 3 | 4 | 5 | 6 |

- **Categories** (adapted from Fudala, 2000): Which category describes how well you understand this child?

    ____ I notice speech sound errors occasionally in continuous speech.

    ____ The speech is understandable, but I always notice that there are errors.

    ____ The speech is understandable if I listen carefully.

    ____ The speech is difficult to understand.

    ____ Most of the time I do not understand the speech.

    ____ I never understand the speech.

- **Comment:** All of these measures are appropriate for clients older than about 3 years and have considerable face validity, but they are nonetheless relatively gross measures. Differences among respondents are expected. Sometimes these differences can provide insight to the client's difficulties.

B. A Measure BASED on Single Words

- **Preschool Speech Intelligibility Measure:** (Wilcox & Morris, 1999): The child client imitates 50 words chosen at random from a master list. Using a four-choice response paradigm, an adult indicates which word was heard. The number correct is expressed as a percent.

- **Comment:** This measure is specific to preschoolers. It is likely to be sensitive to changes in a client's performance and so should be a good measure to repeat at intervals. Its use as a measure of change is enhanced by the fact that learning the test is unlikely because each new word list is selected randomly.

---

## MEASURING SEVERITY

Severity refers to the degree to which speech is deviant or disordered. Severity is not the same as intelligibility, although there is undoubtedly a significant relationship between the two constructs. I once encountered a child in a preschool setting who produced perfectly acceptable /s z/ if you did not look at him; unfortunately, he produced these sounds by protruding his tongue and curling it up over his central incisors. The result was that when he was talking, his tongue flicked in and out of his mouth. This was extremely distracting, and the child had been called "Frog" more than once. In terms of severity, this child was totally intelligible but relatively severe, because there was potential for great distress to arise over his speech.

We tend to measure severity in two very different ways, one a global measure and the other a number derived from transcription of speech. The global measure is embodied in the "severity rating scales" that many state departments of education use to qualify children for services from public school SLPs. These scales are specific to each state.

The more quantitative measures of severity are the **Percent of Consonants Correct** (PCC—Shriberg & Kwiatkowski, 1982a) and the modification of PCC called the **Articulation Competence Index** (ACI—Shriberg, 1993). The PCC measure is based on a transcribed connected speech sample and is quite straightforward. It can also be interpreted in light of data provided by these authors. The ACI is intended to recognize the role played by distortion errors; however, it is more complicated mathematically than is PCC.

---

### MEASURES OF SEVERITY:
### PERCENT OF CONSONANTS CORRECT (PCC)
### and
### ARTICULATION COMPETENCE INDEX (ACI)

| | Background |
|---|---|
| | **Background** |
| **WHO?** | Any client with speech sound problems who can provide a connected speech sample that can be glossed. The PCC is appropriate for children whose error pattern is primarily phonological, while the ACI is used for children who have a number of distortions (residual errors) in their speech. |

*(continues)*

*(continued)*

**WHAT?**     After a connected speech sample is transcribed, the SLP determines which consonants the client produced correctly. To determine the PCC, the rules developed by Shriberg and Kwiatkowski (1982a) are followed to calculate the percent of the total number of target consonants that were correct. To compute the ACI (Shriberg, 1993), the SLP also counts the number of distortions and adjusts the PCC to account for them, using the formula provided by this author.

**WHY?**      Both the PCC and the ACI are reasonable and well-attested estimates of the severity of the phonological disorder.

**WHEN?**     The PCC and ACI are useful at the time of initial evaluation of a client and for re-evaluations at six-month or one-year intervals.

**SUPPORT:**  The PCC was developed by Shriberg and Kwiatkowski (1982a) as a way to describe the severity of involvement of the children they studied who had phonology problems. They reported that the PCC has a moderately low but significant correlation with a direct measure of intelligibility (*r* = .42). PCC is an extremely useful concept, and one that parents and clients grasp intuitively. Its usefulness is enhanced by the use of the category ranges shown below. However, PCC is not always sensitive to short-term improvements in overall consonant production. The reason is that if a child omits phonemes at first and later on substitutes for those same phonemes, both productions are still considered to be errors, although improvement has clearly taken place.

The ACI was developed by Shriberg (1993) as a severity metric for children whose errors are primarily distortions. It also appears to be useful as a change measure taken at half-year or one-year intervals.

## MEASURES OF SEVERITY:
## PERCENT OF CONSONANTS CORRECT
*(PCC—Shriberg & Kwiatkowski, 1982a)*
## and
## ARTICULATION COMPETENCE INDEX
*(ACI—Shriberg, 1993)*
### *Procedures*

### PERCENT OF CONSONANTS CORRECT (PCC)*

The PCC is based on a conversational speech sample. Wherever possible, the clinician who elicits this sample should repeat after the child what she understood the child to say. PCC deals only with consonants, and not with vowels. The following rules are adapted from Shriberg and Kwiatkowski (1982a).

### Determining Which Consonants to Use

1. Use only the intended or target sound in words.
2. When /r/ occurs after a vowel, it is considered to be a consonant. However, the stressed and unstressed "vocalic r," that is, /ɝ ɚ/ are considered to be vowels.

3. If the child repeats a syllable, for example, *ba-baby*, score only the consonants in the first syllable.

4. Do not include consonants in words whose meaning is questionable or in words that are partly or completely unintelligible.

5. If a child repeats a word several times, score only the consonants in the first two, unless the articulation changes.

## Scoring the Consonants

1. Use the following response definition: "Score as incorrect unless clearly heard as correct."

2. If the child speaks a dialect of English, that dialect serves as the standard in determining if the consonants are correct or not.

3. If the child's production is comparable to what an adult would say in casual conversation, then the consonants should be scored against the standards for casual speech, for example, the word *and* said as a syllabic /n̩/. Note that in adult casual speech, the /h/ in pronouns can be deleted unless the pronoun is stressed, for example, *I called him* as [aɪkaldɪm] in contrast to the stressed version *He called me* as [hikaldmi]. Similarly, /ŋ/ may be said as /n/ in unstressed syllables as in *singing* [sɪŋɪn].

4. Incorrect productions (errors) include:
   • Deletion of a target consonant
   • Substitutions
   • Partial voicing of initial voiceless consonants
   • Distortions of a target consonant, even if it is only a slight distortion

## Calculating the PCC

Count up the total number of consonant targets and the number that were correct. Then divide the number correct by the total to determine the PCC.

## Interpreting the PCC

The PCC measure can be interpreted according to Table 2-1.

**TABLE 2-1**   Interpreting the PCC measure.

*The following table is adapted from Figure 1 in Shriberg and Kwiatkowski (1982a, p. 265).**

| PCC Score | Severity Level |
| --- | --- |
| 85–100% | Mild |
| 65–85% | Mild-moderate |
| 50–65% | Moderate-severe |
| Below 50% | Severe |

*Adapted with permission from Shriberg and Kwiatkowsky (1982a).

## ARTICULATION COMPETENCE INDEX (ACI)**

In order to determine the ACI, the values of the PCC and of the Relative Distortion Index (RDI) must be known. The formula for the ACI is this:

$$ACI = \frac{(PCC + RDI)}{2}$$

The PCC is calculated just as above. To determine the RDI, one must count the number of distortions in that same sample, and divide it by the total number of errors. (The RDI can be interpreted as the proportion of errors that are distortions.) Then put the PCC and RDI values into the formula above.

---

** Adapted with permission from Shriberg (1993).

---

## ERROR PATTERNS IN CONNECTED SPEECH

One reason that we emphasize the importance of connected speech is that error patterns in connected speech may not be exactly the same as those that characterize words produced in citation form. Usually, there are more errors in connected speech, and this fact is attributed to the greater complexity of connected speech. This complexity derives from several sources:

- Motor planning for the utterance is complicated by the fact that instead of silence before the first sound of a word and after the last sound of a word, there are adjacent sounds in adjoining words that require rapid articulatory transitions.
- Motor planning for an utterance is made inherently complex by linguistic demands for appropriate content and syntax.
- Motor planning for an utterance must accommodate the suprasegmental aspects of the utterance—intonation contour, loudness contour, and durational variables.

Clients who have well-established error patterns may be able to override those patterns when producing citation forms, but they often revert to those patterns under the complexities of producing connected speech. In addition, some clients may delete syllables or function words in connected speech.

A complicating issue is that English allows certain types of deletions and substitutions in colloquial utterances, which we call contractions. For example, the contraction *don't* changes two syllables (*do* and *not*) to one syllable, and it even substitutes one new vowel for two others (/o/ for /u/ and /ɑ/). Children who are acquiring English hear a lot of contractions, and they also use a lot of contractions. It is possible that some of the excess deletions and substitutions in children with speech sound difficulties may represent an overgeneralization of contraction processes.

Conscientious SLPs have always transcribed and pondered the types of errors represented in a client's connected speech. As was mentioned in Section One, there are computerized narrow transcription systems available to aid in this analysis. These systems are not absolutely necessary, although they certainly can assist in the process. Regardless of how the analysis is done, the SLP should comment in the diagnostic report about comparisons between single-word performance and connected speech performance.

## EVALUATING OTHER ASPECTS OF COMMUNICATION

Speech-language pathologists have known for a long time that variables other than speech sound production can affect intelligibility and severity. These include prosody, voice characteristics, disfluencies, use of unusual registers (manners of speaking) and a large number of language variables, including pragmatics. There are many assessment tools for language at present. However, other than verbal descriptions of prosody, voice, fluency and register, there are relatively few standard ways to take account of these influences.

Shriberg (1993) developed a set of checklist-type indices of register, prosody, and voice (with fluency included under prosody) to use as tools in studying the genetics of speech sound disorders. Although these checklists were developed for research purposes, they are equally applicable to the everyday practice of speech-language pathology, and they have the virtue that they remind the clinician of the range of possibilities within each variable.

---

## *VOICE-PROSODY AND REGISTER CHECKLISTS*
### *Adapted from Shriberg (1993)*

### Background

| | |
|---|---|
| **WHO?** | Children and adults with speech sound disorders |
| **WHAT?** | Checklists to capture characteristics of client's connected speech that may influence intelligibility and severity considerations. |
| **WHY?** | These checklists help to describe the relative contribution to intelligibility and severity of speech production variables apart from speech sound production *per se.* |
| **WHEN?** | Useful at the time of initial diagnostic evaluation and at subsequent annual evaluations. |
| **SUPPORT:** | Developed by a well-respected researcher to give precision to work in genetics and other areas related to speech sound production. This adaptation can also allow practicing SLPs to achieve greater levels of precision in their analyses of performance. |

## VOICE-PROSODY AND REGISTER CHECKLISTS

### *Reproducible Form 2*
### *(adapted from Shriberg, 1993)*

### *Procedures*

Reproducible Form 2 is a checklist adapted from Shriberg's 1993 publication. This checklist allows the SLP to capture all relevant aspects of the child's performance in these areas. This checklist should be regarded as a screening tool, to be followed up with evaluation of any areas that appear problematic.

# THE SEARCH FOR CAUSAL-CORRELATES

Causal-correlates are defined by Shriberg and Kwiatkowski (1982b) as variables that may be related in important ways to the presence of a speech sound disorder. These include anatomic differences, hearing status (both current and previous), linguistic performance (including pragmatics), cognitive level, and social-behavioral issues.

## Oral Anatomy

There are a number of published forms to guide the examination of the oral mechanism, especially with respect to its structure, and a particularly extensive one has been developed by Hall (2000). However, only rarely do we see children with speech sound disorders whose difficulties we can attribute to the oral structures. Somewhat less is known about the functional intactness of the oral and respiratory structures. A recent development in the assessment of oral function is the *Verbal Motor Production Assessment for Children* (*VMPAC*—Hayden & Square, 1999). The areas covered in this assessment include the following:

A. General Motor Control, including tone, respiration/phonation, reflexes, and vegetative functions (chewing and swallowing)

B. Single Oromotor (Non-Speech) Movements, including mandibular control, labial-facial control, and lingual control

C. Oromotor Integrity

D. Double Oromotor (Non-Speech) Movements

E. Single Oromotor-Phoneme (Speech) Movements

F. Multiple Oromotor-Phoneme (Speech) Movements

G. Oromotor Production in Word Sequences and Sentences

H. Oromotor Production in Connected Speech and Language

I. Oromotor Production in Automatic Verbal Sequences

One of the problems in assessing oral nonverbal function in children is that even young, typically developing children have difficulty with many of the typical "oral gymnastics" tasks. So the issue is this: When does a child exhibit so much difficulty with these tasks that her performance is outside of the norm? When the SLP suspects that the child's oral motor function is outside of normal limits, the *VMPAC* should greatly assist in answering this question. It is also helpful for the clinician to note any groping behaviors and whether or not repeated models were necessary for any verbal or non-verbal oral task.

## Hearing

A hearing screening (at a minimum) should be performed every year for most children, and the SLP should have access to those results. Just as important is the child's hearing history. Some authorities claim that if a child has spent considerable time in the early years with hearing loss due to otitis media, then the child is at increased risk of disordered phonology.

## Language

The phonologic system is part of the linguistic system, so it should not be surprising to find interactions with other elements of language. In particular, if a client is having difficulty with complex phonological sequences such as word-final clusters and/or unstressed syllables, this difficulty will affect expressive morphology. Many English inflectional morphemes either form complex sequences, for example, *words* /wɜˑdz/, *danced* /dænst/, *asks* /æsks/, or they introduce weak syllables, for example, *boxes* /baksəz/, folded /foldəd/. Children with phonological problems may also have difficulty with other linguistic functions such as word finding.

## Cognitive Level

During most initial diagnostic assessments with a client, the SLP can estimate cognitive level on the basis of the child's overall behavior. Of course, we do not refer for psychometric assessment if it appears that the child is functioning within typical limits for his or her age. If we have concerns about cognitive levels, and we want to make a referral, we have to remember that parents will need to be convinced that this step is both important and appropriate.

Sometimes we can let language performance serve as a surrogate for the needed information about cognition. For example, in a 4-year-old with poor intelligibility and (as expected) poor expressive language, if receptive language is well within typical limits for the child's age, we probably will not make a referral. However, if receptive language is also depressed compared to norms, then we should be far more likely to refer. For younger children, levels of play can serve as a surrogate for developmental level (Westby, 2000).

From the SLP's point of view, the most helpful information that a psychologist can provide is (a) an estimate of overall cognitive level, (b) separate information on verbal as opposed to non-verbal tasks, and (c) any information about cognitive strengths. Children who are at or below the lower limits of the normal cognitive range overall, and who show similar performance on both verbal and nonverbal tasks, may have difficulty seeing phonological relationships and making the generalizations that are critical to success in treatment. In such cases, the SLP may choose to emphasize functional communication first (for example, intelligible single words or an alternative system) and address systematic phonological issues later.

On the other hand, if the child's verbal performance is below normal limits, but the nonverbal performance is higher, then it may be possible to take advantage of the child's nonverbal skills to remediate phonology. For example, if one of the strengths of a preschooler is in seeing visual patterns, then we can immediately introduce graphic symbols for the child to associate with target sounds. (This is not teaching reading, although it may benefit the child later in learning to read.)

## POSSIBLE DYSPRAXIC ELEMENTS

Most clinicians are aware of the concepts behind the terms Developmental Verbal Dyspraxia (DVD) and Developmental Verbal Apraxia (DAS or DAOS), which will be discussed in depth in Section 8. Despite the controversy over whether such an entity exists, it is useful to delineate any characteristics of the client that represent possible dyspraxic elements. In fact, my experience suggests that many children with phonological problems exhibit one or more possible dyspraxic elements. In our clinic we have some adult speakers of English as a second language who have exceptional difficulty learning spoken English and who also exhibit possible elements of dyspraxia.

In most cases where verbal dyspraxia is a possibility, there is a moderate to profound speech sound disorder plus one or more of the following:

- Difficulty in performing or articulatory groping during speaking attempts, especially elicited imitation
- Difficulty in performing or articulatory groping during elicited oral non-verbal movements

- Vowel errors
- Difficulties with prosody
- Avoidance of speaking situations
- Reliance on gestures
- Reluctance to imitate
- History of feeding problems
- History of tactile sensitivities or aversions (tactile defensiveness in the face or elsewhere)
- If treated previously, slow progress in treatment

The importance of information about possible dyspraxia is that it can alert the SLP to include substantial amounts of motor-based practice in the treatment plan, even if the basic approach is phonological. This information is also helpful in establishing realistic prognoses and expectations for clients and their families.

## PROGNOSTIC INDICATORS

In the preceding pages, I noted that several of the speech-related areas of assessment have prognostic implications, among them cognitive function and possible dyspraxic elements. In addition, there are several assessment procedures that are done primarily because they are related to prognosis. All of them involve trying to determine if there is any variability in the client's phonological patterns, and if so, where the variability occurs and whether it leads to productions that are closer to the target than the usual productions. Phonological variability that we can either find or elicit suggests that the child's phonological system is not yet solidified. For this reason, evidence of variability is a positive prognostic indicator.

One of the issues we need to consider in the diagnostic process is which prognoses we are interested in for this client. One possible prognosis relates to whether the child needs services immediately or is likely to improve without intervention. Another possible prognosis relates to likely progress in treatment. Still another prognosis might relate to the child's likely performance in academic areas.

## PROGNOSTIC INDICATOR—AGE OF CLIENT

Age of the client is sometimes ignored when we establish prognoses or determine eligibility for services. However, age is probably an important indicator because of what it suggests about the client's neurophysiological system. In current speech-language pathology, we rarely hear mention of the concept of a "critical period" during which communication is optimally established. However, the evidence that there is a critical period for phonology seems quite strong.

First of all, every study of how phonology develops shows that the large majority of children, 90–95%, acquire all of the phonological structures under test (except for $/\theta/$) by age 6 or 7. Every set of articulation test norms shows the same phenomenon. Some authorities (e.g., Shriberg, 1993) put the age even lower, at around 5 years of age.

In addition, there are some rules of thumb that are used in other areas of speech-language pathology that are relevant here. For example, in the area of communication development in severely hearing impaired children, one rule of thumb is that if the child does not receive a hearing aid before the age of 2, she is unlikely to acquire intelligible speech. Another rule of thumb is prevalent in the area of autism, where we can hear professionals say that if the child does not start talking by the age of 3, he is unlikely to develop functional oral communication.

All of these pieces of evidence point to the preschool period as a time when the child's neurophysiological system is primed to acquire speech sound systems. The nervous system is still maturing during this time, and it is at its most plastic (malleable) (Netsell, 1986).

It is true that some children continue to improve their phonology up to the age of about 8, but these children are relatively uncommon. Other children who do not have adult-like systems at the age of 7 do not improve spontaneously. It is worth noting that many state education agencies set standards to qualify children for services that assume that all of the children who continue to have errors are likely to self-correct. In fact, this means that children who do not self-correct have to practice their immature patterns for an additional year, or two, or three.

Another concept related to the idea of a critical period is the role of practice in motor learning (Schmidt & Lee, 1999). Repeated production of a motor movement increases the accuracy and speed of that movement until it eventually reaches a level that is considered skilled. Skilled movements are those for which variability in accuracy and speed has reached a minimum. Skilled movements are also less likely to be under cortical control than are less skilled (more variable) movements. Examples of activities requiring skilled movements are the trilling of notes on a musical instrument, fast keyboarding, all kinds of sports—and speaking.

Every time a person produces a sound or a word, that utterance is not only a communicative act, but it is also motor practice. By the time that the child is 6 or 7 years old, many speech movements have been well practiced. Although there are still reductions in variability of speech movements to be achieved up until the teenage years (Tingley & Allen, 1975), nevertheless, the patterns of speech are well on their way to being cemented into the child's phonological system. Unfortunately, error patterns are also well on their way to being cemented into the system.

An important issue in formulating prognoses and recommendations is how to deal with "residual" errors. If the child continues to practice the current error pattern, then if we delay intervention, the child will have that much longer to practice and incorporate the pattern into the system. The pattern then becomes resistant to intervention. On the other hand, the child may be in the process of changing that pattern without intervention. In that case, services may not be needed. Unfortunately, our field has relatively few longitudinal studies of children with speech-sound errors in the preschool years and the eventual outcomes without intervention. A corollary is that we also have few studies of variables that can predict the outcomes.

## Prognostic Indicators—Consistency

Consistency refers to how variable the client's phonological patterns are. Here are several descriptions of consistency (or inconsistency):

**Consistent:** Adult, age 22, produces distorted /s z/ in 100% of exemplars in five minutes of connected speech.

**Consistent:** Child, age 4;0, uses final consonant deletion in all of the 14 exemplars in which the process was tested.

**Inconsistent:** Teenager, age 16, uses unilateral / ʃ ʧ ʤ/ in 85% of exemplars occurring in a three-minute reading passage, with the remaining 15% produced with a central airstream.

**Inconsistent:** Child, age 5;0, uses cluster reduction for initial /l/ and /r/ clusters 50% of the time in a short connected speech sample. The clusters that are not reduced are not necessarily correct because [w] is substituted for the liquids.

Based on these data alone, none of the first three clients is likely to self-correct in the near future, the adult and the teenager because of their age, and the 4-year-old because there is no variation in the productions. Only the 5-year-old is likely to improve without intervention, because he preserves all the elements in 50% of clusters already.

On the other hand, the kind of variability shown when a client is inconsistent like the teenager above is a positive indicator for progress with treatment. This is the best kind of inconsistency because there are some correct productions that occur spontaneously. We can call this type of inconsistency "inconsistency with hits." The clinician can make use of these "hits" (correct productions) early in treatment.

## Prognostic Indicators—Contextual Variation

Contextual variation refers to a particular type of inconsistency in which the nature of the target production depends on the context in which it is produced. In fact, it is safe to say that most inconsistency is not random but is contextually determined. Usually the facilitating context is one in which there is a positive effect of coarticulation between adjacent phones on either side of the target word.

For example, if we examine the transcription of the speech sample from which the data for the teenager above are taken, we may find that all of his correct productions of /ʃ tʃ dʒ/ occur when there is an adjacent /r/, as in words like *shred*, *church*, and *barge*. If he uses a bunched tongue position for the /r/, that tongue placement probably interferes with his usual lateral positioning of the tongue for the adjacent error sounds. Contextual variation for this teenage is a positive prognostic indicator for progress in intervention, but it is not a good prognostic indicator for improvement without intervention because of the client's age.

Contextual variation is considered so important for motoric approaches to intervention that there are both tests and treatment regimes built around it. (See Sections 4 and 7 for more information.) In the area of phonological assessment, the record forms for most formal tests of phonology the data are arranged in such a way that the clinician can easily see if there is contextual variation rather than a seemingly random inconsistency.

## Prognostic Indicators—Stimulability

Of all the prognostic indicators related to variation in production, none has been studied more than stimulability. Stimulability refers to the capacity of the client to produce a speech sound or structure that is otherwise in error when the production is elicited by the SLP. This elicited production must also be repeatable, that is, it cannot be just a lucky accident. Stimulability includes all of the following:

- Imitation of the sound in isolation, with or without phonetic placement cues an models
- Imitation of the sound in a nonsense syllable, with or without phonetic placement cues and models
- Imitation of the sound in a real word, with or without phonetic placement cues and models

The first attempt to study stimulability in a systematic way was made by Carter and Buck (1958). These authors asked children who made speech sound errors to imitate nonsense syllables with the target sound in three positions (initial, intervocalic, final) and with three different vowels in each position. They found that children who were very stimulable under these conditions (75% or more correct) were highly likely to self-correct. This finding has been replicated by others using different research paradigms (e.g., Miccio, Elbert, & Forrest [1999]).

However, there is controversy in the field about what stimulability really means. For example, there is some evidence that children benefit the most from treatment for non-stimulable sounds (e.g., Powell, Elbert, & Dinnsen [1991]). At the same time there is also evidence that treating somewhat stimulable sounds produces faster results in treatment than treating non-stimulable structures, at least when the sounds are stimulable in isolation (Madison, 1979).

It is likely that these findings, which appear to be in conflict, reflect a kind of design artifact. It is well known in psychometrics that there is a relationship between the initial level of performance and the subsequent rate of progress in acquiring a new behavior. That is, the lower the initial level, the farther the client has to go, and steeper the slope of progress. The children who are not stimulable initially have a very long way to go, compared to children who start at a higher level. So their apparent rate of progress is better. On the other hand, stimulable children are likely to acquire the new structure in the short term, while the non-stimulable children will fail to achieve the target in the same period of time.

### Relation of Stimulability to Underlying Representations

There are also questions about the implications of stimulability for the phonological system. For example, if the child is stimulable for a sound that is not otherwise heard in the child's speech, does that mean that the child "knows" about the sound, or is she just acting like a parrot? Another question is this: If we manage to teach a child to be stimulable for previously non-stimulable structures, will the child then make progress without intervention? If so, at what level do we need to teach (isolation, nonsense syllable, or word)?

It is my guess that if the child is stimulable in isolation or in nonsense syllables but not in words, then there is a good chance that the child is simply parroting movements. On the other hand, if the child is reliably stimulable in words whose meaning the child knows, then the child is likely to have knowledge of that sound as part of his underlying forms of those words. This position is consistent with Elbert and Gierut's (1986) setting up of knowledge hierarchies for phonological structures. Knowledge hierarchies are based on the assumption that there are degrees of knowledge of phonological structures. The critical determinant of progress is probably the accuracy of the child's underlying form. We would expect the child with an accurate (adult-like) underlying form to make faster progress than if the underlying form is not accurate.

### Stimulability as Part of Dynamic Assessment

Another reason to assess stimulability is to find a path into the child's system. Perrine, Bain, and Weston (2000) explored ways that an adult can assist a child toward accurate production of a target phoneme. Their research suggests that there is a hierarchy of cues such that children respond more readily to some types of cues than to others. The hierarchy is this, arranged from most facilitating to least facilitating:

- Auditory and visual model plus physical manipulation and/or verbal description and/or instructions (Direct)
- Auditory and visual model plus verbal descriptions and/or instructions (Direct)
- Auditory and visual model (Direct)
- Auditory and visual model (Indirect, i.e., with intervening verbiage such as instructions)
- Auditory model (Indirect)

We may note that the least facilitating cues are the ones that are most often suggested as a way to assess stimulability.

# INTERPRETATION OF DIAGNOSTIC RESULTS

The three important questions to be answered in most initial diagnostic evaluations are these:

1.  Is there a problem with the use of speech sounds for communication?
2.  What are the dimensions of the problem? (In the case of poorly intelligible children, all the contributors to poor intelligibility should be catalogued.)
3.  What is the prognosis for improvement with and without intervention?

Clinical Note 2-2 indicates varying ways in which we can answer this question.

---

CLINICAL NOTE 2-2:  Interpretation of Diagnostic Results

1.  Is there a problem with the use of speech sounds for communication? The answer will tend to be "Yes" if:
    *   The client's speech sound performance is significantly poorer than that of peers.
    *   The client has poor intelligibility.
    *   The client has a poor self-image because of speech.
    *   The client's speech draws attention to itself, thus interfering with communication of content.
    *   The client is frustrated because of inability to communicate.
    *   The client's family is worried about the ability to communicate.
    *   The client exhibits few positive prognostic indicators.

2A. What are the dimensions of the problem? The following, if present, are important issues for intervention:
    *   The client exhibits a cognitive delay.
    *   The client exhibits delay in other areas of language performance, especially receptive language and pragmatics.
    *   The client has or has had a significant hearing loss.
    *   The client has structural or physiological deficits that have an impact on speech.
    *   The client exhibits possible dyspraxic elements.
    *   The client exhibits difficulties with behavioral control.

2B. If intelligibility is poor, what contributes to that poor intelligibility? The SLP should consider the following:
    *   Many errors in speech sound production, usually including deletions and developmental errors
    *   Unusual errors in speech sound production
    *   Difficulties with prosody at both the word and the utterance level
    *   Voice quality deviations
    *   Word-finding difficulties
    *   Difficulties with pragmatics related to topic maintenance
    *   Fast speaking rate
    *   Hearing loss in conversational partners or adverse communication situations in environment in which communication occurs

---

3A. What is the prognosis, without intervention? In most cases the following findings would indicate that the client might self-correct:

- Young age
- Relatively mild disorder (but note that some distortions, such as lateralizations, are unlikely to self-correct at any age)
- Few significant factors impacting speech
- Stimulable in words for one or more of the error sounds or structures
- Positive communication environment in the family, school, and/or work settings, if relevant

3B. What is the prognosis, with intervention? In most cases the following findings would indicate that the prognosis with intervention is very positive:

- Young age
- Normal receptive language
- Variation in production that includes forms closer to the target ("inconsistency with hits")
- Positive motivation on the part of the client and significant others
- No structural or physiological problems, or, if such problems are present, they have been or can be remediated

## RECOMMENDATIONS

Based on all aspects of the assessment, the SLP develops a set of one or more recommendations. It goes without saying that each recommendation should be supported by material elsewhere in the diagnostic report. Additionally, all material in each section that has clinical implications should be noted in the recommendations. If the client has structural or physiological characteristics that affect speech, then the recommendations should include management of those characteristics. If the family environment is not conducive to positive change, then the SLP may recommend several sessions of discussion with family members, or possibly a referral to another professional.

## SUMMARY

Accurate assessment and diagnosis are critical to planning effective intervention. The goal of this kind of assessment is a multifaceted picture of the client and the environment in which he or she functions. Accurate assessment also provides a baseline against which future development and progress in treatment can be evaluated.

# SECTION

## 3

# ASSESSMENT: THE EARLY SCHOOL-AGED CHILD WITH POOR SPEECH INTELLIGIBILITY

● ● ● ● ● ● ● ● ● ● ● ● ● ● ● ● ● ● ● ● ● ● ● ● ● ● ● ● ● ● ● ● ● ● ● ● ● ●

**T**he speech-language pathologist who serves children in the early grades in school needs considerable information about assessment and intervention for children age 5 and younger. There are two reasons to have this information. The first is that many of these SLPs also serve preschoolers, and the second is that some of the children in the early grades are developmentally similar to preschoolers with respect to communication skills, or even to children in the 0-to-3 age range. For these reasons, parts of this section will touch on assessment procedures that are appropriate for 0-to-3 and preschool populations. For an in-depth look at phonological disorders, the interested reader is referred to another book in the [*Singular Resource Guide series, Speech Disorders: Resource Guide for Preschool Children* by Lynn Williams, 2003].

Stoel-Gammon and Dunn (1985) have made a very useful distinction between analyses that treat the child's phonological system as self-contained ("independent" analyses) and those that relate or compare the child's system to an adult standard ("relational" analyses). Relational analyses are familiar to SLPs because most articulation tests explicitly compare the child's production to adult standards.

Independent analyses are more like a linguist's approach to cataloging the speech sounds and syllable structures in a new language. In caseloads that include children in the early grades, only relational analyses need to be completed for most children; however, for very young clients, for example, 0 to 3, or for poorly intelligible children, independent analyses can help us describe the child's capabilities.

## INDEPENDENT ANALYSES

Independent analyses may be performed on a sample of conversational speech, or on a sample of elicited single words, or on both. Crystal (1982) has suggested that any kind of language sample be based on a sample that includes at least 100 different words. This standard also seems to be reasonable for phonological analyses.

There are several issues related to speech samples from children who are in the under-three group chronologically or whose phonological development is comparable to that of children in the under-three group:

- Some of these children may not say much at all in a play situation, so that obtaining an adequate sample may be difficult.

- Conversational speech from some of these children may be very difficult to understand, particularly if the referent or context is not clear.

- Some of these children are too young to be given a formal test based on naming of objects or pictures. Even if they can cooperate and name most items of a standardized test, there is a tendency for typically developing children under the age of three to decline to say many test items (Smit, Hand, Freilinger, Bernthal, & Bird, 1990). We may infer that these children refuse to attempt test words containing sounds that they know they cannot say (Schwartz & Leonard, 1982). Fortunately, this phenomenon becomes far less prominent in children who are older than three years of age and within normal limits cognitively.

Clearly the best approach is for the SLP to record as long a connected-speech sample as possible, gloss it with care (perhaps asking for help from a family member), and if necessary, supplement it with pictures for naming. Narrow transcription is not always necessary, especially if most of the child's productions fall cleanly into adult categories such as "[d] sounds." If, however, the child seems to do a variety of things within categories, for example, aspirating, dentalizing, and frictionalizing the [d] phones, then narrow transcription may be needed.

There are three types of independent analyses. The first is the phonetic inventory, which is a listing of the types of consonants, and sometimes the types of vowels, that the child uses. The list is usually organized by manner of production, place of production, and voicing. No reference is made to the acceptability of these segments, because that would imply a comparison to an adult standard.

The second independent analysis is simply a listing of the shapes of syllables and words that the child has produced. The third is a statement of any sequential constraints that the clinician has identified based on the speech sample. For example, in the case of the child who always reduces clusters, we might state that in this child's phonology, consonants can only precede and follow vowels, not other consonants. Examples of these types of analyses may be seen in Section 9, which presents case studies.

After these analyses are completed, the SLP then makes a general comparison to the phonemes and structures needed in the child's ambient language. Based on that comparison, both immediate and long-term phonological goals can be determined for the child.

## PHONETIC INVENTORIES

### Background

**WHO?**  A child younger than 3 years of age *or* an older preschooler or a child of early school age with severely unintelligible speech.

**WHAT?**  A phonetic inventory is a structured list of the speech sounds that the child uses, regardless of whether they correspond to adult phonemes. There are separate forms for consonant and vowel inventories. Phonetic inventories have been used most often with spontaneous speech samples, which have the best face validity as sources of information. However, a phonetic inventory can also be constructed using responses to single-word tests, if need be. Most research into phonetic inventories has involved consonants only, but vowel inventories can be constructed as well.

**WHY?**  The phonetic inventory is a good way to determine what sounds the client is currently capable of producing in meaningful speech, and it can also be used to determine where there are gaps.

**WHEN?**  The phonetic inventory is used for comparison with normative information about phonetic inventories and to determine the goals of intervention.

**SUPPORT:**  The use of the consonant phonetic inventory as a clinical tool was first proposed by Stoel-Gammon and Dunn (1985). It has been used with older children by Dyson (1988), and with younger children by Robb and Bleile (1994). One commercially available test, the *SHAPE* (Smit & Hand, 1997) explicitly provides for a phonetic inventory of consonants at the clinician's option.

Phonetic inventories for vowels are seen only rarely in the published literature. However, they may have utility as a clinical tool with very young children or with children who have severely disordered speech.

## PHONETIC INVENTORY

*(Reproducible Forms 3 and 4)*

### Procedure

1. Obtain a speech sample from the client. Ideally, this should be a spontaneous conversational sample, usually obtained during play; however, if connected speech is very difficult to understand and to segment, a list of single-word productions may also be used. Crystal (1982) has recommended a sample that is long enough to include at least 100 different words. However, multiple tokens of the same word *should* be included in the inventory.

2. Transcribe each word, lining up the glosses on the left of the page and the transcriptions to the right.

3. Using Reproducible Form 3 for consonants or Reproducible Form 4 for vowels, enter each new type of sound on the form and put a tally mark near it each time that sound is used. If it appears to you that a model spoken by an adult just prior to the client's production might have influenced the production, the tally mark should be differentiated (e.g., written as "m" for "modeled").

4. If the child produces the same word several different ways, tally as if these were separate words.

5. If you do not know the meaning of a word or phonological form that you can nevertheless transcribe, include that word in the analysis. The rationale is that we want to know what kinds of sounds the child is able to say.

6. Establish a criterion for saying that the child "has" a sound, that is, uses it productively. Many SLPs would consider spontaneous use (i.e., not modeled) two to three times to represent productive use of a sound.

7. Make a list of the consonants that the child uses productively in initial position, in final position, and in intervocalic position. If using the vowel list, simply note the vowels used productively.

8. Compare the consonant list to the consonant data in Table 3-1 to determine the client's approximate developmental level. Children older than 3 should be using all the consonants that 3-year-olds are, and more. Note that there is not enough published literature on vowel inventories to make comparisons. However, vowels are generally considered to be acquired early, before most consonants.

**TABLE 3-1.**   Consonant inventories by the ages of 2 years and 3 years. The term "place" refers to place of articulation.

*Adapted from Dyson (1988); Robb & Bleile (1994); Stoel-Gammon (1985).*

|  | *Age 2 years* | *Age 3 years* |
|---|---|---|
| Initial Consonants | Two glides | Three glides |
|  | Nasals at two places | Nasals at two places |
|  | Stops at three places (voiced) | Stops at three places |
|  | One fricative | Fricatives at two places |
|  | Zero affricates | Zero affricates |
|  | Zero liquids | One liquid |
| Final Consonants | Nasals at one or two places | Nasals at three places |
|  | Stops at three places | Five stops |
|  | Fricatives at two places | Five fricatives at three places |
|  | Zero or one affricate | Zero or one affricate |
|  | Zero or one liquid | One liquid |

### *Treatment Goals Based on Phonetic Inventories*

In most cases, the sounds that are missing from the inventory would become the targets of treatment. For example, if a 4-year-old is using only stops, nasals, and glides, then an obvious goal is for the child to acquire one or more fricatives.

---

## SYLLABLE AND WORD-SHAPE INVENTORY, INCLUDING SEQUENTIAL CONSTRAINTS

### Background

**WHO?**  Construction of a syllable and word-shape inventory is appropriate for the same children as the phonetic inventory, that is, a child younger than 3 years of age *or* an older preschooler or a child of early school age with severely unintelligible speech.

**WHAT?**  A syllable and word-shape inventory is a structured list of the types of sound sequences (syllables, words) that the child uses regardless of whether the resulting forms correspond to adult forms. Statements about sequential constraints describe the allowable sequences in the child's phonology.

Syllable and word-shape inventories have been used most often with spontaneous speech samples, which have the best face validity as sources of information. However, an inventory can also be constructed using responses to single-word tests, if need be.

**WHY?**  The syllable and word-shape inventory is a good way to determine what forms the client is currently capable of producing in meaningful speech, and it can also be used to determine where there are gaps. Sequential constraints may also indicate possible goals for intervention.

**WHEN?**  The syllable and word-shape inventory is used at the initial evaluation and perhaps for subsequent evaluations for comparison with normative information about this type of inventory and to determine the goals of intervention.

**SUPPORT:**  The use of the consonant syllable and word-shape inventory and of sequential constraints as clinical tools was first proposed by Stoel-Gammon and Dunn (1985). It has been used with children ages 2;0 to 3;3 by Dyson (1988). One commercially available test, the *SHAPE* (Smit & Hand, 1997) includes the possibility of doing a syllable and word-shape analysis.

## SYLLABLE AND WORD-SHAPE INVENTORY, INCLUDING SEQUENTIAL CONSTRAINTS

*(Reproducible Form 5)*

### *Procedure*

1. Obtain a speech sample from the client. Ideally, this should be a spontaneous conversational sample, usually obtained during play; however, if connected speech is very difficult to understand and to segment, a list of single-word productions may also be used.

Crystal (1982) has recommended a sample that is long enough to include at least 100 different words. Multiple tokens of the same word *should* be included in the inventory.

2. Transcribe each word, lining up the glosses on the left of the page and the transcriptions to the right.

3. Using Reproducible Form 5, enter each new type of structure on the form and put a tally mark near it each time that structure is used. If it appears to you that a model spoken by an adult just prior to the client's production might have influenced the production, the tally mark should be differentiated (e.g., written as "m" for "modeled").

4. If the child produces the same word several different ways, tally as if these were separate words.

5. If you do not know the meaning of a word or phonological form that you can nevertheless transcribe, include that word in the analysis. The rationale is that we want to know what kinds of word shapes the child is able to say.

6. Establish a criterion for saying that the child "has" a syllable or word shape (i.e., uses it productively). Many SLPs would consider spontaneous use (i.e., not modeled) two to three times to be productive use.

7. Compare this list to Table 3-2 to determine the client's approximate developmental level. Children older than 3:3 should use all of these syllable and word types, and more complex ones as well.

8. Statements about sequential constraints are based not only on the syllable and word-shape inventory but also on the phonetic inventories. Some sample statements are indicated here:

"This child does not use syllable-final consonants."

"This child uses [d] only before high front vowels and [g] before all other vowels."

**TABLE 3-2.** Types of word shapes and frequency of clusters produced by children at two different ages. There were 10 children at each age level.

*Adapted from Dyson (1988).*

|  | *Age 2;5* | *Age 3;3* |
|---|---|---|
| Predominant shapes (15% of words or more) | CV, CVC, other monosyll. | CV, CVC, other monosyll. |
| Also used occasionally (5-15% of words) | V, VC, two-syllable words* | V, VC, two-syllable words* |
| Rarely used | Three-syllable words | Three-syllable words |
| Mean number of clusters | 10 | 14 |
| Mean % of lexical types with initial clusters | 12% | 14% |

*Dyson (1988) does not break down two-syllable words. Other literature suggests that the CVCV form with primary stress on the first syllable is likely to predominate in this category.

### *Treatment Goals Based on the Syllable and Word-Shape Inventory*

In most cases, the structures that are missing from the inventory would become the targets of treatment. Typically, these structures would also have been implicated in sequential constraints. For example, if a 4-year-old is using only CV syllables, then both CVC and CVCV syllables would be reasonable goals.

## RELATIONAL ANALYSES

Relational analyses of a child's phonology involve comparison of the child's productions to a presumed adult standard. Relational analyses take two forms. One is a segmental inventory, which is segment-by-segment comparison of the child's version of a segment or phoneme with the adult target phoneme. In this comparison we *do* make decisions about whether a segment is correct or not. Segmental inventories have also been called contrast inventories or phoneme inventories. Most tests of articulation result in a segmental inventory that is based on citation forms of words; however, the segmental inventory can also be based on connected speech.

   The other kind of relational analysis is an evaluation of phonological processes used by the child. This type of comparison with the adult form has a wider scope than in segmental analysis. For example, with respect to the process called final consonant deletion, we can ask this question: "When the adult word has a final consonant, does the child produce a final consonant?" We can then ask similar questions about other phonological processes. There are a number of published tests of phonological processes. Table 3-3 provides an example of errors viewed as segmental and as exemplars of phonological processes.

**TABLE 3-3.** Examples of Relational Analyses

| Segmental | Adult versions: *sew* [so], *sick* [sɪk] |
|---|---|
| | Child versions: *sew* [do], *sick* [dɪk] |
| | Conclusion: Child substitutes [d] for /s/. |
| Phonological | Adult versions: *cup* [kʌp], *ace* [eɪs], *big* [bɪg], *watch* [wɑtʃ] |
| | Child versions: *cup* [kʌ], *ace* [eɪ], *big* [bɪ], *watch* [wɑ] |
| | Conclusion: Child uses the process of final consonant deletion. |

### *SEGMENTAL INVENTORY*

| | **Background** |
|---|---|
| **WHO?** | A child younger than 3 years of age *or* an older preschooler or a child of early school age with severely unintelligible speech. |
| **WHAT?** | The segmental inventory is sometimes called a "phonemic" inventory. It is a structured list that allows comparison of the child's production to that of adults. It is similar to the test forms for most standardized tests of articulation, in which the adult target is in one column and the transcription in the other. |

*(continues)*

*(continued)*

The segmental inventory for consonants typically includes initial, intervocalic (between-vowel), and final consonants. Intervocalic consonants, which occur between two syllables in the same word, are included because accurate intervocalic consonants may be a bridge to accurate production of those consonants in connected speech. The segmental inventory for clusters includes word-initial clusters only. The segmental inventory for vowels includes vowels that occur anywhere in a word.

Segmental inventories have been used most often with responses to citation-form tests. However, a segmental inventory can also be constructed using connected speech samples, which have the best face validity as sources of information.

**WHY?**    The segmental inventory indicates how well the child is progressing toward acquiring the adult phonological system.

**WHEN?**    The segmental inventory can be used when results of standard articulation tests are not available or are suspect, or when the SLP wishes to base decisions on data derived from connected speech. Results can be compared to normative data and used to determine treatment decisions. It should be noted that segmental inventories for vowels are not typically obtained for children, although the *Templin-Darley Tests of Articulation* (Templin & Darley, 1969) include a section that assesses vowels.

**SUPPORT:**    The segmental inventory for consonants has a long history in speech-language pathology, but under other names. Virtually all standardized tests of articulation have test forms arranged to show how the child produces adult phonemes. Use of a slightly different type of segmental analysis ("contrast" analysis) was suggested in 1985 by Stoel-Gammon and Dunn.

## SEGMENTAL INVENTORY

### *Reproducible Forms 6, 7, and 8*

### *Procedure*

1. Obtain a speech sample from the client. Ideally, this should be a spontaneous conversational sample, usually obtained during play; however, if connected speech is very difficult to understand and to segment, a list of single-word productions may also be used. Crystal (1982) has recommended a sample that is long enough to include at least 100 different words. However, multiple tokens of the same word *should* be included in the inventory.

    One issue that comes up frequently with analyses of connected speech is that the child simply may not say any words that have a particular adult phoneme in them. For example, it is easy to imagine that a child would not say any words with /-ð/ in them (e.g., *breathe*, *smooth*). In such cases, the SLP may wish to supplement with a naming task to fill in the gaps.

2. Transcribe each word, lining up the glosses on the left of the page and the transcriptions to the right.

3. Using Reproducible Form 6 for consonants, Reproducible Form 7 for word-initial clusters, and Reproducible Form 8 for vowels, enter each new type of sound on the form and put a tally mark near it each time that sound is used. If it appears to you that a model spoken by an adult just prior to the client's production might have influenced the production, the tally mark should be differentiated (e.g., written as "m" for "modeled").

4. If the child produces the same word several different ways, tally as if these were separate words.

5. If you do not know the meaning of a word or phonological form that you can nevertheless transcribe, do *not* include that word in the analysis, because the adult targets are not known.

6. Establish a criterion for saying that the child "has" a phoneme or structure, that is, uses it productively. Many SLPs would consider spontaneous use (i.e., not modeled) two to three times to be productive use of a phoneme or structure.

7. Make a list of the consonants that the child uses productively in initial position, in final position, and, if desired, in intervocalic position. If using the vowel list, simply note the vowels used.

8. Compare this list to the consonant data in Table 1-4 in Section 1 and the vowel data to Table 3-4 in this section (below) to determine the client's approximate developmental level.

**TABLE 3-4.** Vowels produced correctly by 90% of children at the ages of 3, 4, and 5. *Adapted from Templin (1957).*

|  | *Age 3* | *Age 4* | *Age 5* |
|---|---|---|---|
| High front /i ɪ e/ | All | All | All |
| Mid-low front /ɛ æ/ | All | All | All |
| High back, rounded /u ʊ/ | All | All | All |
| Mid back, rounded /o ɔ*/ | /o/ | /o/ | /o/ |
| Low back /ɑ/ | Used | Used | Used |
| Central /ʌ ə** / | /ʌ/ | /ʌ/ | /ʌ/ |
| Central /r/-colored /ɝ ɚ***/ | /ɝ/ | /ɝ/ | /ɝ/ |
| Phonemic diphthongs /aɪ aʊ ɔɪ/ | All | All | All |

*The vowel /ɔ/ is not used correctly until age 6. However, Templin's subjects were from Minnesota, where the dialect likely conflates [ɔ] with [ɑ].

**Difficulties with /ə/ may be related to Unstressed Syllable Deletion. This vowel was assessed in the words *upon* and *amount.*

***The /ɚ/ (tested in *car*) was not used by 90% of children until age 6.

## Treatment Goals Based on the Segmental Inventory

In most cases, the segments that are missing from the inventory would become the targets of treatment. Priority would be given to omitted segments first, then to substitutions. For those children who produce an adult target in several different ways, it may be important to stabilize the best of these versions.

## Phonological Processes

In the preschool population we generally assume that difficulties with speech sounds production are manifested as phonological processes. Of course, the SLP would not ignore distortions that do not count as phonological processes; however, the vast majority of non-adult productions fit under the rubric of phonological processes.

Fortunately, the SLP has many assessment instruments to choose from when assessing use of phonological processes. Many of these have been reviewed in a systematic way (Bleile, 1995; Bernthal & Bankson, 1998). Some of them are:

The *Assessment of Phonological Processes-Revised* (*APP-R*) by Hodson (1986)

The *Khan-Lewis Phonological Analysis, Second Edition* (*KLPA-2*) by Khan and Lewis (2002)

The *Bankson Bernthal Test of Phonology* (*BBTOP*) by Bankson and Bernthal (1990)

The *Smit-Hand Articulation and Phonology Evaluation* (*SHAPE*) by Smit and Hand (1997)

The *Clinical Assessment of Articulation and Phonology* (*CAAP*) by Secord and Donohue (2002)

All of these tests are based on the naming of single words by the child. All of them use picture stimuli except for the *APP-R*, which uses real or toy objects. All of these tests except the *APP-R* are normed and have acceptable psychometric characteristics. However, the *APP-R* includes a way to determine how severely disordered a child's speech is in comparison with a group of preschool-age children with a range of phonological disorders.

Determining what phonological processes a child uses from a connected speech sample is relatively time-consuming to do by hand. Fortunately, there are a number of computerized phonological analysis systems available. These systems were reviewed in Section 1. The advantages to using computerized systems are these:

- They make an analysis of connected speech possible in a reasonable amount of time.
- Once the input system is learned, that is, the keyboard strokes to represent IPA symbols, the software provides results almost as fast as they can be printed.
- The results are provided in considerably more detail than analyses done by hand.

### *Developmentally Early vs. Developmentally Late Processes*

A clinically useful distinction can be made between processes that are used by most children early in development and those that can persist for some years. Table 3-5 shows some of these processes grouped by the age of suppression (i.e., the age after which most children do not use them). Discrepancies between the two sources of information no doubt reflect differing methodology.

**TABLE 3-5.** Phonological processes grouped by the ages at which they are typically suppressed. Asterisks mark discrepant data.

*Data are from Stoel-Gammon and Dunn (SG-D, 1985) and Smit and Hand (S-H, 1997).*

| *Processes Used Up to 3 Years* | *Processes Used Up to 4 Years* |
| --- | --- |
| Final consonant deletion | Stopping |
| Consonant assimilation | *Velar fronting (S-H) |

| Processes Used Up to 3 Years | Processes Used Up to 4 Years |
|---|---|
| Reduplication | Reduction of clusters without /s/ |
| Prevocalic voicing | |
| *Velar fronting (SG-D) | |
| *Weak syllable deletion (SG-D) | |

| Processes Used Up to 5 Years | Processes Used Up to 7 Years |
|---|---|
| Depalatalization | Gliding |
| *Weak syllable deletion (S-H) | Vocalization |
| Reduction of clusters with /s/ | |

It is important to note that many of the developmentally early processes involve syllable structures, while the later processes include many substitutions. The processes affecting liquids (gliding and vocalization) are extraordinarily persistent.

### Unusual Patterns of Phonology

Children with phonological difficulties may use idiosyncratic processes in addition to the more common or natural processes. Idiosyncratic processes are patterns of sound use that typically developing children rarely use. They often strike the SLP as bizarre. For example, Fey and Gandour (1982) reported on a child who added a syllabic nasal to the end of words that ended in a voiced obstruent (e.g., *bed* was [bɛdn̩]). This is an example of **epenthesis**, or the addition of an element.

Idiosyncratic patterns like this one often have a large impact on intelligibility, because adults are not used to decoding such patterns. In contrast, most adults can decode a substitution like [w] for /r/ easily because it is a very common pattern.

Some children show a pattern of sound use that overrides any of the typical phonological processes. For example, you may assess a child who uses the stopping process in initial position by substituting a [t] or [d] sound for every fricative except the labial ones. You note that the child uses the same substitution for fricatives in other parts of the word. In addition, this child uses fronting, which again involves the use of [t d] for velars, and depalatalization ([t d] again). The result is that the child uses a heavy preponderance of [t d] and very few other consonants. This pattern represents a sound preference, namely a preference for alveolar stops. Preferences such as this are often called "favorite sound," although in this case it is a class of sounds (alveolar stops) that provides default segments.

Any list of idiosyncratic processes is bound to be incomplete. However, the following list of idiosyncratic processes conveys some of the ingenious ways in which children can deviate from the typical pathways of phonological development. The following are examples of idiosyncratic processes have been noted by Stoel-Gammon and Dunn (1985) and by Smit and Hand (1997):

- Fricatives substituted for stops (e.g., *tan* said as [sæn])
- Initial consonant deletion (e.g., *cup* said as [ʌp])
- Glottal replacement (e.g., *messy* said as [mɛʔɪ])
- Atypical cluster reduction (e.g., *school* said as [sul])

- Glides substituted for fricatives (e.g., *zipper* said as [wɪpə])
- Stopping of fricatives in clusters (e.g., *swing* said as [twɪŋ])
- Epenthesis (adding) of segments (e.g., *bed* said as [bɛdn̩])
- Unusual assimilations (e.g., *king* said as [ŋɪŋ]
- Doubling of a single syllable (e.g., *mine* said as [maɪmaɪ])

There is little in the literature to guide the SLP in interpretation of the presence of idiosyncratic processes. By definition, most children do not use such processes, and if such processes do occur in the phonology of a typically developing child, they do not persist for long. However, the presence of idiosyncratic processes in children with phonological delay may be quite significant.

Let us assume that children make hypotheses about how the phonology of their language works. Children then try out the hypothesized forms and note the responses of those in their environment. Based on those responses, they may modify, relinquish, or retain the hypothesized structures. However, if a child retains an idiosyncratic process for a long period of time, say, more than six weeks, this suggests that the child is oblivious to the responses he is getting to his poorly intelligible words, or that the child is incapable of modifying his productions. In any case, the child has veered off the beaten track, so to speak, and has gotten stuck on a path that leads nowhere.

In terms of qualifying children for services, it may be helpful to remember that by definition, persisting idiosyncratic processes are never "normal," as typically developing children do not exhibit them, or at least they do not persist in such children. In fact, based on the arguments presented previously, we may consider the persistence of idiosyncratic processes to be prognostic of a poor outcome without intervention. (It should be noted, however, that Leonard (1985) and others consider the inventiveness shown in some idiosyncratic processes to be a positive sign because the child is generating novel hypotheses.) Finally, because idiosyncratic processes usually contribute to poor intelligibility, these processes might be among the first to be targeted in treatment.

## Other Kinds of Phonological Analyses

Although phonological processes are now enshrined in a number of tests and analysis procedures, there are still other ways to view a young child's phonological system. Typically, these procedures either augment or replace a phonological process analysis.

***Distinctive Feature Analysis.*** One of the older ways to analyze errors is in terms of what distinctive features are missing from the child's production capabilities. McReynolds and Engmann (1975) published a manual for determining what features a child did or did not use and then developed treatment aimed at teaching the missing features. This approach is not used frequently today because it ignored the powerful effects of syllable structure on children's errors. Nevertheless, partly as a result of this work, the use of feature terminology is widespread in clinical phonology. For example, we may describe a child as using only [+labial] consonants in final position.

***Knowledge Hierarchies.*** Elbert and Gierut (1986) have taken still a different tack in looking at child phonology. Their emphasis is on the nature of the child's underlying representation or form, and on how much knowledge of the adult system is embodied in that form. For example, if a child says [dɑ] for *dog*, the SLP does not know if the child realizes that there is a /g/ at the end of the word. In other words, the child's underlying form could be either /dɑ/ or /dɑg/, or even a form in which a consonant is present but its nature is not known, a situation we may indicate as [dɑX], where the X represents an unspecified consonant.

Elbert and Gierut reasoned that if they added a morphological ending, they might be able to discover the child's underlying form. Consider for example, the following two children producing the words *dog* and *doggie*:

|          | Child A | Child B |
|----------|---------|---------|
| dog      | [dɑ]    | [dɑ]    |
| doggie   | [dɑi]   | [dɑgi]  |

At the very least, we can agree that Child B probably knows more about the final /g/ than does Child A.

Based on this approach, Elbert and Gierut have developed an assessment procedure that contrasts the base forms, like *dog*, to forms in which an English suffix has been added to the end of the word (*doggie*). If there is a question about the initial consonant, a prefix might be added to the beginning of the word (*re-dog*). Based on this kind of assessment, one can set up a knowledge hierarchy for the child in terms of distinctive features and syllable structures. The hierarchy is then used to determine the goals of treatment.

This type of assessment is individualized to the child, and it typically involves production of several hundred word forms. Consequently, it is time-consuming, and it also makes use of a mixture of real and nonsensical "words." Nevertheless, even if the SLP does not use these concepts in their entirety, it is often useful to consider the nature of a client's underlying representation (UR). Very likely the child with an adult-like UR will acquire the surface expression of that form more quickly than the child who has little knowledge of the adult target. Moreover, the clinician needs to ask how to help the child who probably has non-adult URs acquire adult-like URs. This question is probably most relevant to children with severely disordered phonology, because we can argue that it is these children who know the least about the adult phonology.

***Nonlinear Phonology.*** A relatively new approach to phonological analysis and intervention based on nonlinear phonology has been taken by Bernhardt and Stoel-Gammon (1994) and Bernhardt and Stemberger (1998; 2000). Traditional phonology carries with it the assumption that phoneme-sized segments are planned and executed in sequences or linear strings. In these strings, structures in one part of the word are independent of structures in other parts of the word. Thus a [d] appearing early in the word *dog* should not influence later segments, and vice versa.

Of course, this implication cannot possibly be true, as there are children who say [dɑd] alveolar assimilation), and other children who say [gɑg] for *dog* (velar assimilation). In addition, work on the motor-planning aspects of speech suggests that planning occurs in chunks that are at least syllable-sized and probably longer. While nonlinear phonology does not explicitly attempt to incorporate this type of information, it is based in linguistic theory and attempts to show relationships among syllables and segments as well as rhythm and prosody. Nonlinear phonology is presented in terms of the formalisms of linguistic theory, which makes it applicable to other languages, but not readily accessible to the practicing SLP.

The English-speaking SLP can take away from nonlinear phonology some important ideas:

- The child's system may operate with constraints on allowable sequences. In fact, these constraints are sometimes called *word recipes*. For example, if the child's system allows only CVCV(C) sequences, then the child will produce the word *sandwich* (adult [sæmwɪʧ]) with only one center consonant (e.g., [sæmɪʧ]).

- Feature spreading from segment to segment can also occur. For example, a child may say the word *smoke* as [fõŭk], where the nasal /m/ is marked only as nasality on the vowel.

- Syllabification and prosody are critically important in production. For example, the production of the /sk/ sequence in the single-syllable word *ask* is very different from the production of the /sk/ in *asking*, in which the /s/ and the /k/ are parts of different syllables, one stressed and the other unstressed.

## MEASURING INTELLIGIBILITY AND SEVERITY IN YOUNG CHILDREN

Section 2 mentioned several global measures of spontaneous conversational speech, and several of these are appropriate for young children. These included measures related to both intelligibility and severity.

### Intelligibility

Intelligibility is an extremely important issue for the preschooler and the young school-age child. Parents of young children as well as teachers are likely to be concerned when a child cannot be understood by themselves or by playmates. Intelligibility is also a more prominent issue in deciding whether intervention is warranted for these young children than it is for their older peers. Fortunately, both the quantitative and the impressionistic estimates of intelligibility that were mentioned in Section 2 can be used with the young child who has delayed or disordered speech. The quantitative measure is **Percentage of Intelligible Words** (PIW: Shriberg & Kwiatkowski, 1982a). In a recent report, Gordon-Brannan and Hodson (2000) have suggested that when Percentage of Intelligible Words (based on audio only) falls below about 66% for a child age 4 years or older, intervention should be considered.

It should be mentioned that because the content of a young child's speech may be highly context-bound, it would be helpful to videotape the interaction. Then if the videotaped sound quality is adequate, the sample can be glossed directly from the videotape, and the PIW calculated. Naturally, we need to recognize that glosses made from videotape are likely to result in higher PIWs than glosses from audiotape alone.

The various rating scales of intelligibility described in Section 2 can also be used with the child's parents and perhaps with the teachers as well. For some children, these scales may constitute the bulk of the information you have about intelligibility because the child is reticent and unwilling to talk with you.

### Severity

The *Percentage of Consonants Correct* (PCC: Shriberg & Kwiatkowski, 1982a), as described in Section 2, is used widely with young children as a measure of severity. The PCC measure is relatively crude because it does not discriminate among types of errors. For example, most SLPs regard omissions as far more damaging to speech than substitutions, and they regard distortions as relatively mild errors compared to substitutions. For this reason, several researchers (including Shriberg, 1993) have offered modifications to the PCC. However, for a straightforward measure that is relatively easy to determine and is readily understood by parents and teachers, PCC is excellent.

## RELATED VARIABLES

In Section 2, we touched on some of the non-speech variables that influence the clinical picture. These included the examination of the oral mechanism, the hearing screening, information about cognitive status and language status, and information about fluency, voice, prosody, general behavior, and possible prognostic indicators. These variables can all influence the diagnostic findings, the prognosis, and the recommendations that the SLP reports. It is probably safe to say that the more findings there are in these related areas, the poorer the prognosis, and the greater the likelihood that we will recommend intervention.

## The Oral Mechanism Examination

Many children are reluctant to have anyone look in their mouths, let alone put a tongue blade in. However, unless there are elements of the speech signal that suggest a problem in the oral mechanism, a relatively cursory look at the structures is sufficient. Elements of speech that would suggest a better look include nasal emission, hypernasal resonance, hyponasal resonance, and unusual fricative distortions.

In most cases the structural findings are less informative than the functional state of the mechanism. So when we ask children to stick out the tongue and touch the nose, and other oral "gymnastics," we observe how quickly and accurately the child can do this. In addition, we may wish to ask the child to repeat syllable trains (e.g., /pʌ/). There are also suggestions in the research literature that among children ages 3 to 5, the *rate* of these movements may be relatively insensitive to differences, but that the *accuracy* and the *consistency* of the movements is a more sensitive measure (Williams & Stackhouse, 2000). In the future, these two aspects of diadochokinetic tasks may turn out to have prognostic value.

## PROGNOSTIC INDICATORS IN THE YOUNG CHILD

The more global prognostic indicators, such as cognitive level and hearing status, function similarly in the preschool population and the school-age population. Other indicators need to be interpreted somewhat differently.

## Consistency

Consistency in this population usually refers to the frequency of use of phonological processes as a percent of the opportunities for use. Hodson and Paden (1991) have recommended that SLPs consider the process to be "productive" for the child only if the child uses it more than 40% of the time. Implied in this recommendation is that processes used less frequently will eventually be corrected without intervention. This implication has not been tested in a controlled manner, although many clinicians use the 40% cutoff for determining eligibility and planning treatment.

## Stimulability

When we are dealing with phonological processes, stimulability takes on the connotation of "stimulability to correct the phonological process." Because phonological processes affect only words, stimulability in this context means stimulability in words. In addition, stimulability may not refer to a fully correct production. If the child who uses final consonant deletion says [kʌk] after your model of *cup*, he is considered stimulable because he inserted a final consonant. Of course, many SLPs would resist reinforcing [kʌk] for *cup* in treatment. However, in most instances, it is possible to find an exemplar of the process that the child is stimulable to produce correctly in every respect. That exemplar can be the starting point in treatment.

## Speech-Sound Discrimination

Speech-sound discrimination is extraordinarily difficult to assess in young children. Tests of discrimination usually have the child pointing to a picture that the SLP has just named. These tests are notoriously susceptible to extraneous variables, among them failure to understand the task, child preference for certain pictures, for example, pictures of toys, child preference for pointing to one position on the page, and fatigue or other internal states of the child. In addition, children with perfect articulation make errors on these tests, as do adults, which suggests that these tests have a substantial cognitive component.

Locke (1980) developed a Sound Production-Perception Task that requires a Yes/No response from the child to many questions about a single picture (e.g., "Is it [θɪp]?" for a picture of a ship). However, this task is difficult for young children with moderate to severe disorders to attend to over time. Instead, they answer randomly, or they consistently respond Yes (or No), or they request to do something else.

In light of these difficulties in assessing speech sound discrimination directly, I recommend that the SLP *not* attempt to assess speech sound discrimination. Rather, we can reasonably assume that in the case of phonological processes, there is almost always an element of unawareness of missing or substituted sound segments. Support for this idea comes from the many reports of successful treatment of phonological processes involving minimal pairs of words. Inevitably, using minimal pairs provides a kind of perceptual training for the child.

It should be noted, however, that in older children, who are likely to have residual errors, we cannot make the same assumption. Speech perception in these children can be assessed, and many of them, if not most, can tell the difference between their error sound and the adult target.

## Potential Dyspraxic Elements

Developmental Verbal Dyspraxia (DVD) is a complex of speech and non-speech symptoms that are usually interpreted as indicating difficulty in sequencing speech movements. Some of the hallmark symptoms are severely impaired intelligibility, inconsistency, difficulty with vowels as well as consonants, difficulty with oral nonverbal movements, and long periods of treatment with slow progress. Each of these symptoms is a potential dyspraxic element (PDE). Section 8 includes an in-depth look at DVD.

We pay attention to potential dyspraxic elements even in children who are not likely to have DVD because a recent study showed that many children with speech sound disorders exhibit one or more of the classic markers for Developmental Verbal Dyspraxia (McCabe, Rosenthal, & McLeod, 1998). The greater the number of PDE, the more severe the disorder, according to these authors. The presence of one or two markers is a negative prognostic indicator.

---

CLINICAL NOTE 3-1: **Not All Potential Dyspraxic Elements (PDE) are Equally Serious**

Sometimes, a given instance of motor difficulty may pose no more than a one- or two-session stumbling block. For example, I once worked with a 4-year-old who had only a few consonants, and the few he used did not include any glides. He exhibited several PDEs. For example, he was not only incapable of imitating [w], but he also could not imitate lip-puckering. He did not round his lips when he tried to hush a baby using a finger in front of his lips, nor did he round his lips when he tried to blow out a candle.

*(continues)*

(*continued*)

After a session spent discovering this information, we decided to provide tactile and gestural cues to increase awareness of the labial area. We started the next session with a gestural cue in which the clinician made a circle with her index finger in front of her own mouth while rounding the lips, then did the same in front of the client's lips when he attempted to imitate. On the second try, he rounded his lips, without even needing the tactile version of this cue. Subsequent progress was not particularly rapid, but at least we could reliably elicit lip-rounding from that point on.

Ordinarily the presence of one or two potential dyspraxic elements suggests that the SLP should plan for more motor practice than would be typical in phonological remediation. For example, if a child who uses the Stopping process is having difficulty putting a fricative into a simple CV word, the clinician might work on the fricative in isolation first, using a lot of drill.

## PSYCHOSOCIAL ISSUES

Shriberg and Kwiatkowski (1982b) have discussed the importance of psychosocial aspects of the child with disordered phonology. They developed assessment checklists that describe issues concerning the types of psychosocial inputs that children may receive and the types of behaviors that may be relevant. Table 3-6 provides examples of inputs and behaviors.

**TABLE 3-6.**

Examples of psychosocial variables—inputs and behaviors.

*After Shriberg and Kwiatkowski (1982b).*

| Inputs | Behaviors |
| --- | --- |
| Appropriate age friends | Affect |
| Parents—Ineffective behavior management | Compliance |
| Parents—Marital instability | Maturity |
| Parents—Sibling comparisons | Responsiveness to SLP and others |
| Parents—Support of treatment | Play modes |

Information about these psychosocial inputs and behaviors comes from the case history and also from the clinician's direct observations. It is not surprising that Shriberg (1997) reports that about 7% of children with speech delay of unknown origin have significant psychosocial issues. We can expect that these concerns will affect the prognosis, and that the effect will be negative.

## PHONOLOGICAL AWARENESS

All of the related variables and prognostic indicators mentioned above are relevant to both young children and older children. However, one area of evaluation that is specific to the young child population is that of phonological awareness.

Phonological awareness refers to the "ability to identify and manipulate the sounds of the language" (Bernthal & Bankson, 1998, p. 369). This ability is often assessed in terms of whether or not the child can segment speech into words, syllables, and sounds, as well as segmenting the parts of the syllable (onset and rime). Stackhouse (1997) has written an excellent review of the research on phonological awareness. An important point that she makes for the SLP working with young children is that these abilities are related to the development of reading. Another point is that children with severe phonological disorders perform more poorly than their typically developing peers on measures of phonological awareness. They are thus at risk for later difficulties in learning to read.

It is important to note that to date, the SLP has no reason to believe that poor performance on an assessment of phonological awareness is a prognostic indicator for improvement in phonology *per se*, either with or without intervention. Rather, this type of assessment indicates potential areas of future difficulty in the academic setting. In order to reduce this risk, the SLP may incorporate activities to enhance phonological awareness into treatment plans.

Published assessment instruments for phonological awareness include the *Test of Phonological Awareness* by Torgeson and Bryant (1993) and the *Phonological Awareness Test* by Robertson and Salter (1995). Additionally, many SLPs use clinician-made materials when assessing phonological awareness.

## SUMMARY

This section has dealt with the aspects of evaluation specific to children who have phonological disorders. The SLP may want to use Reproducible Form 1, the diagnostic checklist, to ensure that the child's performance and life situation has been evaluated in every relevant area. The SLP then describes his findings in clear language, avoiding jargon. The clinical impressions section of the report is particularly important because it is here that the clinician relates all the findings to each other. The recommendations should then flow logically from the clinical impressions.

# SECTION

# 4

# ASSESSMENT OF SCHOOL-AGE CHILDREN AND ADULTS WHO HAVE RESIDUAL ERRORS

● ● ● ● ● ● ● ● ● ● ● ● ● ● ● ● ● ● ● ● ● ● ● ● ● ● ● ● ● ● ● ● ● ● ● ● ●

**T**he clients who are the focus of this chapter are a diverse group. Clients with residual errors tend to differ along many dimensions (McNutt & Hamayan, 1984), some of which are auditory abilities, language skills, academic achievement, and oral sensory acuity. Perhaps the only attribute that they have in common is that they continue to produce speech sound errors well after their peers are using adult-like versions of those speech sounds. For this group of children and adults, intelligibility is often not the primary issue.

We may also have clients who are speakers of English as a second language (ESL), to whom we may provide elective services. Often they are adults, and usually the issue for them is intelligibility of spoken English. ESL clients tend to have difficulty not only with specific phonemes, but also with English stress patterns and prosody. Many of these difficulties are predictable from the characteristics of the first language. For example, a person who speaks

Mandarin as her first language has little experience with syllable-final consonants, tense vowels, and alternating stress, but all of these elements are important in English.

When we are working with school-age children and adults, the division of labor is quite different from when we are working with younger children. Even in play therapy with a 3-year-old, the clinician does most of the work: modeling, encouraging, setting up opportunities, and so forth. In contrast, with older clients, there has to be active participation on the part of the client. In other words, the SLP lets the client know that the responsibility for making changes rests with the client, while the clinician can at best facilitate these changes. Consequently, part of the assessment of school-age children and adults is an estimate of their willingness to commit to the intervention process.

## RESIDUAL SPEECH SOUND ERRORS IN CHILDREN

The residual errors of school-age children and adults are quite different from the error patterns we expect from preschool children, who tend to use well-known phonological processes. By the age of 7 or 8, the large majority of children will no longer use phonological processes except possibly the processes affecting the liquid /r/. For example, an 8-year-old with a residual error on a fricative phoneme is not likely to replace that fricative with a stop, but with another fricative. The child with /r/-errors may use the processes known as Gliding and Vocalization, but sometimes you may detect that the substitute for the /r/ is really not a glide or a vowel, but a somewhat distorted version of the /r/.

Residual speech-sound errors are usually distortions or substitutions of one or more of the "big 10": /s z ʃ ʒ tʃ dʒ θ ð v r/ (Winitz, 1969). These phonemes are typically in error as consonant singletons in all word positions. If the error phoneme participates in consonant clusters, it will likely be in error in those contexts as well. If the phoneme is a member of a cognate pair, for example /tʃ dʒ/, the nature of the error is likely to be the same, except for the pair /θð/, where the most frequent substitution for /θ/ is [f] and for /ð/ is [d].

## THE NATURAL HISTORY OF RESIDUAL ERRORS

One of the interesting questions about these clients is what their speech was like when they were preschoolers. For example, it is unlikely that they ever produced their error sounds any better than they do now. In that case, did these errors co-exist with use of phonological processes? Did some of these clients receive intervention for the phonological processes but not for the errors they now make? Were some of the current errors actually a result of the intervention for phonological processes? A review of the relevant literature shows that our field knows very little about the natural history of speech sound problems. In fact, there are only two studies of the outcomes of specific speech-sound errors in kindergarten and first grade (Sax, 1972; Stephens, Hoffman, & Daniloff, 1986).

In a recent publication, Gruber (1999) used group data from children with speech delay to study the changes over time and the probabilities that the children would normalize. He found two different paths to normalization. In one group, errors of substitution and omission decreased as correct productions increased. The second group, however, appeared to represent children who retain residual errors. For these children, errors of omission and substitution decreased as distortions increased. This finding suggests that at least some clinical distortions result from the "correction" of substitutions and omissions. However, there was no way to predict which children would be in which group.

Lack of knowledge, however, has not prevented the adoption of rules about who may receive services in various settings, especially in schools. In general, school districts and state school boards do their utmost to avoid unnecessary intervention because intervention is very expensive. Consequently, any residual errors that children have when they are younger than the ages of acquisition for those phonemes have generally been declared to be developmental and the children therefore ineligible for intervention. In other words, the assumption is made that most children are likely to correct their errors during the process of maturation.

The assumption that children will correct their errors without intervention is based on extrapolations from cross-sectional data such as is found in the normative studies (e.g., Templin, 1957; Smit, et al., 1990). However, even the cross-sectional data provide inconsistent support for this assumption. Table 4-1 shows estimates of change after age 6 in the cross-sectional age groups for the Smit, et al. (1990) growth-of-acquisition curves for nine of the "top 10" error phonemes.

**TABLE 4-1.** Estimates of changes in proportion of children in error at age 6 and at the recommended age of acquisition for nine of the "Top 10" error phonemes, omitting /ʒ/.

*Data are estimated from the growth-of-acquisition curves and the recommended ages of acquisition are taken from Smit, et al. (1990).*

| Phoneme | Estimated percentage of children in error at age 6 | Estimated percentage of children in error at age of acquisition | How much change? |
|---|---|---|---|
| /s/ | 17% | 10% | Less than half |
| /z/ | 18% | 10% | Less than half |
| /ʃ/ | 11% | 7% | Less than half |
| /ʧ/ | 10% | 8% | Very little |
| /ʤ/ | 10% | 6% | About half |
| /v/ (Age of acquisition is below age 6.) | | | |
| /r-/ | 22% | 8% | Two-thirds |
| /-r/ | 18% | 4% | Three-fourths |
| /θ/ (Females: Age of acquisition is 6 years.) | | | |
| /θ/ (Males) | 23% | 5% | Three-fourths |
| /ð-/ (Females: Age of acquisition is below age 6.) | | | |
| /ð-/ (Males: | 19% | 5% | Three-fourths |

Assuming that the estimates in Table 4-1 mirror faithfully what we would see in longitudinal studies, it is clear that substantial improvement after age 6 occurs only for some of the phonemes shown, namely /r- -r θ ð/, and in some cases, only for males. For the /s z ʃ ʧ ʤ/ we see that more than half of children still in error at age 6 are not going to improve; rather, they get to practice their error for another year or two.

Two longitudinal studies tend to support this finding. In one of them, Sax (1972) followed children in kindergarten, first grade, and second grade for several years. Of the phonemes that many children produced in error in the early grades, the liquids, labial fricatives and interdental fricatives tended to improve markedly, although boys generally lagged behind the girls. The palatal fricatives and the alveolar fricatives were still frequently in error at the beginning of fourth grade.

Another longitudinal study (Stephens, Hoffman, & Daniloff, 1986) also supports a finding that self-correction is questionable for the /s/ phoneme. These researchers followed kindergartners who had /s/ errors. Somewhat more than half of the children with /s/ errors in kindergarten self-corrected by the end of second grade, approximately; however, progress depended on the nature of the error. Children with retracted versions of /s/ (post-alveolar distortions or /ʃ/) were highly likely to self-correct. About half of the children with dentalized versions of /s/ self-corrected. None of the children with lateralized /s/ showed self-correction. However, we should note that the numbers of children in the "retracters" and the "lateralizers" groups were small compared to the number of dentalizers.

There are no data about the average length of time to correction for children who do not receive treatment until after they reach the designated age of acquisition for the phoneme in question. However, it is my experience and observation that some of these children are in treatment for several years. This is embarrassing for the profession, because on the face of it, speech-sound acquisition should not be a matter of slogging through discouraging exercises week after week. After all, these very same children likely acquired most other speech sounds effortlessly.

Clearly, there is a diagnostic issue here. We need to predict which children with one or more residual speech-sound errors will correct them without intervention and which ones will not. The profession has some data on this issue in the school-age group. These findings suggest that children ages five to six years old who are not stimulable for an accurate production will need intervention, while children who are easily stimulable may self-correct.

Given this pattern of results, we might wonder if we could do a short-term intervention with a child who is not stimulable, with the goal of making him/her readily stimulable, and then monitor for change. If this were done with children in the first grade who make errors on /s z ʃ ʒ tʃ dʒ/ and are not stimulable, perhaps we could jump-start the process for the child and prevent later intervention.

## SPEECH SOUND ERRORS IN ADULTS

Adults who seek speech-language pathology services for speech sound errors include at least two distinct groups. One of these groups is adults who had residual errors when they were of school age and did not correct them. A second group includes adults who speak English as a second or even a third language. These adults may have difficulty making themselves understood by the native English speakers around them.

Both of these groups tend to be highly motivated to improve. In the first group we may have people who choose professions where their speech is of great importance (e.g., law, public relations, theater). In the second group we often have people who are students from other countries who want to succeed in their studies, which are conducted in English, and in their professions once they have graduated. They understand that English has become the language common to most of the world.

## ASSESSMENT OF SPEECH SOUND PRODUCTION
## IN SCHOOL-AGE CHILDREN

The assessment protocol for a school-age child is straightforward. Typically, we administer a test of articulation, evaluate connected speech, assess variability and stimulability of production of the phonemes in error, and evaluate other related and prognostic variables. The Checklist for the Diagnostic Evaluation (Reproducible Form 1) can provide structure for this assessment.

Assessment of school-age children typically involves less informal testing than is typical with preschoolers, and a good deal more formal or standardized testing. This difference results from the fact that in the early years of the professional study of speech-sound disorders, very little was done with preschoolers. At that time the emphasis was on school-age children with speech-sound disorders of unknown origin, the so-called "functional articulation problems." Consequently, some of the oldest tests in the field of speech-language pathology are standardized tests of articulation. The term *articulation* indicates the underlying assumption of these tests, which is that speech-sound errors result from problems in the motor speech system.

There are now many standardized tests of articulation. These tests are typically based on single-word naming, are standardized, and provide for a kind of segmental inventory.

## STANDARDIZED TESTS OF SPEECH SOUND PRODUCTION

### Background

**WHO?**  Children who are likely to have residual errors and to use no phonological processes except possibly those affecting liquids.

**WHAT?**  Standardized tests of articulation or speech-sound production that are available commercially. All of these tests require single-word naming of pictures.

**WHY?**  These tests are administered to determine if the child's speech-sound production is within normal limits. The tests mentioned below are normed, and most of them also provide a phonemic or segmental inventory. They are used extensively in public schools because state guidelines for qualifying children for services mandate normed tests.

**WHEN?**  These tests are usually administered as part of a diagnostic battery for speech-sound disorders. They may be used for post-testing also, but an interval of at least one year should be observed.

**SUPPORT:**  Tests of articulation were among the first normed assessment instruments developed in the field of speech-language pathology. The ones listed here are normed, and they conform to accepted principles for diagnostic tests. Because they are based on single-word productions, the information gained from the test must be supplemented with information about conversational speech.

## STANDARDIZED TESTS OF SPEECH-SOUND PRODUCTION
### Procedure

1. The following standardized inventory tests are widely used in clinics and schools. Most of them are normed for ages 3 to 8, but they are most useful with the school-age population.
   - *Goldman-Fristoe Test of Articulation-2* (*GFTA-2*—Goldman & Fristoe, 2000)
   - *Templin-Darley Tests of Articulation* (Templin & Darley, 1969).
   - *Arizona Articulation Proficiency Scale, Third Revision* (*Arizona-3*—Fudala, 2000)

- *Photo Articulation Test* (*PAT*—Lippke, Dickey, Selmar, & Soder, 1997)
- *Smit-Hand Articulation and Phonology Evaluation* (*SHAPE*—Smit & Hand, 1997)
- *Clinical Assessment of Articulation and Phonology* (*CAAP*—Secord & Donohue, 2002)

2. Each test should be administered as specified in the test manual. A child's score can be interpreted relative to peers by referring to standardization tables. In addition, for some phonemes, ages of acquisition for specific phonemes may be available. It should be noted that the *CAAP* also has a sentence form for children age 5 and older.

## Assessing Variation in Production

One of the issues of great interest to the SLP who works with clients who have residual errors is whether or not there is any variability in production. Specifically, we hope that there is the occasional acceptable production, because usually that offers an entry point into the client's error system. This general issue is called *inconsistency*, and *inconsistency with hits* (where the variants include one or more correct productions) is the type we are looking for, although *inconsistency with approximations* (where the variants include productions that are closer to the target than most other productions) can also be helpful. There are several ways to get at inconsistency. One is to analyze the pattern of errors obtained in formal testing. Another is to listen to connected speech to detect any productions that may be acceptable even when most are not, and to note the words in which these improved productions occur. A third is to do a probe that varies the length of utterance in which the target occurs.

We should note that hits (correct productions that occur when most productions are incorrect) are clinically useful only if they are repeatable. If the SLP hears a correct form only once and can never again elicit that form, the hit is probably not going to provide an entry point for treatment.

## HOW TO ASSESS CONSISTENCY/INCONSISTENCY

|  | Background |
|---|---|
| **WHO?** | A school-age child or an adult who has residual phoneme errors. |
| **WHAT?** | Clients with speech-sound disorders often produce variants of their error sounds. They may just use a range of phones, all of which are in error, or they may alternate between correct and incorrect productions. Some variations may be related to coarticulation with surrounding phonemes, while others may occur more often in particular word positions, while still others may occur only in connected speech. |
| **WHY?** | The goal is to determine the range of variation in production of particular phonemes. In particular, inconsistency with hits (where one of the variants is a correct production), may provide the SLP with a starting point for treatment. Inconsistency with hits may also have prognostic value. |

*(continues)*

> *(continued)*
>
> **WHEN?**    We usually assess inconsistency at the outset of intervention or as part of the diagnostic battery.
>
> **SUPPORT:**    One of the earliest ways to evaluate consistency was the McDonald Deep Test (McDonald, 1964). This test assessed contextual variation by systematically placing the target sound in a variety of phonetic contexts. Unfortunately, this test is now out of print, and it would be difficult for clinicians to try to duplicate its procedures and picture stimuli. Since that time, other instruments have been developed to assess consistency, for example the *Secord Contextual Articulation Tests* (*S-CAT*—Secord & Shine, 1997) and the *Contextual Test of Articulation* (Aase, Hovre, Krause, Schelfhout, Smith, & Carpenter, 2000).

## HOW TO ASSESS CONSISTENCY/INCONSISTENCY

### *Procedures*

1. To determine if the phoneme varies with the surrounding phonetic context, a phenomenon known as contextual variation, the SLP can review the results of formal testing and see if the phonetic context might influence the client's production. For example, an /s/ sound might be correctly produced in the /st-/ cluster, but not in the /sk-/ or /sp-/ cluster. The feature of the cluster that appears to make correct production possible is that the /s/ and the /t/ have the same place of articulation.

2. To determine if correct production occurs only in particular word positions, the SLP can again review the formal test data relating to production of the phoneme in syllable-initial, syllable-final, and clustered contexts.

3. To determine if correct productions are less likely to occur in connected speech than in careful speech or single-word speech, the SLP can record a three- to five-minute conversational sample, and note each production of the target phoneme. The percent correct obtained in this way can be compared to the percent correct for citation-form words. The location of any correct variants may also relate not only to length/complexity of utterance, but also to adjacent phonetic context or to position in the word, as noted in (1) and (2) above.

4. The clinician can also administer probes. Two commercially available sets of probes to assess inconsistency and contextual variation are the *Secord Contextual Articulation Tests* (*S-CAT*—Secord & Shine, 1997) and the *Contextual Test of Articulation* (Aase, Hovre, Krause, Schelfhout, Smith, & Carpenter, 2000).

5. The clinician can also construct *Sound Production Tasks* (*SPT*—Elbert, Shelton, & Arndt, 1967), which are probes that include the target sound in contexts from isolation to long sentences. A sample probe developed for /s/ is shown in Table 4-2. One of the virtues of the SPT is that the clinician can develop alternate forms and use the probes to gauge ongoing progress.

6. Assess the repeatability of the hits by trying to elicit them again in the same context.

**TABLE 4-2.** Sample Sound Production Task for /s/. This is one of many possible randomized arrangements that the clinician can devise. Novel items can also be used in these arrangements.

*Elbert, Shelton, and Arndt (1967).*

| | |
|---|---|
| 1. /us/ | 16. Class day |
| 2. Musty | 17. Please breathe softly. |
| 3. /sæ/ | 18. He has on a clean suit. |
| 4. Household | 19. Pass that |
| 5. Glass zoo | 20. Ice room |
| 6. I'm on your side. | 21. Will he be home soon? |
| 7. Placemat | 22. Husky |
| 8. Missing | 23. /is/ |
| 9. The dog sits up. | 24. Will you be up Sunday? |
| 10. House knife | 25. Asleep |
| 11. /s/ | 26. Who took his seat ? |
| 12. I will get some. | 27. I like soup. |
| 13. Bob sent me. | 28. The dress is all silk. |
| 14. /sɑ/ | 29. Icewater |
| 15. Busboy | 30. I lost my red socks. |

## Assessing Stimulability

We assess stimulability in school-age clients much as we do with younger clients. The hierarchy of cues developed by Perrine, Bain, and Olswang (2000) is just as relevant for school-age clients as for younger clients (see Section 2). Typically, therefore, we start with only an auditory model and if the child is not able to correct the sound with that cue, we add explicit visual information. If the client needs more assistance to produce a correct sound, we add phonetic placement instructions.

Stimulability is important to the treatment process because it is best if treatment begins with stimulable sounds. Otherwise the clinician needs to spend treatment time helping the child to become stimulable.

## Assessing Connected Speech—Intelligibility and Severity

Intelligibility is likely to be less of a problem for children with residual errors than it is for children who use phonological processes. Nevertheless, some estimate should be made of intelligibility, whether one depends on the Percentage of Intelligible Words or on one of the rating scales mentioned in Section 2.

The measure Percentage of Consonants Correct (Shriberg & Kwiatkowski, 1982a), the severity measure that was very useful with "phonological" children, is probably less useful for the population who have residual errors, unless a lot of different phonemes are in error. The Articulation Competency Index (Shriberg, 1993; see Procedure in Section 2) was developed for this population, and it can serve as both an initial measure of severity and as a measure of change. In fact, however, there is probably no single measure of severity that does justice to the child's speech pattern when it contains residual errors.

A substitute quantitative measure of severity that has considerable face validity would be the percentage of time that the client uses the error production in a connected speech sample. This kind of measure was proposed a number of years ago by Diedrich (1971), who called it the *TALK* measure. The child talks for three minutes about a topic of interest. The SLP tallies the number of correct and incorrect productions of the target sound and determines the percentage of the total that were in error.

---

## THE *TALK* PROCEDURE (Diedrich, 1971)

### Background

**WHO?**       School-age children and adults who are working on residual errors.

**WHAT?**      The *TALK* procedure is a standardized way of measuring accuracy of production of a specific phoneme or cognate pair in a quantitative way. It can contribute to estimates of severity and can also serve as a measure of change.

**WHY?**       The *TALK* is a measure of how frequently a target phoneme is in error in connected speech. Because the *TALK* is based on conversational speech, it can be administered much more frequently than other types of probes or measures.

**WHEN?**      The *TALK* can be administered at the beginning of intervention and also periodically throughout intervention.

**SUPPORT:**   The *TALK* was first published by Diedrich in 1971 and it has been used extensively since that time. As a measure taken from conversation, it has a great deal of face validity.

## THE *TALK* PROCEDURE (Diedrich, 1971)

### Procedure

1. The SLP engages the client in conversation, or he asks the client to deliver a monologue (e.g., "Tell me how you catch and mount butterflies"). The sample for the *TALK* includes three minutes of client speech. Clinician utterances and long pauses are not included in the three minutes. This sample is recorded on audiotape.

2. The clinician listens to the recording and tallies the number of times that the target phoneme was produced correctly and the number of times it was in error. He then calculates the percentage of the total number of productions that were in error.

3. The percent values from samples elicited during the course of treatment can be plotted on a graph and shared with the client.

4. The *TALK* procedure words best for phonemes that occur frequently in English such as /s z r/ and vocalic and post-vocalic /r/.

---

For estimating severity in the school-age child, we also need to consider the degree to which the speech pattern draws attention to its form rather than its content. We might call this factor "perceived deviance." The SLP can try to evaluate perceived deviance in an impressionistic way. For example, most lateral distortions of fricatives are quite loud (Stephens, Hoffman, & Daniloff, 1986), and they tend to rivet the attention of a person who is not used to the child's speaking pattern. In other words, distortions may actually interfere with the transmission of the child's message.

The perceived deviance factor no doubt interacts with the frequency of occurrence of the error, which in turn is related to the general frequency of occurrence of the phoneme in the spoken language. For example, /s/ is a relatively frequent consonant in English, and a lateral error on /s/ is likely to be quite distracting. On the other hand, a [b] for /v/ substitution will not be nearly so distracting because the /v/ is infrequent in spoken English.

There is yet another issue that relates to severity, and that is the child's reaction to his or her own speech. Some clients are oblivious to their speech sound errors, while others are acutely aware.

---

**CLINICAL NOTE 4-1:**
**Two Very Different Client Reactions to Their Own Speech-Sound Errors**

Two of the case presentations at the end of this book illustrate the two poles of the continuum between indifference and excessive reactivity to one's own speech. Jill, a child of age 9, who had many errors on /r/, chattered away with great abandon, oblivious to the fact of her errors, even when they caused people to misunderstand her. Sean, a boy of age 11, had unilateral errors on /ʃ tʃ dʒ/. He was so acutely aware of these errors that he knew exactly where they were about to occur, and he produced the syllables containing the offending phoneme much more softly than the surrounding syllables. Of course, one may inquire which of these two children had the more severe reaction to his or her own speech. On the one hand, the first child will have to be made aware of her errors. On the other hand, the second child's attempts to avoid making deviant sounds gave his speech a most peculiar quality.

---

We can get at both issues—to what extent the speech is perceived as deviant and to what extent the child reacts to the speech pattern—using checklists that we ask important persons in the child's environment to fill out. We also will be considering these issues as part of our case history and interviews. Finally, the SLP will want to make his or her own rating of severity of the acoustic and visual aspects of the child's error. Visual aspects of an error become important in certain cases (e.g., when the jaw slides strongly to one side during a unilateral distortion of /s z/).

## PROCEDURES TO EVALUATE SEVERITY:

### A Checklist of Responses to Client's Speech

**Background**

| | |
|---|---|
| **WHO?** | Administered to persons who are in contact with school-age children (and adults) whose speech is characterized by residual errors. Teachers and others in the school setting are likely to respond differently from family members, who may not notice distortions or substitutions at all. |
| **WHAT?** | A checklist related to the deviance of the error or errors, to be filled out by one or more listeners. |
| **WHY?** | The use of a checklist for the listener can provide good information about the child's functioning as a communicator. |
| **WHEN?** | Administered as part of an evaluation before the residual errors become targets of remediation. |
| **SUPPORT:** | There is no support in the literature for the use of this particular checklist. However, many authors have mentioned the effect that this checklist attempts to capture, namely that deviant speech can draw attention to itself and interfere with communication. |

## PROCEDURES TO EVALUATE SEVERITY:

### A Checklist of Responses to Client's Speech

#### Procedure

Administer Reproducible Form 9: A Checklist of Responses to a Client's Speech to the child's teachers, and/or parents, or others. This checklist asks about the respondent's own reactions to the child's speech, and about the child's response to his/her own speech. The SLP may be able to compare the responses from persons who see the child in different environments.

A summary of the various ways to assess severity in school-age children is shown in Table 4-3. Information from at least two of these sources should be obtained as part of the evaluation of clients in this age range. A number of the procedures can also apply to older teenagers and adults.

**TABLE 4-3.** Measures that relate to severity in school-age children (and adults). Each measure is described, followed by a comment.

*Percentage of Consonants Correct* (see Section 2)
*Comment:* Not useful if there are only a few residual errors.

*TALK* (Diedrich, 1971): Percent of total productions of the target phoneme that are in error when client talks about a topic of interest for three minutes.
*Comment:* Useful for residual errors *if* they occur relatively frequently in spoken English.

*(continues)*

**TABLE 4-3.** *(continued)*

*Checklist of Listener Responses to Client's Speech* (see Reproducible Form 9): Persons who are in regular contact with the client are asked to indicate their responses to the client's speaking pattern using a checklist.

*Comment:* Considerable face validity. Family members are likely to respond differently from others in the client's environment.

*Checklist of Listener's Impressions of the Client's Reaction to Own Speech* (see Reproducible Form 9): Same format as above.

*Comment:* Considerable face validity.

*Results of Interview with Client and Family:* Clinician notes responses to questions about the speaking pattern, family reactions to the speech difficulties, and reports of the client's reactions to the difficulties.

*Comment:* If the client and family are forthcoming about attitudes, this approach has considerable face validity.

*Clinician's rating of severity of auditory components and any visual components of the error pattern*

*Comment:* Has face validity.

## Related Variables: Speech-Sound Discrimination and Self-Evaluation

As always, we assess potentially related variables as part of the full evaluation of a child or adult with an articulation difficulty. For clients in these age groups, we will want to consider the oral mechanism, along with voice, fluency, rate, and cognitive-linguistic issues, all of which have been discussed in Section 2.

One additional variable to consider is the client's ability to perceive the error as different from the target sound, especially in his own speech. This type of perception is sometimes called "internal" discrimination. As we mentioned in Section 3 with reference to preschool children, perception of errors (also called speech-sound discrimination) is notoriously difficult to assess. However, with school-age and adult clients, perception becomes a critical issue, because usually the changes that need to be made are relatively subtle motorically, and they will need to be guided by the ear.

Sometimes the child can detect "his" error when someone else produces it. This is an obvious first step for the child, but it is insufficient by itself for change to occur. Although there has been research on children evaluating the sounds in their own tape-recorded speech, this research has not been so encouraging that we can recommend using it routinely. One reason is that children may not really think that they said what they hear. Furthermore, there are no formal testing procedures that involve a client evaluating his or her own productions. For these reasons, I recommend one assumption and two observational procedures as ways to approach the issue of error discrimination.

A reasonable assumption about speech-sound perception in the population under study is that if the client has been in treatment for the errors before and has made little progress over a period of perhaps six months, then it is likely (but not certain) that there are some perceptual difficulties. Little progress means that the client remains about as stimulable as at the time of the original evaluation, and that there has been no obvious increase in inconsistency with hits. Lack of progress can be an indicator of Developmental Verbal Dyspraxia (DVD; see

Section 8), also, but both DVD and inadequate error discrimination need to be considered in cases in which clients who are school age or older make little progress.

One observation we can make is of the client's self-evaluative responses to his or her own productions. That is, the clinician provides cues and/or a model, and the client produces a response and then evaluates the acceptability of the production. If the child has adequate internal discrimination, then we expect his judgments of acceptability to concur with the clinician's most of the time. If not, then perhaps the child has difficulty with internal perception.

A second observation we can make is about the client's self-awareness of the presence/location of errors. Sean, the 11-year-old boy mentioned in Clinical Note 4-1, was so aware of errors that it affected his prosody. Other children may give no sign at all that they are aware of their errors.

## Prognostic Variables

The earliest work on prognostic indicators was done with young school-age children who probably had residual errors. The focus of these studies was on stimulability and contextual variation and indirectly on consistency of production. These variables were discussed earlier in this section as methods for finding an entry point to the child's system. However, some of them also may have prognostic implications.

### Prognostic Variable: Stimulability

The early studies tended to show that if the child at ages 5-6 is not readily stimulable at the nonsense syllable level, then treatment is warranted. If readily stimulable, the child might improve without intervention. The latter finding needs to be applied with caution, however. A child of age 12 who is readily stimulable but makes errors on 100% of the target sounds in ongoing speech is not about to make any changes, because if she were going to change, she would have done so already. Even at younger ages, if the child is readily stimulable at Time 1 and has not made any changes by Time 2, say, six months later, it is arguable whether she is going to improve spontaneously.

### Prognostic Variable: Inconsistency

We sometimes think of inconsistency with hits, in which a few correct productions are heard, as being a positive prognostic indicator. To the extent that the occasional correct production provides a starting point for treatment, it is indeed a positive indicator. However, it is unclear that positive inconsistency is a valuable prognostic indicator for long-term improvement when the client is older than 8 or 9 years of age. Again, the argument is that if inconsistency with hits represents ongoing processes toward improvement, the client would have corrected most exemplars of the error phoneme(s) by this age.

---

**CLINICAL NOTE 4-2: Unfortunately, Inconsistency with Hits is Not Always a Positive Prognostic Indicator**

This argument was brought home to me in one of the first clinical failures I ever had. The client was a boy who was 8 years old when he was first evaluated. He used [θ] with substantial tongue protrusion for /s/ about 50% of the time and correctly

*(continues)*

*(continued)*

produced [s] about 50% of the time in conversational speech. When I re-evaluated his situation about three months later, nothing had changed, so he started in treatment. After almost a year of intervention, nothing had changed in the speech that he used outside the clinic room, although within the clinic space he was often 75-95% correct on /s/ for short periods of time. The same was true when I worked with him in the classroom and with some of his friends—he easily achieved 90% accuracy, but then when he turned to talk to other friends, he was back to 50%.

### Prognostic Variable: Potential Dyspraxic Elements (PDE)

As was the case with younger children, school-age children and adults can exhibit one or more dyspraxic elements. Children who have so many of these elements that most SLPs would consider them dyspraxic may have very slow rates of speech and may tend to give equal stress to every syllable. They may attempt multisyllabic words, but they have considerable difficulty producing them. Children who have just a few PDEs may show groping of the articulators when the clinician tries to elicit acceptable phoneme productions, or they may need large numbers of drills to make progress, or they may have a vowel error in addition to consonant errors. In any event, the prognosis is for slow rather than rapid change. Further exploration of Developmental Verbal Dyspraxia may be found in Section 8.

### Prognostic Variable: Speech-Sound Perception

As was mentioned earlier, it is important but sometimes difficult to estimate the child's ability to distinguish between his typical production and the target. Very likely most school-age children and adults can, in fact, distinguish the two types of sounds. However, when they have demonstrable difficulty, this fact indicates a poor prognosis.

### Prognostic Variable: Issues of Motivation and Responsibility

Sometimes children who have been in treatment for a while without a great deal of progress are said to be unmotivated. However, the client's lack of motivation may in fact be realistic. The experience of repeated failure can easily grind away positive feelings about treatment. Although the ideal therapeutic situation occurs when the client can take real responsibility for making progress, it is contrary to human nature to want to be responsible for repeated failure.

In addition, in some cases we find ourselves working with adolescents and teenagers. This is a time in life when children desperately want to fit in with their peers. They do not want to be known as working on their speech. They do not want to leave the classroom to do so. In these cases, the SLP must work hard to enlist the child's cooperation, motivation, and responsibility.

Needless to say, if the client is not intrinsically motivated to improve speech, and if the SLP is not able to establish a contract (whether implied or explicit) about their respective roles and expectations, this fact is a poor prognostic indicator. Sometimes it is better simply to tell the client that there is no point in continuing with treatment but that if he or she wants services at a later date, you will assist in obtaining them.

## INTERPRETATION OF ASSESSMENT RESULTS

When we review the results of our assessments in the many different areas of interest, we try to understand the present clinical picture. The diagnostic checklist (Reproducible Form 1) can help us organize the information. Looking at the whole picture, we try to determine the underlying basis for the speech-sound disorder in order to treat it most effectively. If we suspect that there is a motoric basis for the client's difficulties, then we will plan treatment in that direction. If there seems to be a perceptual component to the difficulty, then treatment will emphasize training perception as well as training production.

The prognostic indicators such as consistency, contextual variation, and stimulability can be helpful to the clinician when trying to enlist the client as an active participant. It is important to be realistic and explicit in these negotiations.

---

**CLINICAL NOTE 4-3: Which SLP is More Credible?**

SLP 1:  "Well, this course of treatment is likely to be a little longer than you might like. The reason is that your ear seems to be unclear about what the /s/ should sound like. We need to work on that first."

SLP 2:  "This shouldn't be too hard to change."

---

## ONGOING ASSESSMENT DURING INTERVENTION

In order to chart progress with a client who has residual errors, we can return to two of the instruments mentioned as part of the initial assessment. The *Sound Production Task* (Elbert, Shelton, & Arndt, 1967; see Procedure in this section on "How to Assess Consistency/ Inconsistency") is a good probe to use in the earlier stages of treatment.

The *TALK* procedure (Diedrich, 1971; see Procedure in this section on "The *TALK* Procedure"), in which the clinician records a three-minute speech sample and determines the percentage of acceptable productions, is more useful in the later stages of treatment when we want to promote carryover. In fact some of the *TALK* samples might be taken in environments other than the usual treatment space.

## ASSESSING THE SPEECH OF OLDER CHILDREN AND ADULTS

Most of the available commercial tests of articulation are not acceptable for use with teenagers or adults. The reason is that the pictures in these tests that the client is asked to name are chosen to be of high interest to young children. The *Templin-Darley Tests of Articulation* (Templin & Darley, 1969) have a sentence version for older children and adults in which two targets are elicited per sentence, for a total of 141 sentences. Unfortunately, many teenagers and adults find these sentences difficult to read because of the unusual vocabulary, for example, *burr*, and because the sentences take on a tongue-twister nature, for example, *They planted shrubs about the shrine*. These difficulties are compounded if the client speaks English as a second language.

For teenage and adult clients, it might be better to provide them with a phonetically balanced reading passage such as part of the "Rainbow Passage" (Fairbanks, 1960). The SLP can then use the transcription of that passage to fill out a Segmental Inventory.

## *EVALUATING SPEECH-SOUND PRODUCTION IN OLDER CHILDREN AND ADULTS*

### Background

WHO?    Older children and adults for whom an assessment of speech-sound production is needed.

WHAT?    Obtain and transcribe a connected-speech sample, preferably one that represents all of the phonemes of English. The sample can be taken from conversational speech, or it can be the reading of text.

WHY?    Tests of articulation intended for young children are not appropriate for these populations.

WHEN?    This procedure is typically done as part of an initial diagnostic assessment, but it can also be carried out to assess progress.

SUPPORT:    The transcription of a conversational speech sample has considerable face validity; however, it may not sample all of the phonemes of English, and it is time-consuming to transcribe. Having the client read the Rainbow Passage eliminates some of the problem because the Rainbow Passage is phonetically balanced.

## EVALUATING SPEECH-SOUND PRODUCTION IN OLDER CHILDREN AND ADULTS (USING THE RAINBOW PASSAGE)

### *Procedure*

The client is asked to read the client copy of the Rainbow Passage (Reproducible Form 10) out loud. The SLP makes an audio or video recording of this sample. Later on, using the clinician copy of the Rainbow Passage (Reproducible Form 11), which has the standard transcription written under the gloss, the SLP notes the productions that are in error. Based on this procedure, the SLP can look for systematic errors and other relevant phenomena. The Segmental Inventory Forms (Reproducible Form 6 for consonants, Reproducible Form 7 for word-initial clusters, and Reproducible Form 8 for vowels) can be used to aid in the description and analysis of errors.

Case Study 11 in Section 9 provides an example of use of the Rainbow Passage with subsequent analysis using the Segmental Inventory forms.

## MOTIVATION IN TEENAGERS AND ADULTS

An important issue for teenagers and adults with residual errors is that some of them have worked unsuccessfully on those errors in the past, and so they may approach remediation with particular caution. Motivation is a complex issue for them, and they often need detailed information about their difficulties, especially information that demystifies the process for them.

If the teenager or adult happens to speak English as a second language (ESL), motivation can also be an issue. Some ESL clients seek services because they have been told to do so by a teacher, mentor, or boss, while others are eager to assimilate and not stand out because of their speech. It is important to keep in mind that services to reduce accent or to improve intelligibility are elective in teenage and adult ESL speakers who usually show no signs of difficulty in learning the first language. Consequently, the clinician's reading of the level of motivation may play into the decision to recommend or not recommend intervention as an option. Of course, motivation will also play into the client's decision to pursue or not pursue SLP services. Additional information about services to ESL speakers may be found in Section 8.

## SUMMARY

At one time in the history of speech-language pathology, a very large part of a typical SLP's caseload in schools was made up of school-age children with "articulation" errors. Such clients still make up a large proportion of children seen for services. Unfortunately, because we sometimes wait a very long time before starting intervention with these children, their errors can become very well-learned. Adult clients, of course, have been practicing errors even longer. Consequently, the more that the SLP can learn about where and how the client can change her speech patterns during the initial evaluation, the more effective and efficient the intervention will be.

# MAXIMIZING OUTCOMES IN TREATMENT OF SPEECH SOUND DISORDERS

● ● ● ● ● ● ● ● ● ● ● ● ● ● ● ● ● ● ● ● ● ● ● ● ● ● ● ● ● ● ● ● ● ● ● ● ● ● ● ● ● ● ● ●

**S**peech-language pathologists are in the business of bringing about behavioral change in clients. In particular, when we deal with speech sound disorders, we help change speech motor behaviors and often the linguistic concepts that underlie them. However, in recent literature on speech sound disorders, very little has been written about the "technology" of this kind of treatment—that is, the moment-to-moment techniques and tools that we use. Used properly, this kind of technology is powerful.

The technology of speech-sound change is equally applicable to phonological disorders, motorically based disorders, and difficulties in acquiring a second language. There may be differences in the direction of treatment and even in the basic assumptions that underlie treatment; nevertheless, change in speaking behavior depends on effective use of these tools.

It is important to note that just because behavioral tools are used in intervention, this does not imply that natural language learning occurs as a result of using such tools. Children acquire natural languages in part because of neurophysiological capacity that supports language, in part because of language inputs, in part because of active hypothesis testing on their part, and in part because of social responses to their attempts at communication.  Classical behavioral principles can account for only a small part of language acquisition, primarily in the area of language use (pragmatics) rather than in language content or form. Certainly, there is little evidence that caretakers reinforce correct sound production directly.

The speech language pathologist uses behavioral methods and tools in cases where natural language acquisition has not accomplished, and probably will not accomplish, the goal of acceptable speech-sound production. These methods are also useful with adults who either wish to improve production in their first language, or with adults who want to be intelligible in a second language. Mowrer (1982), for example, has commented on the power of applying behavioral principles to relatively few responses to change speech behaviors that are extremely well practiced over a period of years.

## SOME GENERAL PRINCIPLES FOR INTERVENTION

What follows are some overarching principles for working on speech-sound change. When a client does not make progress, quite often one or more of these principles has been violated.

**General Principle #1:**    *If you reinforce productions that are not totally accurate,*
*inaccurate productions are what you will get.*

The classic example of violation of this principle occurs when a young child fails to blend a new initial consonant with the rest of the word. The child who substitutes glottal stops for oral consonants is working on, say, /p/ in initial position, where aspiration is required. The clinician models *pie* with exaggerated aspiration. The child says [pʰ//ʔaɪ]. What is the clinician to do? After all, the child said the aspirated [p]. And the clinician wants the child to experience success. So the clinician reinforces the production.

However, reinforcement is one of the most powerful of tools. By definition, reinforcement increases the probability that the behavior will occur more frequently. If the clinician reinforces this type of broken word, the child will continue to produce the broken-word response. Broken words are not understood by others, and probably even the child knows that they are not correct. Therefore, the broken-word response will need to be unlearned later.

Some SLPs might say something like this, "Good! I heard the 'p' sound, but you need to make the word smooth." This distinction is lost on most children. Rather, they hear the positive word "Good," and that serves as reinforcer for the broken-word production.

**General Principle #2:**    *The goal for conducting treatment in most cases is almost error-less*
*learning, with just enough mistakes that the client knows what* **not**
*to do.*

The concept of errorless learning is attributed to Skinner (1954), who defined it as production of a targeted response in 90% or more of trials. However, in our field, Diedrich and Bangert (1980) have studied treatment-outcome data, and they claim that correct response rates of as low as 70% can be tolerated.  The reason that 100% correct production is not the goal is that the client needs to make an occasional error because errors help her define the permissible range for the target production.

**General Principle #3:**    *Reinforce and count only the first production attempt in any one*
*trial, and in general, do not reinforce self-corrections.*

Because the goal of intervention is correct spontaneous production on the part of the client, it follows that we should reinforce the responses that come closest to that goal. Because of the rate at which conversational speech is produced, we usually do not get a second chance at a word. Therefore, only the first production after a model should be evaluated. Self-corrections should be ignored during drill exercises.

Rewarding self-corrections creates two other problems. First of all, there is the issue of differential reinforcement that occurs when the first attempt is in error but the self-correction is acceptable. Clients get confused over what is being reinforced and may not make the same distinctions that the clinician does. Second, when the client hears the positive reinforcement, she may get into a kind of learned superstitious behavior, such as "If I say it wrong and then fix it, my speech teacher really likes me." If the clinician does not insist that the production be acceptable on the child's first attempt, and if he rewards self-corrections, then the client will not achieve long-term goals quickly. Extensive self-correction is simply not practical in ordinary speaking situations.

**General Principle #4:** *Never ask a client to produce a response more than once in a given trial unless you are 100% certain that subsequent productions will be as accurate as the first one.*

Many SLPs think that the way to get a high number of responses in a session is to have the client repeat each response several times. However, we can argue that if models and cues are needed to elicit a correct response, then it is unreasonable to withdraw them for subsequent productions. Moreover, if the accuracy degenerates during subsequent productions, the clinician is in a quandary: Does he reinforce the accurate first response or provide negative feedback about subsequent ones? Will the client understand why the distinctions are being made, given that subsequent productions have wiped out the auditory trace of the first production?

**General Principle #5:** *How the SLP responds to an elicited production that is in error is important to the progress of treatment.*

There are two possible responses to error productions—ignoring them, or providing negative feedback. There is evidence that providing negative feedback is more effective than ignoring the response. Providing negative feedback is the topic of a procedure later in this chapter under the Establishment phase of intervention.

**General Principle #6:** *The SLP should provide feedback non-verbally in the early and middle stages of treatment.*

Most SLPs are aware that feedback must closely follow an elicited response in order for it to be effective. However, if the feedback has a spoken component—and it nearly always does—the effect of the feedback is to erase the auditory trace associated with the production. Thus, even if the immediate feedback is positive, the client is unable to create strong associations among the stored form of the intended production, the movements involved in her successful production, the auditory product of those movements, and the positive feedback. Although no research exists to support this point, it is likely that allowing the client to make these associations by inserting a period of silence after the elicited production would increase the rate of change in treatment.

The reason that the auditory trace is more important in the early and middle stages of treatment is this: Evidence from the motor learning and the speech motor control literatures suggests that internal kinesthetic and auditory feedback is important in the early stages of learning a task. Later on, as the client becomes more skilled at the movements required, immediate feedback becomes less and less important. The literature shows that highly skilled movements are also highly automated movements, meaning that little internal feedback is necessary.

**General Principle #7:**    *The client's focus with respect to intervention is an important variable.*

The term *focus* as used here refers to the capability-focus framework for treatment delineated by Kwiatkowski and Shriberg (1998). In this framework, *capability* captures the linguistic characteristics and the risk factors affecting the client's ability to learn, while *focus* deals with child-based factors such as ability to attend, recognition of need to change, and effort applied in learning. The value of attention to focus is that we recognize the need for the client's active involvement in the process. For example, Kwiatkowski and Shriberg suggest that for highly motivated children, only social reinforcement of responses is necessary. For less motivated (less focused) children, token systems, then tangible reinforcers, and eventually reinforcements for participation may be needed.

**General Principle #8:**    *The clinician controls the client's rate of correct responding.*

No doubt every SLP has learned that taking too big a step can result in complete failure for the client. For example, the child who has just been successful at producing initial [s] in words is probably not going to be able to produce the [s] in sentences containing those words. Intermediate steps are needed, and it is the clinician who provides them.

**General Principle #9:**    *Clients who appear unmotivated or lazy are usually clients who have had little success in treatment.*

This principle indicates that it is possible for a client to lose the focus on intervention that is mentioned above. When the SLP becomes aware that the client is having difficulty with motivation, it is time to examine three areas: appropriateness of the system of reinforcement, appropriateness of the current goals, and rates of correct responding from session to session. Of course, it is possible that variables outside the clinician's control, for example, family problems, are responsible for change in the client's attitude.

In these cases, there are times when the system of reinforcement needs to be made more concrete (cf., Bleile, 1995). Alternatively, the SLP should consider whether the reinforcer is truly reinforcing. Sometimes, however, the most important variable is lack of successful experiences in treatment.

It goes without saying that the word "lazy" applied to a client represents not a judgment on the client, but a judgment that therapy has become ineffective. Ineffective treatment is largely the clinician's responsibility. Clinical Note 5-1 also suggests that parents may need information on this point.

---

CLINICAL NOTE 5-1:
**Counseling Parents about the Process of Learning New Speech Sounds**

Sometimes parents claim that their child is "lazy" because he is not using his newly learned sounds at home. Parents need to be disabused of this idea. In the preschool and early school-age years, the child does not use the new sounds spontaneously because he literally cannot. Spontaneous use of sounds in words and connected speech is an impossible task for a child who is just at the point of saying the sounds under highly structured conditions. For older children, the task is still quite difficult, because they have had many years of practicing those sounds the "wrong" way.

---

**General Principle #10:**     *The distinction between training broad and training deep is an important one because different types of interventions are involved.*

As we noted in Section 1, the two types of speech sound training are based on different conceptualizations of the client's difficulties. Training broad refers to the type of treatment that is appropriate for children with phonological errors (i.e., relating to acquiring a system of phonology). An example of training broad would be the Cycles approach of Hodson and Paden (1991). In this approach, exemplars of a phonological process are taught for a short period of time. Then a different process is chosen. There is no attempt to achieve 100% correct production for any of these exemplars. These kinds of training-broad approaches are the topic of Section 6.

Training deep is appropriate for residual errors and also for work with adults in general, where we assume that the client already knows the phonological system and where motor learning principles are applicable. An example of training deep is the traditional or Van Riper approach (Van Riper, 1978) in which one or two phonemes are taught in isolation, in words, in sentences and finally in connected speech. Training-deep approaches are the topic of Section 7. Clinical Note 5-2 expands on the differences between training broad and training deep.

---

CLINICAL NOTE 5-2:
**Training Broad and Training Deep Are *Not* Interchangeable**

The reason that the distinction between training broad and training deep is important is that these two approaches probably are not interchangeable. These two treatments are designed for problems that are in theory different in fundamental ways.

Unfortunately, there is, so far as I know, no research on this issue. However, time and time again we have had referrals to our clinic of children age 5 or so who are very unintelligible. They have been in traditional ("training deep") treatment, but they have made slow progress with the one or two phonemes they have worked on, and there is little generalization to other phonemes. When we start the "training broad" type of intervention, we start to see changes in the whole system. In addition, we do this type of treatment in a paradigm that is more play than drill, and the parents say that their children respond to it better than to conventional treatment.

Therefore, it is highly likely that training deep is not appropriate for phonological errors because it is far too slow and does not bring about change in the whole system of phonology. At the same time, training broad is inappropriate for residual errors because the basis of the disorder is not a phonological process but a motoric difficulty. Further, training broad is too diffuse and does not really target the motor aspects of the patterns that are already ingrained.

---

**General Principle #11:**     *Effective treatment can occur in a play environment, particularly when training broad is the approach.*

For children whose problems can be considered phonological, intensive modeling is an important part of the treatment. Modeling can easily occur in naturalistic play settings, as Fey (1991) has indicated in his discussion of focused stimulation. Elicitation of responses can also be used in play contexts. A particular virtue of using play contexts is that the child's productions are used in a real-life context, much as they would be in a natural language-learning scenario.

**General Principle #12:**    *There are times in the speech-sound intervention process when we should focus on pragmatics (clear production) rather than correct production.*

It is very easy for both the SLP and the client to become completely focused on correctness. The clinician has a professional responsibility to help the client achieve the best possible production, and the client often becomes intent on whether a response was correct—that is, whether it warrants reinforcement. However, the real reason that the client is receiving intervention is that either the speech is poorly intelligible, or the speech calls attention to itself. Both of these are pragmatic issues because they affect the communicative interactions of the client with a wide variety of people. Clinical Note 5-3 shows how to provide feedback in pragmatic terms.

---

CLINICAL NOTE 5-3:  Maintaining a Focus on Pragmatics

The benefit of maintaining a focus on pragmatics (at least some of the time) is that we remind the client that the ultimate goal extends well beyond the intervention room. The SLP can remind the client of this focus through comments in the early stages of intervention and through discussion in the later stages. When the client is carrying over new sounds into connected speech, the focus might be on saying every word clearly rather than saying every target sound correctly. Below are some comments that a clinician might make.

- "Great! I can understand that word when you say it with a clear /s/."
- "Wow! You said that word just like your brother (friend, parent) says it."
- "If you keep that up, everyone will understand you all the time."
- "Let's show your Mom how clearly you can talk today."
- "How about saying this word as *clearly* as you can?"
- "I like the way you fixed that word to make it clearer." (Said in the early stages of carryover to connected speech and only occasionally—see General Principle #3.)

---

## THE STRUCTURE OF INTERVENTION

Most SLPs have internalized the structure associated with traditional types of intervention (training deep). This structure is described in depth in Bernthal and Bankson (1998). Treatment begins with production of the sound in isolation, in a nonsense syllable, or in a key word. This is the elicitation or establishment phase. Then the client produces the target sound in longer and more complex linguistic structures, a phase which is called generalization (also called transfer). Finally, conversational or connected speech is produced in a variety of situational contexts, and the client takes responsibility for its correctness. This is the maintenance phase. The first two phases, elicitation and generalization, are also relevant for training-broad approaches, and principles relating to these two phases are mentioned here.

## INTERVENTION: ELICITATION (ESTABLISHMENT) PHASE

### Background

| | |
|---|---|
| **WHO?** | A child who is just beginning to work on improving speech-sound production. |
| **WHAT?** | The SLP attempts to elicit the target sound(s) or phonological structures in one, or a few, simple structures such as nonsense syllables or single-syllable words. The goal is stable production of the target in at least one context. Stable production means that the client must easily be able to produce that context with the correct target again and again. |
| **WHY?** | Restricting the linguistic context presumably simplifies the motor speech task for the child. |
| **WHEN?** | This phase typically occurs early in the intervention for each new target, or set of targets, or phonological structure(s). |
| **SUPPORT:** | This structuring of intervention is outlined by Van Riper (1978), and it has withstood the test of time, despite little formal research showing that it is effective. Later versions incorporated behavioral principles, but the basic structure was left untouched. Phonological approaches do not use the terminology "elicitation phase," but there is typically an early phase in which the clinician uses the SLP bag of tricks to elicit the target phonological structure. |

## INTERVENTION: ELICITATION PHASE

### Procedure

The key elements of the elicitation phase appear to be the ones indicated here.

- **The importance of auditory input.** Although traditional treatment, as described by Van Riper (1978), always begins with auditory discrimination or ear training, most clinicians have gotten away from ear training when working with children who have residual errors. One reason is that most of these clients have no difficulty with discrimination. Another reason is a small amount of research suggesting that the kind of informal auditory training that goes on in production training, especially modeling on the part of the clinician, is more effective than direct ear training in producing changes in production.

   However, with phonological children, intense auditory exposure appears to be critical. In fact, Hodson and Paden (1991) pioneered the use of auditory bombardment as an integral part of the cycles treatment. During auditory bombardment, the child plays quietly at a table while listening to words containing the sound or structure targeted for intervention.

- **Use of concrete terminology.** The specificity of concrete language increases the probability that the client's subsequent response will be acceptable. Concrete language also helps clients remember the task from session to session. Finally, use of concrete language helps the SLP avoid telling the client what *not* to do—which is almost always a losing proposition because the client does not know what to do instead. Clinical Note 5-4 shows some alternate ways to express important concepts.

> CLINICAL NOTE 5-4: Ways to Use Concrete Terminology

| Too General | Appropriately Concrete |
| --- | --- |
| *Speech-related Behaviors* | |
| "Put your tongue behind your teeth." | "Put your tongue on that bumpy place behind your teeth." |
| "Say /r/, but don't round your lips." | "Flare your lips and say /r/." |
| "Put your mouth in position and say /f/." | "Bite your lip and blow out while you are still biting." |
| "Say *key* this way: (demonstrates)" | "Say *key* with lots of air and feel the air on the back of your hand." |
| *Non-speech Behaviors* | |
| "Please sit down." | "Please put your bottom on your chair and your feet on the floor." |
| "It's time to put away the toys now." | "It's time to park the truck in its garage (a piece of construction paper) and put the little people up on the shelf." |

- **Importance of models and cues.** During the elicitation phase of any kind of treatment, the models and cues that are provided by the clinician are critically important. The use of effective models and cues sets up circumstances for the client to be accurate and successful, and the lack of effective models and cues leads to a protracted period of elicitation, if not to outright failure. Here are some of my observations on this topic, with as yet no research to back them up:

  - In the early stages of elicitation, multiple models are helpful. I usually start with three models. Then, if the client does well, I reduce the number of models to two, and so on. The client must look at my face while I produce the models, but he must not attempt a production until I cue him.

  - When words are modeled several times in a row, the natural tendency is to use list-order intonation, such as *big big big,* said with upward-going inflection on the first two *big*s and downward-going inflection on the last one. However, a downward-going (utterance-final) inflection on each model seems to be important. When the clinician uses list-order intonation, it seems to make the child anticipate the last word rather than pay attention to the models.

  - Silence between the clinician's model and the child's attempt is important. I want the client to have the auditory image ringing in his ears when he attempts the production, and so I do not speak between the model and the response. Rather, I cue the response with a gesture.

  - Graphemes written on colored paper, articulator positions sketched on a card, and hand gestures representing specific characteristics of a phoneme may be helpful. Even preschoolers can use these effectively.

- **Scheduling models and cues.** The other part of using models and cues effectively is knowing how to schedule them. We should aim for the desired response to be stable at each level before we go to the next step. The most common clinical error is withdrawing models and cues too quickly, before the response is stable. As a practical matter, we might define stability as a high level of correct performance over two to three sessions. Clinical Note 5-5 illustrates this principle.

---

CLINICAL NOTE 5-5: **Maintaining the Model-and-Cue Sequence**

Suppose that the SLP's initial goal is to elicit 10 productions of /s/ in isolation in 12 trials. She starts with a phonetic cue and two models during each trial, with the response definition of a single accurate [s] production. She uses the whole sequence of cue and model for each of the first three trials. The client produces [s] correctly all three times. At this point, she may be tempted to drop the elaborate lead-up to each response. *She should not drop the cue-and-model sequence.* Instead, she should use the sequence until the client reaches the pre-set criteria for stability. If she drops the sequence, the client will likely be in error thereafter and will experience failure.

---

## ALTERNATIVE WAYS TO ELICIT STABLE PRODUCTIONS IN THE ESTABLISHMENT PHASE

### Background

| | |
|---|---|
| **WHO?** | Children who are not responding to a straightforward attempt to elicit the target sound in isolation or in a given word position. |
| **WHAT?** | This section includes suggestions for alternative ways to think about reaching the goal, which is acceptable production of the target speech sound that is stable in some context. |
| **WHY?** | Some children simply are not able to make use of the information that is available in "traditional" elicitation procedures. |
| **WHEN?** | These alternatives should be tried before the child experiences repeated failure and both client and clinician become discouraged. |
| **SUPPORT:** | Several books contain numerous suggestions for eliciting specific speech sounds. Among these are the "Procedures for Teaching Sounds" described in Bernthal and Bankson (1998), the "Facilitative Techniques" found in Bleile (1995), and the whole book by Secord (1981). |

## ALTERNATIVE WAYS TO ELICIT STABLE PRODUCTIONS IN THE ESTABLISHMENT PHASE

### Procedures

*Note: The specific case of smooth or linked production of initial voiceless stops will be used in this section as an example.*

1. Try some of the alternative elicitation procedures indicated in the books mentioned under SUPPORT above.

2. Use a visual image that can represent qualities of the sound you are trying to elicit. For example, to represent a linked production of an initial /k/ (actually /kV/) use a swooping motion of the hand, or any other image that works for the child. Another frequently used image is of cars in a train attached to the engine, not separated from it. Either colored blocks or a picture of a train might be used.

*Note: The techniques below depend on helping the child to generalize from another phoneme (#3) or from the same phoneme in a different word position (#4).*

3. Try another door (phoneme). Find other words with phonemes in the same class of phonemes as the target that have the qualities desired. Call attention to that quality, again using whatever imagery works for the child. In the case of the initial voiceless /k/, look for an initial /p/ or /t/ that is both aspirated and linked, and call attention to the smoothness and continuity of that transition. Then present stimuli alternately, such as /pa/, then /ka/, then /pa/ again, and so on. If no initial voiceless stop is correct, consider initial /h/. The /h/ is all aspiration without the complication of an oral articulation. In fact, if the child does not use initial /h/, then voiceless initial stops are probably not appropriate targets anyway.

4. Go around to the back gate (same phoneme in another word position). In the case of initial /k/, this means that we alter the goal so that the sequence in which we elicit the target sound is final position first, then intervocalic position. Children rarely break the word when producing a final obstruent, but if they do, it is relatively easy to deal with the problem through instruction and demonstration.

When the child is producing the final stop smoothly, go to intervocalic /k/. The intervocalic position shares features of both final and initial consonants. The vowel-to-consonant transitions into the consonant are like those in final position, while the consonant-to-vowel transitions to the second vowel are like the ones that occur in initial position. Again, the SLP repeatedly reinforces the smoothness of the productions. Finally, at this point, go back to initial position /k/, maintaining the emphasis on smoothness.

---

## *PROVIDING NEGATIVE FEEDBACK*

| | **Background** |
|---|---|
| **WHO?** | A child who is in any phase of intervention, although the most important effects are in the elicitation phase. |
| **WHAT?** | Negative feedback is a way to let the child know that her most recent attempt at the target sound was not acceptable. |
| **WHY?** | Negative feedback provides very important information to the client, especially in the early stages of intervention. Negative feedback tells the client to try something different. Negative feedback also helps the client determine the range of productions that are, or are not, considered to be within a phoneme category. |
| **WHEN?** | Like all feedback, negative feedback should immediately follow the child's attempt. |
| **SUPPORT:** | A study by Costello and Ferrer (1976) using a single-subject design showed that negative feedback in the form of "No" was more effective than ignoring the error. |

# PROVIDING NEGATIVE FEEDBACK
## *Procedures*

Giving negative feedback does not have to be devastating to the client. This is particularly true if the SLP is conscientiously planning the treatment so that the client is generally operating at a high rate of correct responding and the occasions for negative feedback are few.

1. Negative feedback can be given in a way that recognizes that the error is an aberration in the context of many correct responses. For example, the exclamation "Oops!" conveys that idea.

2. Negative feedback can be given in a playful way, such as "Nope!," or with a scrunched-up face or a thumbs down signal or even a buzzer.

3. Factual information about what to change in the next attempt can help keep the tone neutral or playful. For example, when eliciting /ʃ/ in a word from a young child, one can say, "Oops! Your tongue slipped," when the child produces [s] instead.

# IMPORTANT CONCEPTS FOR THE
# GENERALIZATION TRANSFER PHASE OF INTERVENTION

The generalization phase of intervention is a formal stage in traditional intervention for residual errors (training deep). During this phase the client learns to use the target phoneme correctly in a variety of phonetic contexts as well as in longer and more complex utterances. In other words, the client transfers this knowledge that was stabilized in the elicitation phase to many more contexts.

It might be noted that there is rarely any need for generalization or maintenance phases when training broad (Elbert, Dinnsen, Swartzlander, & Chin, 1990). Typically, the preschooler's system is so flexible and adaptable that when the child has stabilized production of the chosen exemplars of each phonological process, you very quickly start to hear these productions used spontaneously in other words and in connected speech. In fact, there is usually generalization to other phonemes affected by the targeted phonological process. Occasionally, however, a "phonological" child will require explicit generalization procedures.

## *INTERVENTION: GENERALIZATION PHASE*

|  | Background |
|---|---|
| **WHO?** | Most children with residual errors who produce a target phoneme with stability in only one context, as well as a few "phonological" children who have acquired a phonological target in just a few words and one task, such as picture naming. |
| **WHAT?** | The SLP helps the client maintain almost errorless production in longer or more complex utterances, typically in a series of small steps. |
| **WHY?** | Although most "phonological" children will not require carefully designed generalization procedures, most children with residual errors will require them, as these children are highly unlikely ever to use their new sound productively without explicit generalization training. |

*(continues)*

*(continued)*

**WHEN?** Generalization procedures are used in the early-to-middle parts of the intervention sequence.

**SUPPORT:** Although explicit research support for this phase of intervention is lacking, the generalization phase carries the weight of a long and largely successful tradition that goes back to Charles Van Riper (1978).

## INTERVENTION: GENERALIZATION PHASE

### *Procedures*

The procedures used in the generalization phase of traditional intervention are well known to virtually all SLPs. If the target phoneme was stabilized in isolation at the end of the elicitation phase, then the next step is to produce the phoneme in nonsense monosyllables, then in monosyllables that are real words, then in phrases, sentences and connected speech. Specific principles follow.

1. **We use "scaffolding" to help the child maintain almost errorless production.** Scaffolding is a term used in language intervention (e.g., Paul, 2001) with children who are challenged by the reading of text. That is, the clinician gives the child a lot of information about the contents of the text before the child even approaches the text, which helps the child deal with the print information.

   In treating residual speech-sound errors, we also use scaffolding, but we do it by manipulating models and cues, manipulating the phonetic context, and so on. What we are really doing is asking the child to generalize from something she can do to something she cannot yet do. Taking steps in small increments seems to help most clients accomplish this task relatively easily. Table 5-1 shows some of the variables we can manipulate.

**TABLE 5-1.** Variables that the SLP can manipulate during the generalization phase of intervention.

| Variable | Easier | More difficult |
|---|---|---|
| Position in words | Fricatives, /k/: final<br>All others: initial | Fricatives, /k/: initial<br>All others: final |
| Phonetic context | Maximum coarticulation, facilitating context | Minimal coarticulation, non-facilitating context |
| Length of words | Monosyllablic | Multisyllabic |
| Complexity of words | CVC, VC, CV | Consonant clusters; unstressed syllables in words |
| Position of sound in utterance | Either end | Middle |

| Variable | Easier | More difficult |
|---|---|---|
| Length of utterance | One word | Sentence |
| Presence of other error sounds | Not present | Present |
| Stress on syllable | Syllable containing phoneme is stressed | Syllable containing phoneme is not stressed |
| Communicativeness | Low content; cued generation of speech | High content; spontaneous generation of speech |

2. **Another type of variable we can manipulate is the reinforcement schedule.** Most of us know that 100% reinforcement of correct responses leads to quick acquisition, but we also know that the new behavior can quickly be lost (extinguished). In addition, we know that intermittent reinforcement stabilizes the response so that it does not extinguish, at least in pigeons.

   In practice, it is very difficult to reduce reinforcement schedules and give only intermittent reinforcement, particularly social reinforcement. Human beings are not pigeons, and so clients know when they are getting less of something than they used to get. They may think that they have done something wrong, when in fact, they are improving. Clinicians are sensitive to this issue, and they do not want clients to go without social reinforcement. Clinical Note 5-6 suggests ways to deal with this issue.

---

CLINICAL NOTE 5-6: How to Reduce the Frequency of
Reinforcement to Improve Generalization of Speech-Sound Production—
Without Making the Child or the Clinician Unhappy

Sloane, Johnston, and Harris (1968) suggest that the SLP use tangible reinforcers. Then, when a reduction in frequency of reinforcement is needed, the SLP reduces the frequency of the tangible reinforcer but maintains social reinforcement at 100% for correct responses. This suggestion would be appropriate only for fairly young clients.

With older clients we can, and should, shift some of the evaluation tasks to the client as we go through the generalization phase. This procedure maintains client interest even as clinician feedback (and reinforcement) is being reduced.

---

3. **Client self-evaluation promotes learning of new speech sounds.** A number of writers have commented on the importance of the client assuming some of the duties of the clinician as they together work through the generalization portion of intervention. Having the client evaluate his own productions can be a powerful way to encourage acquisition of the new behavior. As indicated previously, my view is that this should be carried out in a silent way so as not to interfere with the memory trace—after all, that is what the client has to evaluate. For example, a sequence might go like this (target is /r/):

   Clinician:  Right. (Model)
   Client: Right.

Client gives thumbs-up to indicate that production was correct.

Clinician gives thumbs-up or thumbs-down, depending on her evaluation.

---

## ISSUES IN ACQUIRING NEW MOTOR SPEECH SKILLS

Teaching new motor skills is one of the most important goals of training-deep programs, which are appropriate for clients who have residual errors. However, a large number of preschoolers with phonological problems also appear to have at least mild motor difficulties. Consequently, it is important to know how to maximize the acquisition of these speech motor skills.

---

## *TEACHING NEW SPEECH MOTOR SKILLS*

| Background | |
|---|---|
| **WHO?** | Children with residual errors, as well as children with phonological problems who appear to have concomitant speech motor difficulties. |
| **WHAT?** | The SLP uses principles of motor learning to help the child make the correct movements to produce the target speech sounds. |
| **WHY?** | Use of these principles helps the client eventually to produce these speech sounds as skilled, highly automatic movements. |
| **WHEN?** | These principles are typically used throughout the establishment and generalization phases of intervention. |
| **SUPPORT:** | These principles are taken from Van Riper (1978) and also from the motor control literature, for example, Schmidt and Lee (1999). There is, however, no experimental literature that attests to the effectiveness of any one of these principles in teaching speech sounds. |

## TEACHING NEW SPEECH MOTOR SKILLS

### *Procedures*

Some important aspects of teaching motor skills have already been mentioned in this chapter. They include:

- **Almost error-less learning.** The best way to achieve this goal is to redefine it as "maintaining a high rate of correct responding."

- **Immediate feedback.** Ideally, the child should get feedback, preferably non-verbal, before the SLP even tallies the production.

In addition, the motor learning literature suggests that certain other techniques might improve acquisition of speech motor patterns. Among these are:

- **Maintaining a high overall rate of responding.** A high rate of responding is beneficial because it gives the client many opportunities to respond and to receive feedback. That is, high rates of response help motor patterns to become ingrained.

- **Providing multiple short practice sessions as opposed to fewer long sessions.** Multiple short practice sessions can be provided by using the beginning and end of the scheduled session for these motor drills and using the intervening time for other types of activities.
- **Planning for speech-sound speed drills.** Speech-sound speed drills help the client automatize the correct response. It is hardly likely that the child will carry over into connected speech a phoneme that is always produced in a slow and exaggerated manner in single words, or even in phrases. Natural speech is produced at a very fast clip, and the new sound has to fit easily into that stream, or it simply will not be used. The task for the client is to produce these sequences *as fast as possible without sacrificing accuracy.* These drills can be arranged in a hierarchical way, as in these examples with targeted [s]:

| *Number of Variables* | *Sequence* |
| --- | --- |
| Monosyllable, initial position, one vowel | [sa]: [sasasasasasasas…] |
| Same, vary the vowel, one vowel per sequence | [si]: [sisisisisisisisis…] |
| | [so], etc. |
| Monosyllable, final position, one vowel | [es]: [eseseseseseses…] |
| Same, vary the vowel, one vowel per sequence | [us]: [ususususususus…], etc. |
| Disyllable, trochaic, same consonant, same vowel | [sasa]: "SAHsaSAHsa…," etc. |
| Disyllable, trochaic, same consonant, two different vowels | [sasi]: "SAHsiSAHsi…," etc. |
| Disyllable, trochaic, two different consonants, one vowel | [saka]: "SAHkaSAHka…," etc. |
| Disyllable, trochaic, two different consonants, two different vowels | [sifa]: "SIHfaSIHfa…," etc. |
| Disyllable, iambic, one consonant, one vowel | [sasa]: "saSAHsaSAH…," etc. |
| And so forth… | |

## THE ROLE OF PARENTS (AND OTHERS) IN INTERVENTION FOR SPEECH-SOUND DISORDERS

A number of authors have advocated that parents be involved in intervention programs for their children. This idea is appealing because parents may spend more time with the child than anyone else, especially at the preschool level, and because parents may spread the effects of direction intervention. Some have even claimed that parents can be the primary interventionists.

Most of the research on parental involvement has been in the area of physically handicapping conditions or of language development with preschoolers. Several studies have produced positive results, but a few very large-scale studies have not. With one exception, there has been little controlled research in the specific area of speech sound disorders, with parents assuming part of the responsibility for the intervention. The exception is Broen and Westman (1990), who used a highly structured preschool speech program that was successful in incorporating parents.

It is reasonable to think that parents might be more effective with speech sound disorders in preschoolers than in school-age children. One reason is that the nature of the child's errors is likely to be quite different. At the preschool level, the child typically makes errors that everyone recognizes, such as deletion of sounds and obvious substitutions, such as [w] for /l/. Older children are more likely to use fairly subtle distortions, and while listeners know that something seems wrong, they are not sure what it is. Another reason to think that parents may work more effectively with preschoolers is that the nature of the intervention with preschoolers is often different—that is, more language-based.

Parents can be very effective when they are asked to do the following kinds of interventions with their children:

- **Model, expand, and expatiate on what their child says.** Modeling can be helpful for stimulating language and for facilitating fluency. Expanding a word that the child mis-produces can also be useful for parents to do. Furthermore, these types of responses come naturally to many parents.

- **Set aside time for communication.** This is one of the most helpful, most natural things that parents can do. Most interventions go better when the child knows that her communication is valued at home.

- **Provide auditory bombardment.** This is an ideal activity, because the child is not producing the words, and the parent is not evaluating productions.

- **Provide production practice for the generalization of new speech behaviors that are already at a high level of correct production in the clinic.** For school-age children, this assistance can be helpful, even if the child is to monitor her own productions.

Parents are probably most effective in highly structured programs, such as that carried out by Broen and Westman (1990). It is also important that the parents have a great deal of contact with the SLP.

Parents may need some special qualities, also. Certainly, if they are asked to monitor and evaluate correct productions, they must be able to discriminate those productions; unfortunately, anyone who has ever taught phonetics to college students knows that adult learners do not necessarily learn this skill easily. The parent must also have good relationship with the child and be willing to do the work. The parent needs to know the difference between encouraging and nagging. Nevertheless, given a motivated parent who hears speech sounds accurately, intervention with parental assistance can be very effective.

## SUMMARY

The challenge to speech-language pathologists is to accomplish the most in the least amount of time for the client. This is not the kind of challenge that is issued by third-party payers. Rather, this challenge seeks to make the child a fully effective communicator as early in life as possible. To do this, we need to make appropriate choices of type of intervention, and we need to pay attention to the structure and moment-to-moment interactions of our intervention sessions.

# SECTION

6

# INTERVENTION FOR EARLY SCHOOL-AGE CHILDREN WITH PHONOLOGICAL DISORDERS

•••••••••••••••••••••••••••••••••••

**T**he speech-language pathologist who works with school-age children finds that a large proportion of the caseload is children who have speech-sound disorders, with or without language or other difficulties. This SLP also knows that these children vary considerably in the nature and the severity of their speech-sound problems. One child might be age 9 and have lateral distortions of alveolar and palatal fricatives and affricates. Another child may be 5½ or 6 years old and quite unintelligible.

The focus of this chapter is on those children in kindergarten and the early grades for whom intelligibility is a major concern. These children should have a very high priority for treatment for several reasons. First of all, the probability that they will improve substantially if they go another year without service is quite small. Second, there is increasing evidence that children who are still unintelligible at the age of about 5½ are at greater risk of early reading problems than are other children (see Hodson, 1998, for a brief review of this literature). Finally, children who are poorly intelligible may not have typical social relationships with other children (Hadley & Rice, 1991; Rice, Sell, & Hadley, 1991), and as a result, they may not be included in typical learning experiences either. Clinical Note 6-1 reports an example of such a child.

---

**CLINICAL NOTE 6-1: Karen's Atypical Social Interactions**

Karen came to our university speech and hearing center at the age of 6, just before she started school. Her speech was poorly intelligible, and she presented with language learning difficulties as well. She was very talkative, but she was oblivious to the fact that people other than family usually did not understand her. She had never had treatment before. After she had been in school for a month, we did an observation in Karen's class. We found that in her fairly boisterous kindergarten class, with a variety of workstations and peer groups, in a two-hour period no child ever spoke to Karen unless she spoke first, even when she was in an assigned activity group. If she said anything to a fellow student, that child would respond minimally (often only a grunt) and then go back to whatever he was doing.

We also observed Karen on the playground. It was immediately clear that no one was willing either to play with her or include her in a game, with one exception. The exception was a child the same age who had just come from another country and knew little English. Karen and this child played on the swings together and then played over in a corner of the playground by themselves. Here indeed was the perfect companion for Karen—a child with whom little or no oral communication was possible!

Because of Karen's concomitant language problems, we cannot say that her poorly intelligible speech was responsible for her social isolation. Nevertheless, that factor undoubtedly played a large role.

---

## ORIENTATION TO TREATING CHILDREN WHO ARE POORLY INTELLIGIBLE

The most important understanding is that children who are poorly intelligible almost always use a variety of phonological processes, and therefore it is necessary to "train broad." In fact, if we use the traditional one-phoneme-at-a-time approach ("training deep"), we will likely to make the problem worse, because with this population, training deep takes far too long, and the child is still working on being understood years later (Hodson, 1998; Klein, 1996). Training-broad approaches are considered to be cognitive and linguistic in nature because the child learns about the sound system of her language, rather than simply learning a new motor pattern (Bernthal and Bankson, 1998). I encourage the SLP interested in serving children with phonological disorders and who wants an in-depth look at these children read a companion volume in this *Resource Guide* series, *Speech Disorders: Resource Guide for Preschool Children* by Lynn Williams, 2003, which is focused on disorders of phonology.

### Auditory Conceptual Training

A key part of training broad is that the child requires auditory conceptual training. In the Hodson and Paden (1991) Cycles treatment, this auditory component is called **auditory bombardment**. For example, if the child omits final consonants, and the target phonological structure is therefore (C)VC words, auditory bombardment might include these 10 words: *one*, *kick*, *race*, *itch*, *cup*, *tub*, *hive*, *wash*, *ride*, and *path*. All the child has to do is listen, although I often engage the child's attention by asking that he point to a picture as I name it. Auditory bombardment seems to help the child figure out that the underlying representations of these words must contain final consonants and to notice the nature of those final consonants. In the Cycles program, the child hears the words amplified through an auditory trainer, but it is not clear that this is necessary. Nevertheless, Hodson and Paden's development of this form of auditory input was revolutionary.

In Cycles treatment, the child is "bombarded" with these spoken lists of words at the beginning and end of each session. In addition to auditory bombardment during the session, I often pretreat children by having their parents provide auditory bombardment at home for several weeks in advance of any production work on a designated structure or phoneme. In other words, I use auditory bombardment to "soften up" the child's system in a specific area. Specifically, I have seen several children go from not stimulable to stimulable using preparatory auditory bombardment. I should caution that this use of auditory bombardment lacks research support at present (as does its use in Cycles treatment), but it is consistent with phonological theory.

Another, more traditional, way to provide auditory conceptualization training is to use minimal pairs where the contrast involves the target phonological structure. These can be used for both perception and production. When they are used for perceptual training, the clinician typically asks the child to pick up or to point to the picture that she names. Very often, the clinician will use pairs of words in which the target phonemes differ in only one or two features, as in the contrast *bite/bike*. However, several authors, most recently Gierut (1989), have suggested that the clinician start with phoneme contrasts that differ in many features ("maximal opposition") and then move gradually to pairs that differ minimally.

In my view, minimal pairs should be used for production training with caution. The reason is that after many exposures to the minimal pair, the differences in production may begin to seem arbitrary rather than meaningful to children. If the accuracy of production of minimal pairs hovers between 40% and 70% or so, the child may be confused in this way. The best practice is to use the same few minimal pairs for just a few minutes periodically during the session, then switch to a different set.

## Intermittent Treatment

Another revolutionary concept from Cycles treatment (Hodson & Paden, 1991) is that a phonological target need not be completely corrected before moving on to another target. In fact, in Cycles treatment, the clinician may spend an arbitrary length of time, say three weeks, on one or two phonological processes and then move on to different processes. Later on, the clinician comes back to the original targets, re-evaluates, and provides additional treatment if it is needed.

The implication of the Cycles schedule is that for young children, the first go-round alerts the child to a particular aspect of her native language, and after that initial exposure, she may continue to refine the change on her own. This "Aha!" experience is certainly not explicit, as in "Oh, I need to put a consonant at the end of some words." Rather, the structure comes to the child's attention in the way that other phonological structures did when the child was younger, that is, through repeated exposure in meaningful utterances.

## Client Characteristics

The foregoing information makes clear that the child plays a rather active role in figuring out what is needed in his language. The child has to see patterns, must recognize where he needs to make changes, and then must generalize those changes from treated exemplars to untreated exemplars. These capacities all have a heavy cognitive component. It follows, therefore, that a child probably needs to be within the normal range of cognitive function in order to benefit from these cognitive-linguistic treatments.

One caveat is that just because a child is within normal limits cognitively, there is no guarantee that the child will make rapid progress in phonological treatment. In particular, children who have potential dyspraxic elements (PDE) are likely to progress more slowly than others despite adequate cognitive capacity. These children are discussed extensively in Section 8.

## The Words Used as Stimuli when Training Broad

One of the characteristics of phonological intervention (training broad) is that there is *no* role for nonsense syllables or nonsense words. Rather, all intervention is done in terms of real words that the child knows or that can be explained to the child. The reason for this difference from traditional treatment is a powerful assumption, namely that this child does not use particular phonological structures or phonemes because she does not realize that they make a difference in meaning. We need always to remember that phonological intervention is more about discovery than it is about training.

The words used as stimuli when training broad are even more important than the words that we use when treating residual errors. They are important because we empower the child to make changes by making change possible, and we do this by careful selection of words for their phonological content. For example, a child who has few final consonants may have an easier time saying consonants in final position if he starts with the ones that he uses in initial position. If he says only nasals and some stops in initial position, those sounds should be the first final position targets.

We have more choices when it comes to words that are to be used solely for auditory perception training. In auditory bombardment, for example, Hodson and Paden (1991) say that because the child only listens to these words, we can use words that we would not want to use in production training. Consequently, the child mentioned above who uses only nasals and some stops in initial position could listen to many sounds in final position besides stops and nasals.

If we are using minimal pairs for perceptual training, we also have a wider choice of words than if we are using them for production training. This is good because the need to come up with picturable minimal pairs greatly limits our choice of words for production training. For the child with just a few final consonants mentioned above, we can perhaps use *bee/bean* and *hoe/home* in production training, but for perceptual training we can also use *hi/hive* and *bee/beach*.

## WORD CHOICE IN PHONOLOGICAL INTERVENTION

### Background

**WHO?**    Children of kindergarten or early school-age whose speech difficulties are phonological in nature. Often these children are quite unintelligible.

**WHAT?**    Choosing words for production practice so as to achieve maximum effectiveness in the early intervention efforts. In particular, *the words chosen should be fully correct, and therefore fully intelligible, when the child corrects the target structure.* At the same time, there are some targets that should be avoided.

*(continues)*

*(continued)*

**WHY?**  The choice of words can help or hinder the child in improving accuracy of production.

**WHEN?**  Throughout phonological treatment, but especially in the early phases.

**SUPPORT:**  As yet, there is no research support for this position. However, most children with intelligibility problems use very few words that conform completely to adult standards, and they know it. That is probably the reason that many unintelligible children are reluctant to repeat words, or even to repeat what they just said. Therefore, when they do correct the target phoneme, and when they are reinforced for saying the word so clearly that everyone will understand it, this is highly motivating and highly reinforcing to the child.

## WORD CHOICE IN PHONOLOGICAL INTERVENTION

### *Procedure*

The child with intelligibility problems very likely produces few sounds correctly. So the SLP lists the phonemes that the child does use, along with the word position in which the child uses it. Then she takes the correct phonemes and makes words with the same sounds in other positions.

Suppose, for example, that the child uses /w m b p d f/ in initial position and nowhere else, and no other consonants. If we wish to target the process of final consonant deletion, then suitable words for the first production attempts would be:

| | | | | |
|---|---|---|---|---|
| *whip* | *dome* | *puff* | *Mom* | *deaf* |
| *wipe* | *dam* | *poof!* | *map* | *pop!* |
| *mop* | *dim* | *top* | *buff* | *dip* |

Observations about these words:

- **You may notice that none of these words ends in /b/ or /d/.** That is because I agree with Hodson and Paden (1991) that voiced obstruents should never be targets in final position of words. The reason is that the child is likely to overemphasize the final consonant, producing a schwa in the process: *bad* [bædə] or *have* [hævə]. Adding a schwa is the equivalent of adding a syllable, and adding a syllable tends to make words unintelligible, putting the child right back where she was, intelligibility-wise. It is far better to target final voiced obstruents in intervocalic position, such as *buddy* [bʌdi] or *heavy* [hɛvi]. Then, if the child exaggerates the target consonant, she will still learn how to make vowel-to-final-consonant transitions, but without creating a poorly intelligible word. Once children have learned to produce final voiceless obstruents in some words and voiced obstruents in intervocalic position, they usually start using final voiced obstruents spontaneously and correctly, without added schwa.

- **You may also notice that some of these words would not be common in the vocabularies of young children.** However, all of them are explainable (*Mom, deaf, dim*), picturable (*whip, mop, map*), or demonstrable (*buff, dip, poof!, pop!*). Moreover, children are likely to have heard them, even if they don't use them. When starting treatment with a poorly intelligible child, the issue of whether the child can successfully say the word trumps all other considerations such as word familiarity, word frequency, and word relevance. The ability to reinforce a child early for a production that is fully intelligible is worth violating all of these principles, as Clinical Note 6-2 indicates. It gives hope when the child has learned mostly failure. A first intelligible word is also important for parents, who are often discouraged about whether their child will be able to improve.

---

### CLINICAL NOTE 6-2:  Billy's First Intelligible New Word

Billy was the child who first taught me the importance of achieving a fully intelligible word early in treatment. He was exactly 5 years old when he came to the university speech and hearing center. He was about to start kindergarten, and he appeared to be bright, inquisitive, and eager to learn. In fact, his receptive language was excellent. He was also about 100% unintelligible. He used six or seven vowels, but only three consonants: [m w b]. These consonants were all used in initial position. We heard only one other consonant in any other position, and that was in the production [ɛm], which was Billy's version of the word *yes!* (This utterance was accompanied by vigorous head nodding.)

Billy had a rich gesture system, and he was very good at conveying meaning with gestures and onomatopoetic sounds, such as car noises and whooshing sounds. Most SLPs would consider him to exhibit Developmental Verbal Dyspraxia, as did we.

Unfortunately, Billy was not readily stimulable for any other early-developing consonants. So we embarked on a systematic search for stimulable consonants in any word position. We developed a list of CV words and presented them with intensive modeling, along with pictures or explanations. Nothing. We developed a list of VC words and presented them with intensive modeling. Again nothing. Finally, we made up wordlists of the form CVCV where the first consonant was in his repertory ([m b w]) and the second was any consonant, so long as it made a word. This gave us words like *muddy*, *baby*, *water* (the /r/ did not need to be correct*), and *waffle* (the /l/ did not have to be correct*). We presented these words and pictures to Billy, providing three models before he attempted the word. The word *movie* in this list did the trick—Billy said the whole word correctly! Billy knew as soon as he said *movie* that he had done a remarkable thing because first he looked very surprised, and then he smiled broadly. He was highly reinforced by the clinician as well. The clinician stopped presenting the list and made sure that Billy could say *movie* again and again. He went home with instructions to show his family how he could now say *movie*. For Billy, this event was clearly a turning point. In subsequent sessions, he became more readily stimulable for some of the CV, VC, and CVCV words and structures for which he had not been stimulable before.

---

* **We were willing to accept vowels for syllabic /l/ and syllabic /r/ because many children Billy's age pronounce them that way.** In addition, vocalization of liquids is one of the few phonological processes that does not damage intelligibility very much. That is, most adults will understand the child who says *candle* as [kændo] or *butter* as [bʌdɔ].

# DETERMINING GOALS AND OBJECTIVES

Setting goals and objectives for the poorly intelligible child is very different from setting goals and objectives for children with residual errors. For the poorly intelligible child, we target intelligibility and overall accuracy of production rather than absolute correctness of individual speech sounds. We achieve this goal by using patterns of production, usually phonological processes, as the targets of intervention.

---

## DETERMINING GOALS AND OBJECTIVES FOR PHONOLOGICAL INTERVENTION

### Background

**WHO?**  The poorly intelligible child, who is usually the child who uses many phonological processes.

**WHAT?**  Choose long-term goals and short-term objectives for intervention that will maximize effects on intelligibility.

**WHY?**  Traditional treatment, with its focus on correct production of individual sounds, does not produce rapid changes in intelligibility. The theoretical basis of traditional treatment is that the problem is basically one of motor difficulty. Although "phonological" children may have minor difficulty with motor sequences, the underlying problem is conceptual: The child has not learned key features of the phonology of his/her language—for example, that the language has consonant clusters.

**WHEN?**  Intervention should begin as soon as the child is identified as being outside of normal limits or as a child whom few people understand. This child is at risk for later reading difficulties as well as social difficulties, and it is imperative that the child become intelligible as soon as possible.

**SUPPORT:**  There is now a large literature on the effectiveness of phonological intervention for bringing about relatively rapid change in intelligibility. Similarly, there is a substantial literature on the risks associated with poor intelligibility.

## DETERMINING GOALS AND OBJECTIVES FOR PHONOLOGICAL INTERVENTION

### Procedures

I. Long-Term Goals

Long-term goals for phonological intervention target either overall intelligibility of conversational speech or the overall accuracy of speech sound production. Sample long-term goals might be:

- "Elly will increase the percentage of intelligible words in conversational speech from 60% to 75%, the percentage to be determined from a sample of her conversational speech which is at least 100 unduplicated words in length, and which is transcribed by a listener unfamiliar with Elly who is allowed to listen only once. The number of intelligible words is taken as a percentage of the total number of words."

- "Elly will increase her Percentage of Consonants Correct (Shriberg & Kwiatkowski, 1982) from 52% to 70%, the percentage to be determined from a sample of her conversational speech which is at least 100 unduplicated words in length, and which is transcribed by the clinician. The PCC represents the number of correctly produced consonants taken as a percentage of the total number of consonants."

II. Initial Short-Term Objectives

To determine initial treatment objectives, we may start by examining the phonetic inventory and the syllable-and-word shape inventory. Where we begin depends on the answer to questions such as these:

- Are there gaps that ought to have been filled by this child's age? Does the child use at least one stop, one nasal, one glide, and one fricative in word-initial position? If the answer to this question is "Yes," then we can ask if the number of stops, nasals, glides, and fricatives needs to be augmented. Sample short-term goals might be:

  - "Elly will spontaneously produce at least one fricative in four to five meaningful CV words in response to a picture or a cue." Note that which fricative is taught depends in part on stimulability. Note also that if [f] is chosen, English does not have four to five /fV/ words that children can reasonably be expected to know. In that case the SLP can either attempt to teach [s] (*see*, *say*, *sew*, *Sue*, and *saw*) or can use the giant's incantation from the story "Jack and the Beanstalk": "Fee, fie, foe, fum," with the clinician saying the "fum" if the child cannot manage it.

  - "Elly will spontaneously produce two stops at different places of production in four to five meaningful CV words in response to a picture or a cue." Note that if a velar stop is not readily stimulable, it may be better to wait and elicit a velar stop later in final position. Typically developing children appear to learn a velar stop, usually the voiceless cognate, in word-final position before word-initial position.

- How complex are the child's syllables? Does she use CV, CVCV, and VC? If one or more of these structures is missing, then sample short-term objectives might be:

  - "Elly will spontaneously produce four to five VC words in response to a picture or a cue. The final C in these words will be ones that Elly has in initial position, where possible."

  - "Elly will spontaneously produce four to five CVCV words in response to a picture or a cue." Note that if Elly does not already produce words that have reduplication of the consonant, such as *Mama*, *Daddy*, and *baby*, then we will first target CVCV words in which the two consonants are the same. Otherwise, we will target CVCV words in which the two consonants are different.

- If the child seems to be developing the variety of speech sounds and the variety of syllable shapes mentioned above, then the clinician can consider phonological processes as targets. The top priority would be targets that greatly affect intelligibility, including processes that affect syllable structure (e.g., weak syllable deletion) and idiosyncratic processes. Note that although cluster reduction is a syllable-structure process, the SLP may want to wait to target that process because it is one of the last processes that typically developing children suppress.

- Once the syllable structure and idiosyncratic processes have been targeted, then the SLP can consider the substitution processes, particularly the ones that are typically suppressed early, such as stopping.

Finally, most clinicians who work with young children have had the experience of needing to depart from their planned sequence of short-term goals because of what I call "treatment yeast." The process of paying attention to speech sounds in this way seems to spread and expand like yeast, and we begin to hear occasional new structures or speech sounds, including some that have not been targets of intervention.

---

## Role of Stimulability in Phonological Goal-Setting

In the procedures outlined previously there are several references to whether or not a child is stimulable. When we consider stimulability, we should again consider the work of Perrine, Bain, and Weston (2000). In particular, these authors have developed a hierarchy of cues to use in assessing stimulability. This hierarchy is discussed in detail in Section 2. The initial phonemic targets or exemplars for intervention will likely be sounds that are stimulable with an auditory model only (Perrine, Bain, and Weston's top level) rather than sounds that require considerable modeling, cueing, and instruction (lower levels of stimulability).

## Looking for Openings

Most SLPs develop a feel for each client's speech patterns, and they notice when a child does something unexpected given her current phonology. Very often these unexpected events are surprisingly accurate productions that the clinician has never heard before or are not entirely accurate but are surprisingly close.

    For example, a child might exhibit 100% cluster reduction at the onset of treatment. A few weeks later, after the child has learned to say a few words with initial /tw/ and /kw/, you may hear her attempt the word *squeeze*, which she says as [θkəwið], even though she usually says the word as [kið]. This change may be an opening. At that point it is very appropriate to depart from the lesson plan and see if you can elicit that /skw/ cluster several times, ignoring the dental substitutions for /s/ and /z/. If so, you may decide to add some words to your treatment list that begin with /skw/.

## How Many Words (Exemplars) Are Enough?

In the procedures outlined above, we indicated that a suitable goal would be four to five spontaneously produced words of a particular type. This number is probably sufficient for the child to discover that the target structures are needed in his language. Most children will not backslide on these words. Instead, they will continue to make the necessary changes in other words similar to these in length and presence of the target structure.

## Alternative Goal-Setting Procedures

There are at least two alternative ways to set short- and long-term goals for poorly intelligible children. The first of these is the method of Elbert and Gierut (1986) that is based on the child's presumed knowledge of phonological structures. These authors have provided an extensive list of words for the child to produce with and without morphological endings. Based on the child's performance on this test and on stimulability measures, the clinician can determine the degree of knowledge that the child has about specific phonemes in specific word positions.

Gierut, Elbert, and Dinnsen (1987) as well as Gierut, Morrisette, Hughes, and Rowland (1996) have reported that based on a number of replications of single-subject designs, children who begin treatment on the *least*-known phonemes or structures show faster change in the entire phonological system than children who start with more conventional targets, which would likely be those that the child knows more about. These authors would categorize a phoneme for which a child is readily stimulable as one about which the child knows quite a bit. However, the first large-scale study of this hypothesis, carried out by Rvachew and Nowak (2001), showed that selection of targets on the basis of their being the phonemes least-known by the child did *not* produce better results than traditional selection based on typical sequences of phonemic acquisition. In fact, the subjects receiving "minimal-knowledge" treatment made significantly less progress than subjects receiving treatment based on more traditional criteria.

The second systematic look at phonological targets is that of Bernhardt and Stemberger (2000), which is based on nonlinear phonology. Nonlinear phonology stresses the relationships among the elements that make up a syllable and the relationships among the syllables that make up a word. In terms of intervention goals, these authors discuss what they call "old stuff" and "new stuff." "Old stuff" refers to the phonological structures, segments, and distinctive features that the child already knows. "New stuff" refers to the structures, segments, and features that are generally missing from the child's system.

Bernhardt and Stemberger (2000) recommend that the clinician analyze a speech sample from a nonlinear perspective, and they provide numerous worksheets to assist in this process. The analysis proceeds in four major areas. These areas are summarized in Table 6-1. A key point for these authors is that children are more likely to be successful in learning new structures if they first put "old stuff" in new forms, such as a new word position or a new sequence of segments. A corollary is that if the child is learning totally "new" structures, it is best to learn them with "old" segments, or features. Table 6-1 shows an overview of how their analysis proceeds.

**TABLE 6-1.** Goals in a Nonlinear Phonological Intervention Plan.

*Reproduced with permission from Bernhardt, B. & Stemberger, J.P. (2000)* Workbook in Nonlinear Phonology for Clinical Application *(Table 4.1, p. 51.). Austin, TX: Pro-Ed.*

| *Phonological Level* | *Syllable and Word Structure* | *Segments and Features* |
|---|---|---|
| Totally new stuff | Type 1<br>(Phrases)<br>Word lengths<br>Stress patterns<br>Word shapes | Type 2<br>Individual features<br>(and related segments) |
| Old stuff in new places *or* in new combinations | Type 4<br>1. New word positions for old segments<br>2. New sequences of segments | Type 3<br>New combinations of old features |

Once the analysis is completed, Bernhardt and Stemberger recommend that the SLP adopt at least one goal for each box in the table. The following examples are taken from their work:

- **Type 1 goal ("New syllable/word structures"):** If the child has no consonant clusters in the syllable onsets, then clusters can become a goal.

- **Type 2 goal ("New features and segments"):** If the child has no fricatives, then [+continuant] is a reasonable goal.

- **Type 3 goal ("New simultaneous combinations of 'old' features"):** If a child has labial stops [p b] and alveolar fricatives [s z], but no labial fricatives [f v], then a suitable goal would be to target the [f v], which combine the labial and continuant features.

- **Type 4 goal ("New places for old segments"):** If a child uses velars at the end of a syllable but not in the onset of a syllable, then a reasonable goal is the production of velars in syllable onsets.

## INTERVENTION PROCEDURES

There is a variety of approaches to the actual treatment procedures used during phonological intervention. For example, several different authors advocate the use of minimal pairs for production training. One or two advocate systematic auditory exposure as part of the treatment process. Some approaches are rather traditional, while others occur in the context of naturalistic play.

## Minimal Pair Approaches

In virtually all therapies that use minimal pairs, the child is reinforced for differentiating between the two members of the pair. For example, if the child uses final consonant deletion, she might be asked to imitate the pair *bow/boat*. Weiner (1981) does not even provide a model for the child. Rather, his goal is to frustrate the child slightly by not reinforcing her when she says [bo] and means *boat*. At that point, the clinician tells the child what she has to do to make the word sound right.

Minimal pair approaches are widely used. However, as mentioned earlier, they run the risk that when the same stimuli are used over and over again, the words may lose their meaning for the child, and they may in fact seem arbitrary to the child. In addition, this is primarily a sit-at-the-table-and-pay-attention activity, and very active youngsters may not be able to cooperate.

---

### *MINIMAL PAIRS INTERVENTION*

| | Background |
|---|---|
| **WHO?** | Children with moderate-to-severe phonological disorders and poor intelligibility. |
| **WHAT?** | Minimal pairs are words that differ by only one phoneme. They are typically used to draw the client's attention to the fact that meaning is signaled by the difference between those two phonemes. There are |

*(continues)*

*(continued)*

several different variants of minimal pair intervention, depending on whether the actual phonemic contrasts are themselves minimal (differing by only one distinctive feature) or maximal (differing by several distinctive features). They also differ in terms of whether there are only two contrasting phonemes or multiple ones.

**WHY?**    Most authorities assume that the underlying problem with disordered phonology is a failure to "break the code." That is, the child has not figured out how to make differences in sounds that result in differences of meaning.

**WHEN?**    Minimal pairs intervention is appropriate for children who can perceive the relevant distinctions or can be taught to do so in a relatively short period of time.

**SUPPORT:**    There is research support for the effectiveness of minimal-contrast minimal pair treatment (Weiner, 1981). There is single-subject research suggesting that maximal-contrast minimal pair treatment is more effective than minimal-contrast treatment (Gierut, 1989).

## MINIMAL PAIRS INTERVENTION
### *Procedures*

I. Selection of Phonological Targets

Phonological targets can be chosen in a variety of ways, depending on one's theoretical orientation.

- Many researchers appear to choose a minimal-contrast approach using at least one phoneme that the client can already say (e.g., Blache, 1982; Weiner, 1981).

- Others choose a maximal-contrast approach in which sounds that the child knows least about are chosen for practice (Gierut, 1989; Elbert & Gierut, 1986). In this approach, a child who uses no fricatives or liquids but is stimulable for /f/ might actually work on /ʃ/ in contrast to /l/. The child "knows" the least about these two classes, and the chosen exemplars also contrast maximally. The /f/ is not used because the child presumably knows more about /f/ than the other fricatives.

- Still others use multiple oppositions (Williams, 2000). Multiple oppositions are used when the child collapses a number of phoneme contrasts to the same surface form, such as when *tip*, *sip*, *ship*, *Kip*, and *chip* are all pronounced as [tIp] (example taken from Williams, p. 282).

II. Training Procedures

Typically, in minimal pair approaches, the clinician chooses 5-10 pairs of words that contrast the chosen phonemes. These pictures are used for both perception and production training. There are three ways in which minimal pair training can proceed, the first two involving mild frustration for the child.

- Weiner (1981) used minimal pairs such as *bow/boat* for a child who used final consonant deletion and asked the child to tell him what card to give her. When the child persisted in saying *bow*, when she clearly meant *boat*, Weiner instructed her how to say *boat* so that he would understand. The child's frustration created an opportunity for learning.

- Blache (1982) uses the picture pairs first for ear training, choosing them so that the child can say one members of the pair relatively easily.
  - First the clinician shows the child the pair of pictures, says one of the words, and has the child point to the appropriate picture. This auditory exercise continues through all the word pairs.
  - Then the clinician tells the child to be the teacher. When the child persists in saying the one member of the pair that she can say, the clinician persists in pointing to that picture. The child becomes frustrated, and at that point, the clinician models the word for her. This kind of production practice continues until the child can readily name all of the pairs accurately. (Incidentally, Blache [1982] emphasizes that the clinician should reward production of the chosen distinctive feature rather than the exact sound. For example, if the child does not usually use the tongue-back feature in the minimal pair *tea/key*, but on one attempt she produces /ʧi/, she should be reinforced because /ʧ/ is a tongue-back sound also.)
- The third way to implement minimal pair intervention goes by the name of "Metaphon" therapy (Howell & Dean, 1994). In this program, the emphasis is on the child's metaphonological knowledge. This approach uses metaphors to talk with children about the properties of speech sounds (distinctive features) and to label those properties, often with pictures, such as Mr. Noisy for voicing and Mr. Whisper for voicelessness. The intervention proceeds in stages.
  - Stage 1: Developing awareness of phonology at the concept level, the sound level, the phoneme level, and the word level (minimal pairs).
  - Stage 2: Using the knowledge from Stage 1 to recognize when misunderstandings occur and why they occur, and to repair those misunderstandings. This stage also incorporates sentences that use the minimal pairs.

## The Cycles Approach

The Cycles approach of Hodson and Paden (1991) is perhaps the most widely known phonological intervention. There are three key elements: auditory bombardment using the targeted structure at the beginning and end of each session, use of minimal pairs to train production, and the "cycling" of phonological targets. All of these elements have been described previously in this Section, but it is well to remember that Hodson and Paden put them all into the same package. Although this approach is widely used, there is relatively little research support for it. It has not, apparently, been used in systematic controlled intervention studies.

### CYCLES INTERVENTION

| Background |
| --- |

| | |
| --- | --- |
| **WHO?** | Children who have severely impaired intelligibility. |
| **WHAT?** | Cycles intervention (Hodson & Paden, 1991) has as its goal the emergence of phonological targets that are not yet in the client's repertory. This intervention includes a number of innovative procedures, |

*(continues)*

*(continued)*

including auditory bombardment and the use of cycles of intervention. Cycles refer to periods of intervention for one set of multiple phonological targets, followed by a period of intervention for another set of targets, and so forth, eventually returning to the targets from the first cycle. Cycles are typically several weeks long. There is no attempt to reach a certain level of proficiency within each cycle.

**WHY?** The premise of Cycles therapy is that phonological acquisition is gradual. It is also known that children can show development of multiple phonological targets in the same period. An unstated premise of Cycles treatment is that when phonological structures become available to the child as a result of Cycles training, the child will generalize their use.

**WHEN?** Cycles intervention should be instituted immediately after the child has been identified and evaluated as having a severe phonological disorder.

**SUPPORT:** Hodson and Paden (1991) have reported that this intervention is highly effective with children in their clinics. However, these studies were not carried out with controls.

## CYCLES INTERVENTION

### *Procedures*

- The clinician identifies phonological processes, syllable structures, and idiosyncratic processes used by the child.

- For the first cycle, the clinician selects patterns or processes that are typically early developing, such as words with two syllables, early-developing syllable-initial consonants, and early-developing final consonants. However, liquids are stimulated in every cycle if they are not present.

- Select two to three exemplars for each pattern identified. For example, if the child does not use CVCV words but does have [m b d], the initial exemplars might be *Mommy*, *baby*, and *Daddy*. If final consonants are the target, then the clinician might choose final /p k/ if these sounds are used in other word positions.

- The SLP targets each exemplar for 60 minutes per cycle. The clinician prepares stimulus picture cards, including minimal pairs, where possible.

- Each session starts and ends with auditory bombardment for the pattern and the exemplars targeted during the session. In auditory bombardment, the child plays quietly while wearing amplification and listens to the clinician, who reads 10-15 words that contain the target pattern.

- Model-imitation procedures are used for production practice, followed by production practice in play or game situations.

- After the criterion of 60 minutes per exemplar per cycle is reached, the clinician selects a completely different set of phonological targets and exemplars for the next cycle.

- After two or three cycles, the clinician "cycles back" to the first cycle and assesses how the client is doing with those targets. If necessary, Cycle 1 is repeated, possibly with new exemplars.

## Naturalistic Play

Many interventions for phonological disorders use traditional types of treatment activities for intervention sessions. For example, the minimal pair interventions involve attention to picture representation and correct choices, whether in perception tasks or production tasks. Although the SLP can use these words to model and elicit utterances longer than a word, nevertheless, the target words are very much divorced from a meaningful, sustained context.

Both Hoffman (1993) and Camarata (1993) have argued forcefully for a type of phonological intervention that is based on social interaction during play. Hoffman, working from the background of whole language, incorporates phonology into the larger language context, encouraging all aspects of language to develop simultaneously, and providing corrective feedback that maintains the conversational interaction.

Camarata (1993) also advocates for phonological work to occur during naturalistic play interactions. However, his intervention is more focused on phonology and specific phonological targets. The technique is simply to model back the child's error word as part of the interaction and without any special emphasis on the target form. Camarata reports on a single subject multiple baseline study replicated across two children. Both children made relatively rapid progress when each new target was introduced, leading Camarata to conclude that "...many children with communication disorders simply require an increased number of relevant models, compared to the number available in the ambient communication environment..." (p. 180).

Finally, Hodson and Paden (1991) have described an alternative form of intervention for children who are not able to tolerate structured activities such as work on minimal pairs. This alternative involves play as well as focused stimulation similar to that advocated by Fey (1991) to stimulate one process at a time, although several processes may be targeted in one session.

## Pressure Points Intervention

Still another type of naturalistic intervention is called Pressure Points intervention (Smit, 2000). The idea behind this intervention is that the clinician finds spots in the child's system where change can occur quickly with treatment, and she leads the child to change the system at those points. Pressure Points treatment can be done in either a relatively structured intervention program or it can be done in a naturalistic play setting using focused stimulation, a concept borrowed from Fey (1991). Focused stimulation occurs when the SLP repeatedly says target words in a play situation, but without asking the child to imitate them. At least one study using focused stimulation (Giromaletto, Pearce, & Weitzman, 1997) has shown that children (late talkers) expand their syllable- and word-shape inventories and their phonetic inventories when exposed these models.

---

### *PRESSURE POINTS PHONOLOGICAL INTERVENTION*

| | Background |
|---|---|
| **WHO?** | Very unintelligible children up to children with moderate phonological disorders. |
| **WHAT?** | Pressure Points intervention (Smit, 2000) is a type of treatment conducted in a play setting. The clinician makes a best guess as to which |

*(continues)*

*(continued)*

phonological structures or exemplars are likely to change most quickly and presents those to the child, modeling specific target words repeatedly in play.

**WHY?**   Most phonological interventions require that the child sit and attend to pictures of minimal pairs. Pressure Points intervention makes use of auditory bombardment, naturalistic play, words that will be intelligible when the child corrects the target structure, focused stimulation, and reinforcement for intelligibility rather than correctness. The child's newly accurate productions are used right from the start in a meaningful context, which is thought to promote generalization.

**WHEN?**   Pressure Points intervention is appropriate for most children from the beginning of treatment.

**SUPPORT:**   At present, this type of intervention has no published research support. However, it is well grounded in both phonological theory and learning theory. The role of auditory bombardment is to help the child develop adult-like or near adult-like underlying representations of the phonological structures that are targeted. The presentation of multiple models in a play context is similar to the focused stimulation discussed by Fey (1991). Intensive modeling is intended to show the child that the missing structures make a difference in meaning and to jump-start generalization to meaningful speech in other settings. The attention paid to points where the child might be able to change easily and to ongoing change in the child's system comes from Vygotskian or dynamic systems theory (Vygotsky, 1978), which emphasizes the guiding role that alert adults can play in showing the child how to take the next step.

## PRESSURE POINTS PHONOLOGICAL INTERVENTION
### *Procedures and Example*

I. Selection of Phonological Targets

- The phonological targets are chosen in much the same way as indicated in the procedures mentioned earlier, except that the SLP tries to select a process or structure that the child is likely to be able to change quickly. This selection is done on the basis of knowledge of developmental sequences, on the basis of knowledge of the sounds and structures already present in the child's repertory, and on the basis of stimulability.

- At the same time as he selects the target process or structure, the clinician also selects two or more exemplars for that structure.

II. The Use of Auditory Bombardment

- At the same time as selecting the exemplars for starting treatment, the clinician selects another 7–10 words with the same target for use in auditory bombardment and finds pictures to represent them. These pictures are pasted or taped onto a sheet of cardboard.

- The clinician presents the first auditory bombardment set at the first treatment session with the parent observing. The child is asked to point to each pictured word as it is said, but is required only to listen and not to say any of the words. Then these pictures are sent home and the parent provides auditory bombardment once a day at home until the phonological target changes. After the first exemplar is targeted, the clinician tries to stay one to two weeks ahead of the next exemplar, so that the child gets one to two weeks of auditory bombardment on a structure or exemplar before ever attempting the target in production.

*Note: It is critical that the child not attempt any of the words during auditory bombardment. The goal of bombardment is to shape the child's underlying representation, and if the child produces the word, it will inevitably be wrong, besides interfering with the auditory trace of the clinician's or parent's model.*

III. Production Practice in a Play Context

- Production practice can occur in play, and the child is given a number of different activities from which to choose. The SLP models one of the chosen words intensively during play, without encouraging the child to imitate. This procedure is similar to the focused stimulation mentioned by Fey (1991). If the child does not imitate the word spontaneously after 10–12 models, the clinician may ask the child to try the word.  The clinician focuses on one word for a period of minutes and then goes to a second word for several minutes. Feedback to the child is brief—"I understand you!" or "Oops! You have to put your lips together."

  *Note:* For the child who can tolerate it, production practice can occur in drill-type work. In these instances, the productions are initially elicited with intense modeling and cueing, which is faded later, depending on the child's accuracy levels.

IV. Stability and Change in Pressure Points Intervention

- In Pressure Points intervention the targets and exemplars change much more quickly than in most conventional and even most phonological treatments. The clinician tracks each production, noting those productions that could have been direct imitations or slightly delayed imitations and which productions were relatively spontaneous in the context of the session.

- As soon as the clinician hears 80-90% of the spontaneous productions being correct during the focused stimulation for that word, and he hears several correct productions of that word in other contexts (no matter how many are incorrect), he chooses another exemplar. If the parent can detect changes readily and report them, then that information is also used to determine whether to stop emphasis on that word. In other words, the child shows the clinician that she is starting to generalize. At the same time, the clinician remains alert to potential for change in the child's speech, that is, pressure points. Clinical Note 6-3 illustrates this approach.

---

**CLINICAL NOTE 6-3: Pressure Points Intervention with Tony**

The example used here is a 4-year-old named Tony. He had not had previous treatment. At the time of evaluation, he was about 100% unintelligible. He used very few consonants in connected speech, but he used glottal stops freely where consonants should be. He also had a variety of vowel errors. He used very few CVCV words, and in fact, he said his own name as [ʔʌiʔ]. His phonetic repertoire was smaller than that of most 18 month olds. He had difficulty with many oral motor

*(continues)*

*(continued)*

tasks. He was reluctant to imitate speech. Many SLPs would consider him to have a number of potential dyspraxic elements.

Tony was an alert child and interested in the world around him. He was learning to read, and sometimes when he was attempting to produce single words, he would approximate a true consonant, pause, then follow up with his usual production, such as [p//ʔɪʔ] for *pin*.

The SLP selected the idiosyncratic process of glottal replacement in word-initial position to start treatment with Tony, along with his maladaptive behavior of attempting a true consonant in isolation before saying a word. She decided to tackle this process in two ways. First of all, Tony would learn the two glides [w] and [h], which he did not have. Then the characteristics of the /h/ ("Listen to all that air!") would be continued in teaching initial voiceless stops, and the characteristics of /w/ ("Listen to how your voice keeps going") would be continued with initial nasals. Because Tony had no real consonants in his inventory, choosing appropriate words was a challenge, and in the end, mostly CV words were used.

The clinician presented words with initial /h/ (*hay, he, who, hi, hoe*) to Tony and asked him to point as she said them. Then she asked him to point, and she would say the one that he pointed to. At a different point in the session, the clinician presented /w/ words: *weigh, we, woo* (as an owl sounds), *whoa!* (as for horses). At the end of the first session, she asked Tony's parent to participate and provide some of the models. Tony's parent then agreed to do this task at home once a day until the next week's session. At the second session, the clinician presented one set of words with initial /p/ for auditory bombardment, and another set of /d/ words. Tony's parents took both sets home to provide auditory bombardment for several weeks before these sounds were targeted in intervention.

Because Tony liked quiet activities, the clinician used conversation about books, toys, and games interspersed with large motor activities. At first, the clinician used intensive modeling of one of the two phonemic targets during each activity, without asking for imitations, waiting for Tony to attempt one of the target words. It was not until the third session that Tony attempted an [h] in a word, and when he did, it was separated from the vowel. He needed another session or two to link the consonant and the vowel, and in these sessions, some traditional drill was used. However, his first attempt at /w/, which came later, was linked.

After Tony began to stabilize on the /h/ and the /w/—for example, could say them in an elicited production (not modeled) in four or five words—the intervention shifted to initial /p/ and initial /n/, with the shift occurring later for the /n/. Tony's first productions of /p/ words were broken, but he soon made the analogy to his work with /h/ and smoothed out the productions. At this point he knew he was on his way to more intelligible speech, and he wanted to bring his books in for the sessions. In about the seventh session, Tony spontaneously produced a word with initial /d/ that was linked to the following vowel, much to his and the clinician's surprise. The clinician took a few minutes to make sure that this word was repeatable, and thereafter incorporated some modeling of /d/-words. Within about 10 sessions, Tony was readily able to produce all of the stops, voiced and voiceless, in initial positions of two to five words each. In other words, he was stabilizing these sounds.

*(continues)*

*(continued)*

The SLP then shifted to word-final consonant targets, starting with nasals. As was becoming typical of Tony, he took several sessions (including some with traditional motor drills) to get the idea of ending with a nasal rather than a glottal stop, but once he figured this out, he was able to expand his final consonant repertory relatively quickly.

Over the course of a year, Tony filled out most of the segmental (phonemic) inventory. He had some difficulty with retroflexing the tongue for /r/ and with the suprasegmental aspects of two-syllable words (he stressed the syllables equally); however, again with the aid of some motor drill, he was able to sort out the /r/ and the stress patterns of two-syllable words.

At the end of the year, not all words that Tony said were correct, but his intelligibility had improved greatly. One of the most important indicators of Tony's increasing intelligibility was that he started to be willing to talk to people he did not know, even to the point of insisting that only he, and not his parents, could tell new people what his name was.

## Techniques to Promote Motor Learning

Many kindergarten and school-age children with phonological disorders appear not to have motor difficulties sufficient to account for their phonological difficulties. At the same time, many of them exhibit at least a few potential dyspraxic elements (PDE). For example, you may see a child who has extraordinary difficulty producing velars, or surprising difficulty with the /f/. In these cases, there is undoubtedly an interaction between the motoric system and the abstract linguistic system.

The SLP working with such a child may wish to add in some practice for the motor system requirements for particular sounds, as we did for the child Tony, whose case was used as an example in the previous Procedure section. Motor practice usually means drill, and it may mean drill on the target phoneme in isolation or even in nonsense syllables. The idea is to bring the child to the point where she can easily produce the sound or the syllable on command and without a model.

In addition, some of the children with PDE may have real difficulties with vowel-to-consonant or consonant-to-vowel transitions, or with connecting two syllables in a two-syllable word. In these cases, the clinician may need to devise practice sequences that systematically pair a variety of vowels with the consonant target. Sequences such as these would need to be modeled by the clinician, possibly with increasing rate of production as the child becomes more skilled.

## Promoting Intelligibility Rather than Correctness

When we are working with children who have phonological disorders, our goal is usually to promote intelligibility and to help the child realize that she has it in her power to produce speech that others readily understand. Consequently, what we say as part of our social or verbal reinforcement should sometimes reflect that orientation. The traditional way to reinforce is to say "Good" or some other positive word, and we can do that for the "phonological" child also. Nevertheless, much of the reinforcement should come in the form of continuing the conversation, which lets the child know that we understood her.

Another reason to reinforce in terms of intelligibility is that it lets the child know that we value communicating as much as, or more than, merely saying something correctly. This emphasis may be particularly important for severely unintelligible children, who are known to be at risk for stuttering. These children may well have constitutional or biological predispositions toward motor coordination difficulties that can affect both speech sound production and fluency. Such children may initially have mild disfluencies.

The mechanism by which stuttering can develop in these children relates in part to environmental feedback that suggests to the child that his talking is not "right" (Guitar, 1998). The child may try to fix the talking problem without knowing how to do so, in the process doing things that are counter-productive such as holding his breath or clamping his tongue to the roof of his mouth. As clinicians, if we reinforce only in terms of correctness, we may inadvertently feed into the idea that talking can be right or wrong. If we put the emphasis on intelligibility and communication, on the other hand, we direct the child's attention to the interaction, which is healthier.

## Incorporating Phonological Awareness Activities

After the child has begun to show definite progress, the clinician may wish to incorporate activities to promote phonological awareness. Alternatively, the child's clinician and teacher might collaborate on phonological awareness training for the whole class. In any event, children with phonological disorders that persist into the early school years are at risk for difficulties with phonological awareness and with reading, which appears to depend in part on adequate phonological awareness.

Section 1 notes some commercially available programs for phonological awareness. Many clinicians also do this type of teaching using clinician-made materials. The types of tasks might include word segmentation into its sound components, and synthesizing components into words, segmenting longer words or utterances into syllables, and rhyming games, as well as games in which the goal is to come up with as many words that start with the same sound as possible.

## DOCUMENTING PROGRESS

For our discussion of documentation, we need to go back to the long-term and short-term goals. We need to recognize that measures of intelligibility or of overall accuracy are likely not going to change for a considerable period of time. The short-term goals that we have written are much easier to document, but there seems to be a large gap between the long-term and short-term goals.

## Charting with the Segmental Inventory

One way for the clinician to track progress and to share it with the parents and teacher is to use Reproducible Form 6: Segmental Inventory—Consonants. This inventory shows all of the consonant singletons that the child will need to be a competent speaker. I often use colored pencils to write in three categories of sounds: the phonemes that were stable at the onset of treatment, the phonemes that are stabilizing (using the Pressure Points definition of stabilizing), and the phonemes that we are starting to hear either because we are eliciting them or because the child is trying them out spontaneously. Naturally, some of the colors on the inventory will change from one documentation point to the next. Parents and teachers seem to understand the idea of this chart, and they also understand the incremental nature of progress. In most cases, they also get to see that quite a lot of change can occur in several domains, once phonological treatment is started.

## Probes of Phonological Processes

Because we most often target individual phonological processes when training broad, it makes sense to probe the processes that we have selected on a biweekly or monthly basis. The clinician can devise several different probes of the same phonological process by making a list of picturable or explainable words that could be affected by the process and randomly assigning them to each of the probes. Probes of 10 words each are the easiest to track or graph in terms of percentage correct. Clinical Note 6-4 provides an example.

CLINICAL NOTE 6-4:
### Three Probes of Cluster Reduction Affecting /s/-Clusters

| Probe 1 | Probe 2 | Probe 3 |
| --- | --- | --- |
| spike | spin | spot |
| screen | screw | scrape(r) |
| snow | snore | snap |
| stove | stump | stick |
| sled | slip | slide |
| sweater | swing | swim |
| smell | smile | Smurf |
| ski | skate | school |
| Sprite | spray | sprinkle |
| spark | spare (tire) | sports |

## DISMISSAL CRITERIA

In our discussion of dismissal criteria, we need to keep in mind that the goal of treatment is not 90% or 100% accuracy of all phonemes or structures in all contexts. If our goal is improved intelligibility, then children may be dismissed before they are 100% intelligible. It is reasonable to expect that children will maintain their phonological achievements and continue to build on them. We really do not expect children to relapse, because cognitive/linguistic improvements tend to be permanent, just as we do not expect the child who has learned to read fairly well to forget how to read. On the other hand, continued improvement is not guaranteed. For this reason, if we dismiss a child who is 85% intelligible or whose PCC is 82%, we should commit to follow up in six months or so.

If a child who has been dismissed from treatment with follow-up does not continue to progress, then intervention may need to be reinstated. On the other hand, if we observe actual relapse in a "phonological" child, this would be highly unusual. In such cases, all possible causes should be investigated, including neurological events or processes, depression, and abuse.

## EFFICACY OF PHONOLOGICAL INTERVENTION

There have been a number of case studies, group reports without controls, and single-subject studies (with internal controls) that have been reported in the literature. All of these suggest that the "training broad" approaches are effective with preschoolers who have phonological disorders. This is true whether the approach is based on minimal pairs or cycles or some other factor. It is also true for the many varieties of goal-setting procedures.

The gold standard for efficacy studies is randomized control designs based on groups. As a practical matter, in the United States it is now impossible to compare intervention groups with no-intervention groups because of public laws mandating services. However, it is possible to carry out group studies that compare two or more different phonological approaches. There is apparently only one of these to date, namely that of Rvachew and Nowak (2001), which showed that both minimal- and maximal-knowledge approaches were effective but that the maximal-knowledge approach produced more far-ranging results and increased satisfaction on the part of parents.

## SUMMARY

The goal of this chapter is to give the SLP some ways to think about intervention for children with phonological disorders. There are many possibilities, all of them very different from traditional treatment methods for articulation disorders. These methods are different because they target the speech-sound system, rather than individual speech sounds. This kind of intervention can also be very rewarding for the clinician, because when these methods are used appropriately, children typically make rapid progress.

# SECTION

# 7

# TREATMENT WITH CHILDREN WHO HAVE RESIDUAL ERRORS

●●●●●●●●●●●●●●●●●●●●●●●●●●●●●●●●●●●●●●●●●●●●●●●●●

Treatment with children who have residual errors is one of the most neglected research areas in our profession. At the same time, there is substantial research suggesting that this is a very heterogeneous group of clients. They vary in perceptual skills, language competence, oral structures, oral motor abilities, developmental history, and personality. If this variability means anything, it means that treatment needs to be tailored to the child's abilities, yet I know of no research that attempts this matching, except in the case of suspected Developmental Verbal Dyspraxia. As a consequence, the profession seems to operate with a statement like this: "Whatever the child's background that led to persistent speech sound errors, the fact remains that he or she presents with an inappropriate motor pattern for particular phonemes." We then treat the motor pattern, but we often operate in a vacuum with respect to variables that might influence the course and rate of progress.

This Section is no different, as I view treatment of the motor patterns associated with residual errors as appropriate. I also argue that precision-oriented treatment is usually the most effective kind of treatment. Along the way, we will discuss the influences of some of the client variables on treatment. The framework for this discussion is the treatment continuum put forth by and Bankson (1998), which has three phases: establishment (sometimes called elicitation), generalization (sometimes called transfer), and maintenance.

Precision-oriented treatment has a focus on efficiency—that is, bringing about the maximum possible change in the shortest period of time. In fact, we should bring a sense of urgency to this work because we generally are working with school-age children who have already had too many years of being identified on the basis of their speech. It is safe to say that every school SLP has had the experience of treating a school-age child for years without the child reaching dismissal criteria. We need to find a better way, and precision-oriented treatment can help. Some of the principles relevant to precision-oriented treatment are noted in Section 5.

## SETTING GOALS

After the SLP has completed assessment of the child's communication skills, the immediate issue is selecting the goals of intervention. If the child has several of the typical phoneme errors, the clinician may ask the child about his or her preference. Or the clinician may target all of the error sounds and spend time on each error sound in the treatment session. Alternatively, the therapist may target stimulable sounds.

In addition, there may be other elements of communication that need attention, quite apart from those revealed in formal assessment. For example, some children have become quite self-conscious about their speech, and as a result they speak softly, or they avoid talking, or they do not look at the person with whom they are speaking, or they manage to get one hand up near the mouth whenever they talk. These issues will also need attention, although perhaps not initially.

There is no reason why several sounds should not be targeted in a single session. In fact, this may be desirable because there may be a spread of benefits from working on different articulatory patterns. That is, the child may become more alert to articulatory distinctions in general. In addition, the treatments for multiple sounds will not all proceed at the same rate, so that there is usually at least one target on which the client experiences success, at least compared to the other targets. The only caveat about working with multiple targets within one session is that some children may become confused. Confusion is more likely when there is cognitive delay.

## THE ESTABLISHMENT (ELICITATION) PHASE

The goal of the establishment phase is that the client will be able to produce the target in at least one context, and he will do so with stability. Stability means that the client is able to produce the target correctly and repeatedly without a model. The reason for a requirement of stability is that this production must be readily repeatable in order for it to serve as the springboard for putting the sound in other contexts. Of course, stability can be determined operationally in a number of ways. One possibility is this: "The client will produce the correct target in isolation on command, without a model, 9 out of 10 times over three sessions."

One of the most common clinical errors is for the clinician to attempt transfer a production that is correct in one context to other contexts before the target is stable. Moving to additional contexts before the target is stable virtually guarantees that the child will have a low rate of correct production in the next phase. Furthermore, because the next step is generally more difficult than the current one, low rates of accuracy will require a lot of rehearsal before a new level of stable correct production is reached.

### Perceptual Training

In the traditional or Van Riperian type of intervention, production training would not begin until perceptual training is completed. At the present time, however, most SLPs do not routinely provide perception training prior to production training because of evidence that many children with residual errors do not need it. However, if it is needed, then there are preferred ways to do it.

## *PERCEPTION TRAINING FOR RESIDUAL ERRORS*

<table>
<tr><td colspan="2" align="center">Background</td></tr>
<tr><td>WHO?</td><td>A school-age child or adult who has one or more residual speech sound errors and who also appears to have difficulty perceiving the target forms.</td></tr>
<tr><td>WHAT?</td><td>Systematic exposure to the acoustic differences between sounds, culminating in the contrast between the client's own error type and the target phoneme. Perception training is sometimes called ear training or discrimination training.</td></tr>
<tr><td>WHY?</td><td>The goal of perception training is to help the client hear the difference between his current production and the standard production. The client can then monitor his own production, which may be a crucial component of intervention.</td></tr>
<tr><td>WHEN?</td><td>Perception training may carried out prior to production training. Alternatively, if the SLP starts with production training and the client does not make progress, then perception training may be needed.</td></tr>
<tr><td>SUPPORT:</td><td>Perception training has been a part of traditional approaches since Van Riper first described it in 1939. Winitz (1975) has presented a systematic way to structure such training. However, the evidence relating speech sound disorders to problems in auditory perception is equivocal, and there is no evidence that perception training for all clients is critical to the overall success of intervention.</td></tr>
</table>

## PERCEPTION TRAINING FOR RESIDUAL ERRORS

### *Procedures (after Winitz, 1975)*

Although the eventual goal of this training is for the client to perceive the difference between her own error type and the target, the training should start with sounds that share few features with the target. For example, if the child substitutes [s] for /tʃ/, the first contrasts might be [sa] - [ka], then [sa] – [na], then [sa] – [ta]. Only after this point would the client be trained on the [sa] – [tʃa] distinction.

The child should be given many opportunities to make perceptual judgments at each level, with the last contrast—between error and target—reached only after systematic training to that point. Then this type of sequence can be repeated with real words.

The next step is for the client to discriminate the target sound in running speech. Thus the client raises a finger or marks on a paper when he hears the target sound while the SLP talks or reads to him. When the child can do this successfully, production training can begin.

Which clients need this type of "ear training"? Locke (1980a, 1980b) has presented evidence that most children have no difficulty in discriminating their target sound from their error sound, but it is difficult to know which child does and which child does not have difficulty. General-purpose tests of discrimination are not useful first of all because they are not phoneme-specific. Second, they are subject to a wide variety of extraneous influences, ranging from external noise to a child's preference for certain types of pictures.

Locke's (1980b) *Sound Production-Perception Task* was designed to be phoneme-specific. The clinician shows the child a single picture (e.g., *ship*) and asks her these three types of Yes/No questions repeatedly:

Is it ship? (Target phoneme is /ʃ/.)

Is it sip? (Error production is [s].)

Is it dip? (Control phoneme is /d/.)

However, some children do not tolerate such 30-question tests well, probably because of their abstract and repetitive nature. The child may respond accurately for the first 15 questions but not for the second 15, or may respond randomly, or may respond with all Yes or all No answers. As a result of such problems with even a phoneme-specific measure, many clinicians start production training first and then go back to perception training if the child does not respond well to the production training.

## The Establishment Phase: Eliciting Correct Productions

There are many ways to get to a stable production. If the child is stimulable for the target or if the target can be elicited in a specific word, then treatment usually can proceed rapidly. Quite often the successful context is isolation, although sometimes a child has an easier time with words in which there is a considerable degree of coarticulation related to the target sound. For example, if the target is [s], words like *stop* or *stick* might be helpful. Sometimes a nonsense syllable with a facilitating vowel will do the trick. As with all elicitation procedures, the more concrete the SLP's instructions and feedback, the more accurate the client's attempts will be. Figure 7-1 shows the three phases of treatment along with some of the variables that the SLP can manipulate to help the client move across the continuum.

If the target phoneme is stimulable in isolation, in a nonsense syllable or in a facilitating word, then the clinician attempts to stabilize the production by gradually reducing the number and frequency of models. A specific technique that also helps to stabilize a new production is to introduce delays between the model and the response. This can be done by telling the client not to attempt a production right after the model but to wait until you hold up your finger.

This is also the time to observe scrupulously the relevant principles at the beginning of Section 5. By way of reminder, they are these:

- If you reinforce productions that are not totally accurate, inaccurate productions are what you will get.
- The goal for conducting treatment in most cases is almost errorless learning, with just enough mistakes that the client knows what *not* to do.
- Reinforce and count only the first production attempt in any one trial, and in general, do not reinforce self-corrections.
- Never ask a client to produce a response more than once in a given trial unless you are 100% certain that subsequent productions will be as accurate as the first one.
- How the SLP responds to an elicited production that is in error is important to the progress of treatment.
- The SLP should provide feedback non-verbally in the early and middle stages of treatment.

**Figure 7-1** The phases of intervention for residual errors, along with variables that may be manipulated in each stage. (I am indebted to J. Bruce Tomblin, personal communication, for sharing the basic formulation of continua for these variables.)

| | | Phases of Intervention | | |
| --- | --- | --- | --- | --- |
| | | Establishment | Generalization | Maintenance |
| Property of Speech Units | **Length** | Isolation    Syllable    Word | Phrase/Sentence | Discourse |
| | **Syllable Structure** | CV   CVC   CVCV    CCVC | | |
| | **Position in Syllable/ Word** | Initial    Final    Intervocalic | | |
| | **Adjacent Context** | Facilitative | Less facilitative | |
| | **Presence of Error Sound** | Error absent from context    Error present in context | | |
| Property of Speaking Situation | **Attention** | Attention to sound form | Attention to form and meaning | Attention to communication and meaning |
| | **Communi- cation** | Non-communicative speaking activities | Quasi-communicative speaking activities | Typical communicative activities |
| Training Activities: Antece- dents | **Phonetic Placement** | | | |
| | **Models/Cues** | | | |
| | **Modification of Other Sounds** | | | |
| | **Shifting Production** | | | |
| | **Use of Delays** | No delays    Short delays    Long delays | | |
| Training Activities: Conse- quences | **Reinforce- ment** | 100%    Fixed ratio    Variable ratio | Fixed interval | Variable interval |
| | **Negative** | 100% social "No" | Nonverbals and cues to self-monitor | |

- The client's focus (motivation, ability to attend) with respect to intervention is an important variable.
- Clients who appear unmotivated or lazy are usually clients who have had little success in treatment.

Finally, with most clients, this is the time to begin the process of self-monitoring or self-evaluation. Most experts agree that self-evaluation is an extremely valuable tool. Typically, the SLP tells the client that after the next response, she is to evaluate her own production, and then the clinician will evaluate, and they can compare their evaluations. In my view, it is critical that this all be done wordlessly so that no auditory interference degrades the client's memory of the just-produced sound. Thus a typical sequence for having the client self-evaluate a production of /ɝ/ might be this:

1. SLP:   [ɝ] (model)
2. Client: [ɝ]
3. Client silently indicates the thumbs-up sign if the production was accurate.
4. The clinician does the same and afterwards provides verbal feedback on the accuracy of the self-evaluation.

If the child is not stimulable for the target selected by the SLP, then the clinician has a number of choices. If the child has residual errors on other sounds, the clinician can see if any of those sounds are stimulable. If not, then below are some directions to consider:

1. Consult one of several texts that deal with elicitation procedures for particular sounds, such as Bernthal and Bankson, 1998; Bleile, 1995; Bauman-Waengler, 2000; or Secord, 1981.
2. Administer appropriate sections of the *Contextual Test of Articulation* (Aase, Hovr, Krause, Schelfhout, Smith, & Carpenter, 2000), the *Secord Contextual Articulation Tests* (Secord & Shine, 1997), or the *McDonald Deep Test* (McDonald, 1964a) to find a context in which the target is produced correctly.
3. Consider variant placements. For example, acoustically acceptable [s] can often be elicited as a bladed (tongue-tip down) production, and the [r] can be either retroflexed or bunched.
4. Consider a shaping procedure, in which closer and closer approximations are reinforced. Be sure to achieve a degree of stability at each level. Shaping procedures can be used to get from one sound to the target sound or from an oral, non-verbal posture to the target sound. Clinical Note 7-1 illustrated just such a shaping procedure.
5. If there is competition from a non-involved articulator—for example, the lips keep rounding during attempts at /r/—teach a competing behavior. In the case of /r/, the instructions might be:

   Flare your lips (or push your lips out).
   Keep your lips flared and pull your tongue tip back.
   Etc.

6. Use tactile feedback to help cue the client. Lemon-glycerin swabs, a toothbrush, a tongue blade, and even peanut butter (if the client is not allergic) may be used.

In most of these alternatives, the clinician will need to devise a stepwise sequence to follow, a sequence that includes stabilizing the production at every step. Clinical Note 7-1 shows a sample shaping procedure for /ɝ/, taken from Shriberg (1975).

**CLINICAL NOTE 7-1: A Model Program
for Devising Elicitation Sequences for Specific Phonemes**

The following elicitation program includes various elements to elicit a difficult sound, in this case, the /r/. It includes a number of steps, with a criterion at each step for passing to the next step. It also includes elements of shaping as well as modeling and cueing. Adapted with permission from Shriberg (1975) Copyright American Speech-Language-Hearing Association. Used with permission.

| Goal | Step | Instruction | Response Definition | Reinforcement | Pass Criterion (Consecutive) |
|---|---|---|---|---|---|
| I. Part names, basic mobility | 1. | Stick your tongue out. (Model) | Tongue extends behind lips. | "Good" (or "Not right" and re-instruct) | 3 |
| | 2. | Stick your tongue out and touch the tip with your finger. (Model) | Touches tip with index finger. | Same | 3 |
| | 3. | Put your finger on the bumpy place right behind your top teeth. (Model) | Finger placed on alveolar ridge at midline. | Same | 3 |
| | 4. | Now put the tip of your tongue lightly on that bumpy place. (Model) | Very tip of tongue placed on alveolar ridge. | Same | 3 |
| II. Tongue control, sustained phonation | 5. | Put your tongue tip up there again, and say /l/. (Model) | Produces /l/ for 2 seconds | Same | 3 |

*(continues)*

*(continued)*

| | | | | | |
|---|---|---|---|---|---|
| | 6. | Say /l/ each time I hold up my finger. | Produces /l/ for 2 sec. | Same | 3 |
| | 7. | Now say /l/ for as long as I hold my finger up, like this: (Hold finger up for 5 sec.) Ready, go! | Produces a 5-sec. /l/ with no phonation breaks and minimal tongue movements | Same | 5 |
| III. Evoke /ɝ/ | 8a. | Say a long /l/, but this time as you're saying it, drag the tip of your tongue slowly back along the roof of your mouth—so far back that you have to drop it. (Model hand gesture.) | Tongue tip is dragged back slowly sustaining phonation until tip has dropped and a good /ɝ/ is heard. Jaw should not drop during movement. | "Good, that's the sound that I want—exactly like that." | 5 |
| Branch | 8b. | Let's practice pulling the tip of your tongue back across the roof of your mouth. Pretend you are licking whipped cream off the roof of your mouth. Do it without making any sound. | Child's report. | "Did you..." | 3 Return to 8a |

## Unusual Clients

No doubt every SLP encounters the client who is so out of the ordinary that it is unclear where to start or how to conceptualize progress. Quite often these clients will have more than one complicating area that needs to be taken into account in planning treatment. For example, you might have a child with traumatic brain injury on the caseload who not only has the expected cognitive and memory deficits, but also has severe articulation difficulties. Or you may have a child who is so reluctant to be "wrong" about anything that you are concerned about giving negative feedback.

In these complicated cases, the team is critically important. The team may decide, for example, that the child with the head injury needs functional communication more than accuracy of production, so you may work on speech sounds only in the context of single, useful words. In the case of the child who is reluctant to be wrong, the team may recognize underlying issues that need to be explored. In addition, the SLP may decide to design the intervention to proceed in such small, achievable steps that the child can receive positive reinforcement almost all the time.

There are other types of unusual cases as well. Clients who make sounds in unusual ways sometimes pose the issue of whether to intervene or not. In most cases, these unusual productions will have a distracting visual component, and both the auditory and the visual aspects of the production must be managed. Clinical Note 7-2 illustrates just such a case. The critical procedure for this young man was that his productions of fricatives had to meet not just an acoustic criterion for acceptability, but also a visual one. In other words, the client was held to two criteria every time he produced a fricative or affricate. That is, the production had to sound right and it had to look right (jaw moving in the midline only).

---

### CLINICAL NOTE 7-2: Correcting a Case of Jaw Slide

At age 14, Danny knew his career goals. He wanted to go into theater, acting in particular. Unfortunately, Danny had very prominent unilateral [s z ʃ tʃ dʒ] distortions. Whenever he said these sounds, his jaw would slide to the left and then back. Consequently, his errors had both a distracting auditory component and a distracting visual component. Attempts to elicit a centrally produced [s] resulted in an acoustically adequate production, but with the same prominent jaw slide. He had received treatment in the school setting for a number of years. He was discouraged and not highly motivated.

Much to Danny's surprise, treatment began with non-verbal exercises. Danny was to practice in front of a mirror, opening and closing his mouth repeatedly, with his fingertip or thumb placed lightly on the point of the jaw. He was to keep the jaw movement relaxed and absolutely in the midline and to concentrate on the sensations associated with the movements. At his second session, he combined this exercise with soundless postures for [t n d]. At the third session, he added a vowel (e.g., [ta ta ta ta]) while still maintaining the midline movement. Finally, at the fourth session, he was allowed to combine the opening and closing movements with any kind of centrally produced tongue-tip fricative that he could, provided that the movements were relaxed and in the midline.

Finally, Danny was ready to refine the acoustic qualities of the centrally produced [s]. In this work, and in subsequent work with him on this and the other targets, the

*(continues)*

*(continued)*

clinician maintained a focus on the midline production of these fricatives. Specifically, Danny was not reinforced for an acoustically acceptable fricative unless the jaw also stayed in the midline. Danny required a large amount of rehearsal of this type—after all, he had been practicing the unilateral distortions for many years. Each time we introduced a new target, he would revert somewhat to the unilateral slide, but he also corrected this tendency quickly.

## THE GENERALIZATION PHASE

The goal of the generalization phase is that the client will be able to produce the target phoneme in many different contexts, but still with conscious attention. This is the phase in which scaffolding is most important as the child goes from levels of reduced complexity to levels of higher complexity.

## *THE GENERALIZATION PHASE*

### Background

**WHO?**  The client who has at least one stable context in which the target phoneme is produced correctly.

**WHAT?**  The generalization phase of intervention immediately follows the establishment phase. Then at the end of the generalization phase, the client goes into the maintenance phase. The generalization phase is probably the longest phase involving the clinician. During this phase, the target behavior—correct production of the selected phoneme in a linguistic unit—is transferred to more complex linguistic structures, while the accuracy of production remains high. The clinician manipulates many variables in order to achieve this goal. Typically, for example, the client moves from production of the target in syllables, then to words, then to phrases, then to sentences, and finally to discourse.

**WHY?**  Clients who are past the preschool years hardly ever make wholesale changes in sound production once they have gotten through the establishment phase. In fact, it is typical that the client makes *no* changes in spontaneous speech at that point. Therefore the client needs assistance in getting from acceptable production of the target in a very limited context to acceptable production in discourse. The generalization phase is intended to help the client bridge that gap.

**SUPPORT:**  The generalization phase has been a part of traditional intervention for many years, although not under that name. Bernthal and Bankson (1998) gave us the concept that the intervention regime can usefully be divided into establishment, generalization, and maintenance phases.

## THE GENERALIZATION PHASE
### *Procedures*

- In the generalization phase, the SLP manipulates the complexity of the target response. The most commonly mentioned variables are the phonetic context and the length of the linguistic unit. There are other variables too, however, and these were shown in Figure 7-1. In any case, the idea is to provide a graduated sequence from less complex to more complex linguistic structures. Stable performance at one level, together with appropriate cues and/or models, provides the basis for proceeding to the next level.

- *Continuum: Phonetic Context*

  The phonetic context in which a sound is produced can be facilitating or non-facilitating. For example, for most clients, the word *stay* would represent a facilitating context for the /s/ because the /t/ is also made at the alveolar ridge. Early in the generalization period we try to use phonetic contexts that facilitate correct production of the target, but in the latter part of the generalization period, we try to expose the client to many words in which the phonetic context is not facilitating.

  Phonetic context can also include the presence of additional instances of the error phoneme, such as for target /r/, the two /r/ sounds in the word *rubber.* Alternatively, the client's substitution may be present—for example, if the child substitutes [w] for target /r/, the word *rewind* would contain the error production as well as the target. Early in the generalization phase, such words would not be used, but later in the generalization phase, they should be used. After all, the client will eventually need to produce such words accurately.

- *Continuum: Properties of Speech Units*

  - **Position of target in the syllable.** For most phonemes, the word-initial position is the easiest. The one exception to his rule affects fricatives, which often occur first in word-final position and are often easier to elicit in that position. The medial or intervocalic position is probably most difficult regardless of phoneme. Early in the generalization period, the easier word positions would be used, and later in the generalization period, the more difficult positions would be used.

  - **Syllable structure.** In the early generalization stages, we use simple syllable structures such as CV or VC syllables. Later on, more complex structures, including consonant clusters and multisyllabic words, should be used.

  - **Length of the speech unit.** In the establishment phase of treatment, typically either a sound in isolation or a single syllable was used to elicit the target. As we take the client through the generalization period, the length may change from single syllable to word to phrase or short sentence to long sentence and then to discourse.

- *Continuum: Properties of the Speaking Situation*

  - **Communicativeness.** The speech activities in the establishment and early generalization phases (for example, sounds in isolation and nonsense syllables) are clearly not communicative. As we assist the client through the generalization period, we go to quasi-communicative speech activities (naming of pictures, sentence frames) to typical communicative activities such as discourse or a conversation.

  - **Locus of attention.** Locus of attention is a description of where the client directs her focus. In the establishment phase of intervention, the client clearly has a focus on the sound form, whereas during much of the generalization phase, the focus is on both form and meaning. In fact, in the generalization phase, we often go back and forth between attention to form and attention to meaning. Finally, in the maintenance phase, the client's attention is on meaning, communication, and form.

- *Continuum: Antecedents*

Antecedents are the events that precede the client's response. Typically, we manipulate the antecedent events to increase the probability of a high rate of acceptable responding. Later in the generalization phase we reduce the presence of antecedents because we want the acceptable response to stabilize, that is, become more automatic.

  - **Phonetic placement instructions, shifting production, modification of other sounds, and use of delays (between model and response).** These techniques are prominent in the establishment phase, and we continue to use them occasionally during the early generalization phase.

  - **Models and cues.** During the generalization phase we often continue to provide models for the child to imitate, although we also fade them as quickly as possible. Cues can refer to almost anything that assists the child to produce an acceptable target. Possible cues might include:

    - A hand-cue to indicate when the client is to make a response

    - An iconic gesture indicating some aspect of the placement or manner of production of the target phoneme

    - A printed symbol corresponding to the target sound

    - A picture to be named or described

    - A printed word together with the grapheme corresponding to the target phoneme underlined

- *Continuum: Consequences*

Consequences are the events that follow the client's response. They can be positive ("reinforcement") or negative ("punishment"). Consequences are very powerful tools to help the client achieve high levels of acceptable responses.

  - **Nature of the feedback.** Positive reinforcement increases the probability that the acceptable response will occur again. SLPs have many ways of providing positive feedback, most of which depend on the maturity and needs of the client. These ways can range from a thumbs-up sign to a spoken "Good!" to a plus mark on a data sheet. It is usually helpful to provide positive feedback non-verbally so as not to erase the client's auditory and sensory trace of the correct production.

    Research suggests that the most effective way to provide negative feedback is simply to say "No," even though saying "No" is extremely difficult for most clinicians. However, one can say "No" in a playful manner ("Nope!" or "Oops!" or an exaggerated thumbs-down sign). It is also important to give concrete information about what to fix, for example, "Oops! Your tongue slipped down." The second way to deal with incorrect responses is to ignore them, although ignoring is less effective than saying "No." Nevertheless, ignoring incorrect responses may be acceptable for the occasional client who cannot tolerate even a playful approach to saying "No."

  - **Schedule of feedback.** Psychologists have known for a very long time that the schedule of reinforcement is a powerful conditioner for almost any type of behavior. When we want to elicit a target phoneme quickly, then we use a 100% reinforcement schedule for acceptable responses. However, this new behavior will quickly extinguish (disappear) unless we reduce the schedule of positive reinforcement. Consequently, when we start a new task or a new level, we often reinforce on a 100% schedule, but in order to maintain that new behavior we reduce the schedule of reinforcement. (Section 1 gives some examples of how to reduce the schedule of reinforcement.) At the end of the generalization phase, we need to be at a sparse level of positive reinforcement.

### The Clinical Question: With so many variables, how do we know which ones to manipulate?

The primary variables to manipulate are undoubtedly the length of the speech unit, the presence of models and cues, and the reinforcement, both nature and schedule. However, the other variables can be useful when the client comes up against a roadblock. Suppose, for example, that a client is working on /r/ and has been successful in CV(C) words that have front, mid, and low-back vowels, such as *read, rip, rake, wreck, rat, run,* and *rock*. However, when you introduce words with back vowels, especially the rounded ones, the client produces heavily labialized /r/. The sample words you have tried include *room, root,* and *road*. No doubt the lip rounding for the vowel has an influence on the /r/ production.

There are several ways to take a side branch in this case, but all of them involve having the client pay more attention to the sound form than to the meaning of what he is saying. Back at the nonsense syllable level, he either did not experience this problem, or it was dealt with there, so the clinician can take him back to the nonsense syllable level and gradually shift. For example, the instruction might be, "After I say these items, you say them, and make sure that the first part of each one sounds the same: /ru/.../ru/.../ruːm/." You would use a 100% schedule of positive reinforcement until these types of productions have stabilized, then you would back down to 50%. The next step is to eliminate the two preceding /ru/ syllables, first using just one, and then eliminating both, moving back to 100% reinforcement if needed. Finally, you acknowledge that /rum/ is a real word (*room*), model it, and ask the child to imitate with the same type of /r/ as was just practiced.

### Procedures that Promote Change over Establishment and Generalization Phases

There are certain procedures that promote change and that remain constant over the first two phases of intervention, that is, establishment and generalization. They are:

- Maintaining high numbers of correct responses per session
- Scheduling multiple short treatment sessions rather than fewer long sessions
- Maintaining high levels of correct production
- Incorporating client self-evaluation
- Incorporating speed drills
- Working in a variety of physical locations

As with so many aspects of intervention that have been presented so far, these procedures generally lack research support. However, some of them have been used in large-scale interventions, while others enjoy widespread agreement among published authorities.

### *Maintaining High Numbers of Responses per Session*

If we think about the process that the child went through in learning the error response, and if we consider her every utterance of a word with that error response as a unit of practice, then it is clear that the child usually has had several years and probably tens of thousands of units of practice on the old sound. Consequently, when we are working to lay down new motor patterns for the articulators, it is important that the client have enough practice to interfere with the "old" motor patterns. In the past, this idea has been called "drill," sometimes even with a sneer. I prefer, like Hoffman, Schuckers, and Daniloff (1989), to call this kind of practice "rehearsal." We have every reason to think that providing for rehearsal (many repetitions of a new speech sound pattern) is critically important to success in treatment.

Unfortunately, how many responses constitute the bare minimum undoubtedly depends on a number of factors, including some that characterize the child herself. Nevertheless, it is clear that high numbers of responses per session are likely to result in greater gains than low numbers of responses. Therefore, the clinician is challenged to organize the treatment session so that high numbers of responses are possible.

The necessity for extensive rehearsal is a variable that separates children with residual errors from children with phonological errors. Children whose errors are phonological and whose treatment is based on phonological processes typically do not need quantities of repetitive practice. Because their learning is at least partly cognitive-linguistic in nature, and because they are typically preschoolers who have not practiced their errors for a long time, they often start to generalize even without extensive motor practice.

### Scheduling Multiple Short Treatment Sessions Rather than Fewer Long Sessions

The motor learning literature appears to be unequivocal about the usefulness of distributed practice, that is, practice that is carried out in multiple short sessions rather than fewer longer sessions over the same time span (Ruscello, 1984). There is also evidence that distributed practice is beneficial for school-age children who are working to change residual errors. Consequently, if the SLP can schedule multiple short sessions, or arrange for someone else with a good ear to practice with the child for frequent short periods of time, this will very likely produce faster results than if the child is seen for just two sessions per week, however long those sessions are.

### Maintaining High Levels of Correct Production

One of the procedural goals that the SLP sets for himself is for the client to achieve almost errorless learning of motor patterns. In order to do this, the clinician must manipulate variables along certain continua so that the client consistently achieves high levels of correct production. In the *Monterey Articulation Program* (Baker & Ryan, 1971), the client is to perform at about 90% correct production in all steps of the program, and if she drops below 80% for three sessions, then remedial procedures are instituted. The Monterey Learning Institute, which has reportedly used its procedures with thousands of clients, claims that maintaining these high levels of production accuracy is critical to the client's success (Stan Dublinske, personal communication), although the Monterey authors have not published controlled studies on this topic. Nevertheless, when we are in the business of changing well-ingrained motor patterns, high levels of correct motor patterns would seem to be important.

### Incorporating Client Self-Evaluation

Many authors recommend incorporating self-evaluation into treatment procedures in order to promote rapid generalization of acceptable productions to additional linguistic structures or to additional situations. The research on the effectiveness of self-monitoring is equivocal. It is worth noting that the heavily operant systems of intervention, such as those from the Monterey Learning Institute (Baker & Ryan, 1971), include no self-evaluation procedures.

My own sense of the issue is that if self-evaluation is built into treatment from early on, it will promote generalization. Moreover, self-evaluation procedures can be defended on logical grounds with clients who are older than early school age, because the client will eventually have to serve as his/her own clinician during the maintenance phase of treatment. The use of self-evaluation requires that the child be able to make a metalinguistic decision correctly, a skill that likely develops after the preschool years.

Another consideration is that when the client is of school age or older, we assume that most of the residual errors are due to difficulties with the motor sequence, and not with the sound system of the language. With school-age clients we need to achieve at least a minimum of intentionality in speech sound production, and self-evaluation procedures can help to achieve this end.

Incorporating self-evaluation early means that even in the establishment phase, the client will be asked to make judgments of her own productions. Hopefully this task can be accomplished using nonverbal indicators, so that there is no interference with the client's sensory awareness of the motor and auditory pattern that was just produced.

### Incorporating Speed Drills

Consider the child who has to prolong and exaggerate a correctly produced phoneme in order to use it in a linguistic unit such as a sentence or discourse. This child, it is safe to say, is unlikely to generalize the correct target to connected speech outside of the clinic room. The child's production is just too effortful, and the prosody of the utterance is typically distorted. The difficulty arises because the child is not yet skilled (i.e., fast) at producing the new motor pattern or at adapting the new pattern to its phonetic environment.

One way to help the client acquire the skill is to provide speed drills. A speed drill is an exercise in which the client utters the correct target as fast as possible without compromising accuracy. This can happen at most stages of intervention, as follows:

- In the establishment phase, if the client is successful at the isolation level, such as for /s/: Ask the client to repeat the sound whenever you hold up your finger. The clinician starts somewhat slowly at first and then speeds up the task gradually.

- At the nonsense syllable or CV(C) word stage, the client can repeat syllables with a variety of vowels. For example, when working on /s/, the clinician might elicit sequences such as [sasasasasa] or [isisisis] or [koso koso koso] or [sasisasisasi] faster and faster until the child's accuracy of production threatens to erode.

- At the multisyllabic and phrase/sentence stages, these linguistic units can be said faster and faster until the client approximates a typical speaking rate with prosody and accuracy intact.

There is apparently only one published research study supporting the idea that speed drills might improve generalization (Bankson & Byrne, 1972). However, the motor learning literature strongly suggests that a skilled motor activity is not skilled until it can be done fast and automatically. The typical way to acquire this degree of skill is to start slowly and accurately, and gradually to increase the rate while maintaining accuracy. This is how musicians learn a new and difficult piece of music. Many athletic skills also need to be practiced this way.

## *Working in a Variety of Physical Locations*

The Monterey Learning Systems (Baker & Ryan, 1971) incorporate the idea of moving the physical location of the treatment session to other locations besides the usual treatment room. The idea is that the clinic room becomes a discriminant stimulus which is capable of eliciting improved productions of a target phoneme, while the rest of the client's life is conducted in spaces that do not promote improvement. Consequently, the more varied the spaces in which the clinician conducts treatment, the better the client's generalization, in the long run. There has been little research on this issue published in refereed journals. However, the idea of moving the place of the session around is a logical one.

In the Monterey programs, when the child is ready to work on maintenance, the move away from the treatment room is systematic. First, a session is conducted in the hallway right outside the treatment room. Then the next session is conducted down the hall. Then the next one might be in the child's classroom. SLPs can certainly think up other systematic progressions for their clients. Additionally, there is no reason why we would have to wait until the maintenance phase in order to shift treatment locations.

## THE MAINTENANCE PHASE

In the maintenance phase, the client assumes major responsibility for sound change, and client contacts with the SLP decrease in frequency. This phase can be considered the later part of the more traditional carryover period. The client is typically using the correct target phoneme in discourse most of the time in the clinic session. Generally, the client and the clinician plan together for the kinds of activities the client will engage in to help maintain awareness and accurate production of the target phonemes. Often the schedule of sessions drops from once a week to once every two weeks and then to once-a-month sessions. The clinician may talk with the client over the phone during the intervening periods of time to see how the client is doing.

The kind of generalization that needs to occur in the maintenance phase is primarily situational generalization, which has also been called carryover. Getting to this phase has already required a variety of types of generalization. The interested reader may wish to review Bernthal and Bankson (1998), pages 351–361, where the topic of generalization is explored. A key finding from Bernthal and Bankson's review is that while generalization can be expected under known conditions, individual children vary widely in the *rate* at which they show any type of generalization. Children also vary in the *extent* of generalization that they show.

My own view is that while situational carryover is a frequent bugaboo of practicing SLPs, these difficulties can be made a bit easier by incorporating motor learning principles early in remediation. That is, at the end of the generalization stage it is too late to turn to these principles. In particular, we can emphasize the importance of high rates of production within a session, high levels of correct production, early and frequent self-evaluation, and use of speed drills at all stages.

## NOVEL APPROACHES TO INTERVENTION FOR RESIDUAL ERRORS

In recent years, several authors have looked at the issue of providing treatment for phonetic disorders in light of an overall emphasis on communication and real-world activities. Hoffman, Schuckers, and Daniloff (1989) consider four domains to be appropriate for rehearsal: non-symbolic syllables, words and word pairs, sound-in-context sentences, and narratives. Their non-symbolic activities are much like the nonsense items presented earlier as part of speed drills, but without the emphasis on speed.

These authors advocate spending a great deal of rehearsal time on nonsense items that vary in a systematic way in order to ease their way into real speech. At the same time, they do not follow a linear progression from isolation to nonsense syllables to words to phrases, and so on. Rather, they may work on all phases in the same session. The child is engaged in an active way (e.g., in writing a skit in which he is to say words that he has or will practice intensively ahead of time). In other words, there are elements of whole language approaches in this paradigm.

Finally, Ertmer and Ertmer (1998) have presented a novel orientation to the issue of carryover. They posit that the child who achieves carryover easily is the child who displays "the directedness, motivation, and goal-orientation of self-regulated learners" (p. 70). They are also the children who are able to make use of metacognitive knowledge to achieve metacognitive control. That is, they are able to recognize when they are or are not performing as expected, they recognize that they have strategies to deal with the issue, and they are able to monitor subsequent performance. These authors suggest that children may need to be actively involved in planning of therapeutic activities and in developing strategies to carry the new behaviors into other settings.

Ertmer and Ertmer (1998) emphasize the importance of authentic communication tasks to help children achieve metacognitive control. These authors appear to agree with Hoffman, et al. (1989) that a strict linear progression through treatment need not be followed. They suggest that children be engaged in such performance activities as telling jokes and riddles, telling stories, and giving oral reports. The rehearsal process for such activities provides for multiple repetitions at the same time that the child is highly motivated to engage in them. The child can also develop strategies to use when needed. These authors also point out that many performance activities are likely to include speech that is not planned, and the child may be able to apply previously practiced strategies to this unexpected event.

These novel approaches to intervention for residual speech sound disorders are intriguing, not least because they make sense in terms of current thinking about the development of competent communicators. At the same time, we need to note that there is little, if any, empirical research to back up these approaches to intervention.

## Dismissal Criteria

As in most areas relating to treatment for speech sound disorders, there are few data to guide the SLP about when to dismiss a client from treatment. We do know that there is a substantial risk of regression associated with residual errors. Consequently, clinicians are likely to err on the side of caution and perhaps keep clients in treatment longer than necessary. On the other hand, it seems reasonable that clients should be performing at a very high level of acceptable productions both inside and outside the treatment room before we consider dismissal. In addition, we would expect the client who is ready to be dismissed to show high levels of retention between treatment sessions.

## DOCUMENTING PROGRESS

Speech-language pathologists have at their disposal several ways to document progress in treatment for residual errors. One of these ways is to graph or map the session-by-session treatment data. Another way is to probe the client's production system every so often. In Section 4 we described 30-item Sound Production Tasks (Elbert, Shelton, & Arndt, 1967), which are appropriate for use in the establishment and early generalization phases. Later on, three-minute conversational samples known as TALK samples are useful (Diedrich, 1971). TALK samples were also described in Section 4.

## Efficacy of Intervention for Residual Errors

Diedrich and Bangert (1980) published a series of studies of what was most likely "traditional" intervention coupled with operant behavioral techniques. However, these studies, while they generally found efficacious results, did not involve control groups. There have been few, if any, controlled studies of the effectiveness of traditional intervention, except for a few studies of specific aspects of this type of intervention. Nevertheless, this type of program is the treatment of choice for most clinicians when working with clients who have residual errors. It appears that most clinicians have seen for themselves that the traditional treatment "works."

## SUMMARY

Children with residual speech sound disorders often constitute a large proportion of a speech-language pathologist's caseload, yet in this area of practice, we have paid relatively little attention to making the process as efficient as possible. It is embarrassing for me to recommend practices that have little research backing, despite the fact that the recommended practices make sense from a motor-learning-for-communication point of view. I hope that over the next few years we can generate evidence that will lead our profession to best practices with residual speech sound disorders that have adequate research support.

**8**

# APPLICATIONS TO PARTICULAR POPULATIONS: DEVELOPMENTAL VERBAL DYSPRAXIA, ENGLISH AS A SECOND LANGUAGE, AND DEVELOPMENTAL DELAY

The focus of this chapter is on how we might apply information about speech-sound disorders to speech-sound difficulties in particular populations. Specifically, this chapter concerns clients who have Developmental Verbal Dyspraxia, in which the speech-sound system is clearly disordered, clients who speak English as a Second Language (ESL) and are poorly intelligible, and clients who have developmental delays.

## DEVELOPMENTAL VERBAL DYSPRAXIA

**Developmental Verbal Dyspraxia (DVD)** is a term used to designate children with a relatively severe impairment of speech-sound production (including prosody) that appears to have an important component of difficulty in planning and sequencing speech sounds. DVD is also called **Developmental Apraxia of Speech** (abbreviated **DAS** or **DAOS**) by some authors.

In order to understand dyspraxia, we need a clear understanding of praxis. **Praxis** is "the ability to select, plan, organize and initiate the motor pattern (for a particular action)" (Velleman & Strand, 1994). We become most aware of praxis when it "goes wrong." For example, adults who have sustained neurological damage may exhibit apraxia. Consider this man who has had a stroke resulting in apraxia: When you hand him a comb, he may be unable to demonstrate its function even though he correctly combed his own hair in front of a mirror just an hour before. In adults, a discrepancy between ease of performing so-called automatic tasks and performing the same task volitionally is a hallmark of apraxia.

In adults, difficulties with praxis that affect speech manifest themselves as groping, inconsistency of production, and severe limitations on the length of an utterance. Again, there is often a discrepancy between the patient's ready use of automatic or reflexive speech, such as swearing or saying the names of the days of the week, and the ability to say the same words volitionally. This disability is usually attributed to difficulty in sequencing movements to form words in a volitional way.

Most speech-language pathologists would agree on the existence of a group of children who have severe difficulty producing speech and whose disorder appears to have components of **dyspraxia**, that is, difficulty in planning and sequencing articulatory movements. They would agree that these children have more than just a severe phonological disorder. They would also agree that some of the signs of apraxia in adults would be missing because children have never been skilled users of speech and language. For example, in children there would not be a difference between automatic and volitional speech. And there the agreement would end.

The disagreements about Developmental Verbal Dyspraxia have been going on for many years. In the early years, the arguments concerned whether or not DVD existed as an entity separate from severe phonological disorder. At present, the arguments revolve around issues of definition—that is, how we determine which children belong in the group that has DVD. The issues are not trivial, because advances in our understanding of DVD may have been delayed due to lack of uniform definitions. At the same time, this is a rare disorder, and each researcher's pool of potential participants in DVD research is typically small and therefore likely to be unrepresentative of the whole.

Another factor to consider is that Developmental Verbal Dyspraxia may not always be a difficulty that is confined to the oral mechanism. Our colleagues in occupational therapy have worked with children who have problems in developing motor coordination (dyspraxia) for many years (Ayres, 1972; Portwood, 2000). The *DSM-IV-TR* Manual (American Psychological Association, 2000) labels these types of motor difficulties as Developmental Coordination Disorder. The criteria for diagnosing Developmental Coordination Disorder include performance on activities requiring motor coordination that is below expectations for the child's age and intelligence. This lack of coordination must be severe enough to "interfere with academic achievement or activities of daily living" (p. 56–57). In addition, there must not be any general medical condition such as cerebral palsy that could account for the difficulties, there must be no diagnosis of Pervasive Developmental Delay, and if mental retardation is present, it cannot be sufficient to account for the coordination difficulties.

We should note that there appears to be high co-morbidity (co-occurrence) between generalized dyspraxia and autistic-spectrum disorders. That is, many children with autism and similar disorders exhibit substantial generalized dyspraxia. However, dyspraxia can also exist by itself without being related to any kind of autistic-spectrum disorder.

## Recognizing DVD

Developmental Verbal Dyspraxia is usually diagnosed in otherwise healthy and cognitively normal children, although in some cases there may be a more generalized dyspraxia as well. Table 8-1 shows characteristics of DVD that have been mentioned in the literature. The material in Table 8-1 is also available in checklist form as Reproducible Form 12 in Appendix A.

**TABLE 8-1.** Characteristics of Developmental Verbal Dyspraxia that have been mentioned in the literature. Characteristics which have widespread support, and which some authorities consider to be strong indicators of DVD if they are present, are indicated with an asterisk. (This book calls the asterisked indicators *potential dyspraxic elements*.) It is well to note that Marquardt and Sussman (1991) consider the severity of reported DVD behaviors to be as diagnostic as their presence. A checklist version of this table is available as Reproducible Form 12.

### *Speech and Oral Behaviors*

1. Significant disturbances in intelligibility or naturalness* (Poor intelligibility is a common characteristic in young children who have DVD. Some older children who have undergone treatment have speech that is mostly intelligible, but slow and deliberate.)

2. Severely limited consonant repertory, with many omission errors*

3. Reduced syllable-shape inventory*

4. Assimilation and metathetic (transposition) errors*

5. Vowel errors*

6. Presence of an oral, non-verbal apraxia*

7. Groping for articulatory contacts*

8. Inconsistency in production, especially within the same word*

9. Increase in errors when word length increases or when word complexity increases*

10. Errors in prosody*

11. Increase in errors in connected speech compared to single words

12. Occasional well-articulated word that is not heard again*

*(continues)*

**TABLE 8-1.** *(continued)*

---

*History*

---

1. Poor feeding in infancy and/or persistent drooling after an age when most children reduce drooling

2. Sensory aversions such as tactile defensiveness in infancy and early childhood—that is, unwillingness to put certain textures or tastes in the mouth or to encounter certain textures on the skin

3. Relative silence during infancy

4. Generalized clumsiness

5. Slow progress in treatment*

---

*Non-Speech Indicators of Difficulty in Speaking*

---

1. Unwillingness or refusal to imitate modeled words

2. Well-developed gesture system to supplement speech*

3. Avoidance of speaking situations

4. Reliance on parent or older sibling as a translator

---

*Concomitant Characteristics*

---

1. Expressive language depressed in comparison to receptive language

2. Specific difficulty with vocabulary, especially word-finding

3. Signs typically associated with central neuromotor disorders: perseveration, difficulty inhibiting gestures or behaviors that interfere with production attempts, and evidence of fatigue relatively early in a task

---

It is no doubt obvious from the list in Table 8-1 that the "symptoms" of DVD are not always unique to DVD. For example, children who have severe phonological disorders often have very restricted consonant inventories, inconsistency in production, an increase in errors when word length increases or when word complexity increases, and an increase in errors in connected speech compared to single words. In addition, many children who have phonological disorders perform better in receptive language tasks than in expressive language tasks. Children with cerebral palsy or some other form of dysarthria may exhibit poor feeding in infancy, including persistent drooling after an age when most children reduce drooling, generalized clumsiness, and slow progress in treatment, as well as some of the central signs. Medically fragile children may experience sensory aversions, including tactile defensiveness, in infancy and early childhood.

We can raise other issues about some of the characteristics of DVD. For example, many writers consider inconsistency of production to be a hallmark of DVD. However, a young child with DVD who has very few speech sounds does not have much room to vary—that is, to demonstrate inconsistency. Consequently, inconsistency may be relevant only when the child has at least a small variety of consonants and vowels. Another example is the criterion of slow progress in treatment. We cannot always assume that the treatment offered to the child has been appropriate. If treatment is ineffective, then slow progress may not be exclusively a function of the disorder, but also a function of the therapy regime.

Finally, it is probably a mistake to talk about DVD as if it is an all-or-nothing diagnosis, because there appear to be degrees of difficulty with oral motor coordination (Bradford & Dodd, 1996; Crary, 1993; Strand & McCauley, 1999). For example, one 6-year-old child in my experience was making slow but regular progress on several sounds and had started to work on /θ/, for which he substituted [f]. The plan was to work for a short time on the sound in isolation and then go immediately to CVC words. However, we could not elicit /θ/ in those words, even if we helped him line up the tongue-tip posture before attempting the word. He would assume the [θ] posture, start the word, lose the posture, and say an [f]. It is true that many children do this kind of insertion of the old sound for a while, but most children manage to inhibit the old production in a short time, especially when dealing with sounds that are easy to see in a mirror. This child did not seem to have any ability to inhibit the [f], with or without a mirror. This difficulty in inhibiting an unwanted movement was so persistent and unusual that I considered it to be a potential dyspraxic element.

**Potential dyspraxic elements** are the kinds of behaviors that lead an experienced clinician to suspect that the child has unusual difficulty in planning and sequencing speech movements. In fact, we can think of the top two parts of Table 8-1 as a list of potential dyspraxic elements. These elements may not add up to a picture of DVD, but they nonetheless suggest that the clinician should incorporate some of the methods used for DVD into treatment. They also suggest that the clinician should be cautious about stating a prognosis.

## Theories of Developmental Verbal Dyspraxia

There are at least two types of conceptualizations of the origin of DVD (Davis, Jakielski, & Marquardt, 1998). One conceptualization is that DVD is purely a motor disorder in which the key deficit is difficulty in planning, initiating and carrying out motor sequences (e.g., Robin, 1992; Hall, Jordan, & Robin, 1993). An alternative conceptualization is that the underlying deficit is an inadequacy in the underlying representations of speech segments and suprasegmentals, so that there may be cognitive and linguistic difficulties as well as motor sequencing difficulties (e.g., Velleman & Strand, 1994). The latter is supported by findings that children with presumed DVD have difficulties with auditory perception of speech (Bridgeman & Snowling, 1988) and that these children may also have deficits in vocabulary (Velleman & Strand, 1993). Still another conceptualization is that of a motor-linguistic deficit that includes the translation from idea (meaning) to planning and executing the required motor movements (e.g., Crary, 1993).

Aram (1984) proposed a definition of what she called Developmental Verbal Apraxia as a syndrome complex. By this she means that "diagnosis (would) not depend on identification of *the* distinguishing characteristics, and any single characteristic may overlap with other developmental speech and language disorder" (p. 3 of Preface). Instead, there is a cluster or constellation of difficulties that leads to the diagnosis of developmental verbal apraxia.

My own view of the source of DVD is a hybrid of all of these conceptualizations. In particular, I consider DVD to be primarily a disorder in the planning and execution of sequences of movements, but I also think that the expressive vocabulary deficits that frequently accompany DVD are in fact attributable to the DVD. Even receptive vocabulary is often depressed in these children, that is, *if* the investigator actually assesses it rather than relying on clinical judgment. The same disordered motor processes that may impinge on expressive vocabulary can also influence the child's receptive vocabulary.

One way to think about the vocabulary deficit is to hypothesize that in normally developing children, their productions of a word provide kinesthetic, auditory, and other sensory information from their own articulators to the brain, which in turn uses the information to form a kind of phonetic template for the word. This template has connections with an underlying and abstract representation of the segments in the word (based on phonemes), with the meaning (or meanings) of the word, with semantic features associated with each meaning, with a coding for syntax (part of speech) and another for morphology (such as regular or irregular plural), and often, with non-linguistic information about the context in which the word was learned. All of these bits of information have connections with each other as well. If the information generated by the child's motor system is variable or inconsistent, as we might expect in a child with DVD, then the phonetic template will be "fuzzy," that is there may be numerous overlapping templates with varying strength of links to the underlying phonological representation. For example, if the child says the name *Ken* as [kʌm], [kɛd], [dʌŋ], and [gʌŋk], the kinesthetic and other sensory feedback is going to be quite variable. There may be some overlap in representations, because at least the child always knows that he is attempting to say *Ken*, but the individual versions are not going to converge on just one template.

The connections between this child's fuzzy phonetic templates and the phonological, semantic, syntactic-morphological, and contextual representations will not be strong because the child does not repeatedly access the same neural networks. Rather, the child may access one or another of the multiple versions that that he has produced while intending the same word, or he may come up with a new version. Unfortunately, when this child next intends to say his friend Ken's name, the pathways between the intent (semantic domain) and any one of these many phonetic versions will be weak. If the child does finally come up with an approximation to say when naming Ken, then there is no way to predict which version eventually will come out of his mouth.

In formal expressive vocabulary testing of children with DVD, we would expect their performance to show not only delays due to accessing problems, but also frequent substitution of semantically related words because weak connections may lead them astray and into forms that have stronger connections with semantics. For example, if internal monologue were involved in naming a picture of a *goat,* it might go like this: "That's an animal with horns. I saw one once on Aunt Kay's farm. It must be a – a – a [dok]. No, it's a – a – a – a [gat]. Can that be right? Animal with horns, animal with horns—DEER!"

How do we account for *receptive* vocabulary deficits under this conceptualization? Presumably, what happens in typically developing children when they respond to language receptively is that they try to match the form that they hear to a phonetic template stored in the brain. From that, they determine the meaning by accessing the links between the stored template and the underlying phonological representation, and from there to the meaning, syntax, and so on. If the child has a fuzzy phonetic template (capable of generating a variety of forms that are mostly incorrect by adult standards), then there will first of all be difficulty in making the match. The second difficulty will come in trying to access the phonological form because the links between each phonetic template and the corresponding phonological form will be weak.

It is interesting that one of the most robust findings concerning the adult lexicon is that words that have many similar-sounding words in their "similarity neighborhood" take longer to access receptively than words that occupy sparse similarity neighborhoods (Charles-Luce, Luce, & Vitevitch, 2000). We may assume that the similarity neighborhood would exist at both the phonetic and the phonological levels. For example, the word *pot* is in a dense similarity neighborhood of words such as *cot, hot, not, lot, shot, rot, got, pock, pom, pod, pop, spot, pit, pat,* and many, many more. In contrast, the word *job* is in a sparse similarity neighborhood—for example, *jot, jock, john, joss, bob, lob, knob,* and so forth. Theories of the lexicon suggest that a person would access the word *job* in a shorter time than the word *pot*. This access time is considered to be an index of the work involved in retrieval. Children also show effects of density of the similarity neighborhood (Jusczyk, Storkel, & Vitevitch, 2000).

So we may suppose that when a child with DVD tries to access a particular word receptively, she finds a number of phonetic templates that she has generated for the same word in the neighborhood, as well as legitimate words that are similar sounding, perhaps including the target word. If we take the example of *pot* above, the child might know a number of the words in the neighborhood as well as having several forms for *pot*—for example, [paʔ], [bat], [ba], [pap], [βa], and other variants. In fact, the similarity neighborhood is made denser by the addition of the child's numerous variants. Given the confusion that this arrangement could engender, we can make two predictions for performance of children with DVD on a receptive vocabulary test:

1. For words that we have reason to believe the child has been exposed to, we would expect to see (a) slow response times for correct choices, and (b) error choices that are semantically related.

2. For words that the child probably does not know, she points at random, just as a typically developing child would do.

We might wonder about whether there really is any role at all for kinesthetic feedback to the brain in the development of vocabulary. After all, some babies who have had tracheostomies near the time of birth and have been on ventilators for a long time catch up quickly to their peer group in vocabulary and talkativeness when the tracheostomy tube is removed. Thus, we could argue that oral motor experience of a word cannot play the major role in laying down a word's neural connections—rather, auditory information, which such babies typically have had, is far more important. However, it is worth noting that such babies typically do not produce words right away when the normal airway is restored (Ken Bleile, 2001, personal communication). Rather, they go through a babbling period and then an acquisition period. In other words, they are getting feedback from the articulators and the ear at the same time, and this seems to be a necessary precursor to producing meaningful words.

## Diagnosis of Developmental Verbal Dyspraxia

Because of the long history of disagreements over the definition (hence the diagnosis) of DVD, there is no generally agreed upon list of characteristics. Some authors, such as Shriberg and colleagues (Shriberg, Aram, & Kwiatkowski, 1997a and 1997b), have tried to find a "diagnostic marker" for DVD—that is, a symptom that is shared by a substantial proportion of children with DVD. The importance of a diagnostic marker is that if one can be found, then it is possible to study a group of children with DVD that is relatively homogeneous. We can then interpret results with more confidence than if the group under study is inherently heterogeneous. Shriberg, Aram, and Kwiatkowski (1997a; 1997b) found that disorders of prosody appeared to characterize a subgroup of children with DVD, but not all children with DVD.

In contrast to the efforts of Shriberg and colleagues, other investigators appear to use a definition of DVD based on "the preponderance of the evidence." For example, Hickman (1997) has constructed a test of DVD, *The Apraxia Profile*, in which the clinician asks the child to perform a large number of oral non-verbal and speech tasks. The clinician then goes through a long list of possible characteristics of DVD and determines whether or not the child exhibits DVD. Definitions based on preponderance of the evidence are actually the most commonly used definitions in the research literature. They are also the bases for diagnoses derived from administering such tests as the *Screening Test for Developmental Apraxia of Speech* by Blakely (1980) and the *Verbal Motor Production Assessment for Children* by Hayden and Square (1999).

However, we have reason to be cautious about checklists. The reason for the caution is that the longer the checklist, the more opportunities there are to check off potentially deviant behaviors, and it will soon start to look like the client actually has DVD. For example, if we check only three behaviors in a list of 10 possibilities, we are likely to be more cautious about declaring that the client has DVD than we are if we check 15 behaviors in a list of 50, even though the percentage checked is the same—30%. In addition, the application of a rubric about "the preponderance of the evidence" will clearly result in heterogeneous groups of subjects in any investigation of DVD.

In recent years, some investigators have become quite cautious about diagnosing DVD for purposes of research. Davis, Jakielski, and Marquardt (1998), for example, consider high levels of variability to be diagnostic, assuming that the client has a severe phonological disorder. Shriberg, Aram, and Kwiatowski (1997a, 1997b) have implicated prosody as a diagnostic marker.

Given the lack of agreement even among researchers who know a great deal about Developmental Verbal Apraxia, what is the concerned SLP to do about a child who appears to have DVD? First of all, the SLP should be aware that this is not the thorny problem that the controversy would suggest. After all, the child clearly has some behaviors or characteristics that raise concerns about DVD. Those characteristics need to be taken into account in planning intervention regardless of whether or not a diagnosis of DVD is warranted. Table 8-2 provides a way to think about these diagnostic issues.

**TABLE 8-2.** Strategies for assessment of potential Developmental Verbal Dyspraxia and similar disorders. These strategies are based on the purposes of the assessment.

---

A. If the purpose of the evaluation is clinical—that is, the results are to be used in diagnosis and planning of treatment—then use a rubric based on the preponderance of the evidence. Many references and several tests of verbal apraxia provide such lists, as does Table 8-1.

B. If the purpose of the evaluation is clinical, as in (A) above, but there is a possibility that this client might participate in a retrospective study at some time in the future, then document as many criteria as possible, including at least the more generally accepted characteristics from Table 8-1 and the criteria used in restrictive definitions, such as that of Davis, Jakielski, and Marquardt (1998). Their definition assumes severe phonological impairment, including these key characteristics (p. 41):

- Variability of productions of both C and V

- Vowel errors

- Suprasegmental variability (including possibly vocal quality, syllable and word stress, word and sentence intonation, and loudness dynamics)

---

Table 8-2 is based on the purpose of the evaluation. If our purpose is exclusively clinical, then we need a portrait of the child's strengths and weaknesses. Consequently, we will be interested in how to take these strengths and weaknesses into account, and documenting "the preponderance of the evidence" is a good way to do this. Sometimes we may even find the label of DVD useful in counseling parents and recommending appropriate types and levels of service. Finally, if this clinical case could possibly be used in research in the future, then the clinician should document all generally agreed-upon indicators of DVD, including particularly the ones used in restrictive definitions.

There is sometimes a question about which professionals can legitimately diagnose DVD, and some clinicians seem to think that only a child neurologist can do this. However, I maintain that the SLP is the only professional who will have all the critical information for making the diagnosis of Developmental Verbal Dyspraxia. Having said that, I also think that referral to a child neurologist is often appropriate as follow-up to the diagnosis because the child may have related deficits that need to be documented and possibly treated. The SLP who is interested in learning more about diagnostic issues and procedures with children who are suspected of having DVD should consult the excellent work by Hall, Jordan, and Robin (1993), Hodge (1994), Hodge and Hancock (1994), Crary (1993), and several chapters in the book by Caruso and Strand (1999).

## PROCEDURES TO EVALUATE AND DOCUMENT DEVELOPMENTAL VERBAL DYSPRAXIA

### Background

**WHO?**    A child of almost any age who is severely delayed in developing speech or who is having exceptional difficulty making progress with treatment.

**WHAT?**    A series of assessments designed to assess the possibility that the child has Developmental Verbal Dyspraxia, which is usually defined as difficulty in planning and executing sequences of articulatory movements for speech.

**WHY?**    Children who have Developmental Verbal Dyspraxia often need different procedures from children whose speech-sound disorder is regarded as phonological in nature.

**WHEN?**    This type of assessment is done when the clinician suspects DVD based on a speech-language pathologist's observation of the client. Failure to make progress in treatment also may trigger this type of evaluation.

**SUPPORT:**    A great deal has been written about assessment of DVD for the purpose of providing appropriate types of intervention. Some examples include Hall, Jordan, and Robin (1993), Davis, Jakielski, and Marquardt (1998), Strand and McCauley (1999), Hodge (1994), and Hodge and Hancock (1994).

## PROCEDURES TO EVALUATE AND DOCUMENT DEVELOPMENTAL VERBAL DYSPRAXIA

### *Procedure*

The assessment procedures for possible DVD include a very thorough evaluation in many areas. Nevertheless, the judgment that the client does or does not exhibit DVD is, in the end, a clinical judgment.

I. Obtain a careful clinical history, including questions about the presence/absence of at least the following characteristics:

- Poor feeding in infancy, including persistent drooling after an age when most children reduce drooling

- Sensory aversions such as tactile defensiveness in infancy and early childhood, including an unwillingness to put certain textures or tastes in the mouth or to encounter certain textures on the skin

- Relative quiet as an infant
- Generalized clumsiness
- Slow progress in treatment
- Unwillingness or refusal to imitate modeled words
- Well-developed gesture system to supplement speech
- Avoidance of speaking situations
- Reliance on parent or older sibling as a translator

II. Screen or assess hearing.

III. Assess speech production, and make the best audio or video recording possible. Most often this assessment would include an inventory test of articulation and/or a test of phonological processes, with special attention to idiosyncratic phonological processes.

IV. Make a good recording of spontaneous conversation. Gloss and transcribe this recording, being as complete as possible. The related analyses and measures that are typically made with this information should be carried out for the child with possible DVD:

- Percent of Consonants Correct (Shriberg & Kwiatkowski, 1982a).
- In addition, determine the Percent of Vowels Correct (Shriberg, 1993) from this sample.
- Percent of Intelligible Words (Shriberg & Kwiatkowski, 1982a)
- Ratings of voice and prosody (see Reproducible Form 2). For prosody, pay special attention to word-level and sentence-level stress patterns. Make notes about any variability in vocal quality and variability in suprasegmentals.
- Ratings of the child's speaking rate and fluency. Note that for speaking rate, poor intelligibility often makes listeners think that the speaker is talking fast, probably because the listener needs more time to process the speech. Consequently, an objective measure is needed. Note that for fluency, a child with very severely disordered speech may produce many syllables that sound the same. It can be very difficult to determine if these are disfluencies or not.

V. Using the client's responses to a formal speech assessment instrument, supplemented with information from the connected speech sample and any other formal or informal observations about the child's productions, develop the following:

- For preschoolers and children with very restricted sound systems:
  - Phonetic Inventory for Consonants (Reproducible Form 3)
  - Phonetic Inventory for Vowels (Reproducible Form 4)
  - Syllable and Word-Shape Inventory (Reproducible Form 5)
- For all children:
  - Segmental Inventory for Consonants (Reproducible Form 6) and for Clusters (Reproducible Form 7)
  - Segmental Inventory for Vowels (Reproducible Form 8)

VI. Although some authors consider inconsistency of production to be a hallmark of DVD, there is no generally accepted procedure for determining that a child is or is not consistent. Consequently, the SLP should be alert to inconsistencies in production, especially inconsistencies that occur when the same word is produced multiple times, as well as inconsistencies that affect the same phoneme in the same word position. These inconsistencies should be documented by listing them. The clinician should also note the degree to which these inconsistencies make the child's pattern unpredictable.

VII. Although some researchers consider groping movements during speech and non-speech tasks to be an important indicator of DVD, there is no standard way to evaluate these behaviors. Therefore the SLP should make careful notes about any such behaviors that are observed.

VIII. Administer a normed assessment of the child's motor speech system. Two possible instruments include the *Apraxia Profile* (Hickman, 1997) and the *Verbal Motor Production Assessment for Children* (*VMPAC*—Hayden & Square, 1999). If the assessment instrument does not include sequences of non-speech oral movements, such as "smile, then stick out your tongue," be sure to include some in your evaluation.

IX. Evaluate receptive and expressive language, as well as pragmatics. Many children who have severe phonological disorders are unable to produce the unstressed syllables and morphological endings required in English morphology. Consequently, evaluation of spoken language needs to be made cautiously. However, the mean length of utterance can provide important baseline information on development in this area. In addition, a test of expressive naming may be important because children with DVD often have difficulty with this type of task.

At the end of all these assessments, go through a checklist such as the one in Reproducible Form 12. Based on the preponderance of the evidence, determine a diagnosis, such as "definite DVD," "probable DVD," or "phonological disorder with potential dyspraxic elements."

## Treatments for Developmental Verbal Dyspraxia

It should come as no surprise that there are numerous treatments for DVD. It should also come as no surprise, given the controversial nature of the area, that the various treatments for DVD tend to have strong advocates, that is, professionals who write about or give workshops on their preferred treatment. Further, despite the emphasis of some investigators on linguistic deficits being an inherent part of DVD, there are few interventions that are directed at the proposed linguistic components. Rather, almost all treatments are directed at the motor speech system. Finally, it is clear from report after report that traditional treatment, with its emphasis on remediating one sound at a time, is *not* appropriate for children with DVD unless they are older and have only a few residual errors.

The various treatments for DVD are of several types: those that emphasize principles of motor programming, those that incorporate touching or manual molding of the child's articulators, those that impose speech on a suprasegmental pattern, those with a sensorimotor focus, those that are basically phonological interventions, those that are both motor and linguistic in orientation, and those that seek to increase strength and agility of the oral musculature. There is, of course, considerable overlap in emphases and techniques among all these approaches.

### Treatments Based on Motor Programming Principles

Treatments for DVD that are based on motor programming have been carefully articulated by several authors (e.g., Hall, Jordan, & Robin, 1993; Strand & Skinder, 1999; Marquardt & Sussman, 1991; Velleman & Strand, 1994). Typically, these approaches resemble traditional intervention in their use of a bottom-up approach (syllables, then CV or CVC words, then more complex words, then phrases, and so on), and in their reliance on clinician models and client imitations. Some of the authors cited above rely on normal developmental sequences in choosing targets.

Where these motor programming approaches for DVD differ from traditional treatment is in their use of inputs from multiple modalities, in their emphasis on accurate vowels as well as accurate consonants, in their manipulation of prosody, and in their careful attention to principles of motor learning. For example, most of these authors emphasize the need for intensive drill distributed over many short treatment sessions.

Strand and Skinder (1999) have called these approaches "integral stimulation methods," after Milisen (1954), and their terminology and emphases will be reported here. One area that Strand and Skinder discuss is the number of stimuli, such as syllables or words, to be trained at any one time. These authors use the severity of the child's disorder as their guide. Thus the child with very severe DVD may work on only five or six different stimuli at one time, whereas a child with less involvement could deal with eight to ten stimuli. These authors also echo Velleman & Strand (1994) in their incorporation of functional vocabulary (e.g., *no, mine*) into the stimulus materials whenever it is feasible. Functional vocabulary is important because many children with DVD have speech so unintelligible that they are routinely frustrated in trying to communicate their wishes.

Finally, Strand and Skinder (1999) discuss the issues relating to keeping a young child motivated when massive amounts of drill are needed. They point out that careful planning to keep the child working at a high level of success is critical. They also report that making minor changes in the procedures every so often is helpful, even such minor alterations as shifting body position every 10 responses, or having the child do 10 responses with an altered hand position.

## Treatments that Incorporate Touching or Molding of Articulators

There are several variations on treatment for DVD in which the clinician cues oral positioning by touching or molding the articulators, including Prompts for Restructuring Oral Muscular Phonetic Targets (PROMPT—Chumpelik, 1984; Square, 1999) and the Touch-Cue Method (Bashir, Grahamjones, & Bostwick, 1984). The PROMPT technique will be used as an exemplar of approaches that require touching or molding of articulators. In PROMPT treatment, the clinician cues a child about the articulatory placement of a speech sound using a well-defined system of cues that are implemented by touching the child's face or neck while providing a model of the desired response. Sequences of sounds are similarly cued using sequences of touch cues. Specialized training is needed for speech-language pathologists who want to use PROMPT techniques.

## Treatments that Impose a Suprasegmental Pattern on Speech

One treatment that has shown promise with children who have DVD is a variant of Melodic Intonation Therapy (MIT), which was originally developed for adults with aphasia. Helfrich-Miller (1984) modified MIT for use with children and has reported considerable success for two children with DVD. Thus the child is asked to produce speech with a particular intonation contour and rhythm, and this attention to prosody appears to facilitate phoneme production. It should be noted that the Helfrich-Miller adaptation also has an emphasis on the linguistic components of speech, in that the stimuli are chosen precisely because they represent syntactic forms and vocabulary needed for effective communication.

## Treatment with a Sensory-Motor Focus

One of the earliest well-defined interventions for articulation disorders was that of McDonald (1964a). Although McDonald did not mention a condition like DVD or DAS, his approach has two areas of focus that are helpful for DVD. The first of these is the idea of starting every session with a kind of "babbling" practice, in which the child is encouraged to produce strings of syllables containing phonemes that are already in his repertoire. These syllable strings are produced with a variety of stress and intonation patterns, always with an emphasis on accuracy of the speech-sound productions. The syllables might be CV or VC syllables, and they would typically be nonsense syllables. McDonald's goal appears to be an increase in the child's ability to sequence the motor patterns of phonemes with normal timing and coarticulation. It is precisely a deficit in this ability appears to be at the heart of Developmental Verbal Dyspraxia.

The second aspect of sensorimotor therapy that is helpful with children who have DVD is its emphasis on facilitating contexts. It should be noted that the McDonald Deep Test (1964b) was developed to aid in discovery of facilitating contexts for various phonemes; however, that test is probably far advanced for many children with DVD. (In any event, it is out of print at this time.) Nevertheless, McDonald's emphasis on moving from more facilitating contexts to less facilitating contexts is very useful concept in the treatment of DVD.

## Phonological Treatments

Preschool children who have DVD may have the same kinds of difficulties in figuring out the phonological system of the ambient language that other children of similar ages exhibit. In such cases their poor intelligibility may stem from a general phonological disorder *and* from a specific difficulty in sequencing commands to produce speech. That said, we should remember that these two sources may produce similar effects. In other words, most of the standard phonological processes appear to simplify the child speaker's task, but so do many of the errors attributed to children who have DVD.

In any event, aspects of phonological treatments that help the child to learn the patterns of the language should be helpful to preschoolers and early school-age children with DVD. These include auditory bombardment (Hodson & Paden, 1991), simultaneous work on multiple exemplars of the same phonological process (a feature of several phonological approaches), use of minimal pairs to demonstrate phonemic contrasts, and work with meaningful words and phrases as much as possible.

## Treatments Based on Both Motoric and Linguistic Considerations

Crary (1993) and his co-authors have articulated the importance of including a linguistic planning component in treatment programs. By this they mean that not only does the child practice sounds in isolation, words, and phrases, but she also has experience in slotting appropriate word forms into sentences and experience in formulating narratives using newly learned sounds and words. Crary regards a motor planning component as intrinsic to linguistic aspects of communication.

The Pressure Points intervention (Smit, 2000), as described in Section 6, is another approach that combines motor and linguistic aspects of intervention for preschoolers with severe phonological delays (some of whom undoubtedly have DVD). The stimuli for this approach are chosen so that when the child produces a sound in a word correctly, the word will be completely correct and intelligible to others and can be used immediately in communication. Although this early intervention has not been expanded to further stages of intervention, a logical expansion of this concept is that the child would be expected to produce appropriate syntactic forms, such as plurals, in naturalistic drills and in conversation.

## Oral-Motor Exercises

Oral-motor treatments constitute yet another possible route for intervention for Developmental Verbal Dyspraxia. There is no uniform definition of what constitutes an oral-motor treatment; however, for purposes of this discussion, oral-motor treatments include all interventions intended to increase strength and agility of the structures of articulation and respiration. These exercises are often presented not only as ways to increase strength and agility, but also to promote normal oral-facial tactile sensation, increase functional differentiation of the head and face from the rest of the body, build muscle tone, and heighten proprioception (e.g., Boshart, 1998). Many of the concepts and techniques used in oral-motor therapy have been borrowed from the field of occupational therapy.

Oral-motor treatments have been promoted for both phonological disorders and for DVD. They have a certain intuitive appeal, because it seems obvious that the muscles must be strong enough to be used for the complexities of speech, and the articulators must be agile enough to reach specified positions quickly. There are a number of assumptions that follow from this intuitive position, as Forrest (2002) has noted. One assumption is that a complex behavior can be broken down into its parts and that practice on the parts will improve learning of the whole pattern. Another assumption is that speech activities emerge from the structures used for vegetative functions such as swallowing; consequently, oral-motor exercises may improve the basis or substrate for speech.

Unfortunately, there is little evidence that oral-motor exercises do what they are intended to do—namely, improve speech production. Furthermore, there is evidence from the few studies that have incorporated controls that these exercises do not, in fact, improve speech. Forrest (2002) has recently undertaken a review of the role of oral-motor exercises with children who have phonological disorders and has also related this work to the motor learning literature. She notes a much-replicated finding in the rather large literature on acquisition of complex behaviors, namely that training on constituent parts of such behaviors actually reduces the learning of these behaviors.

When it comes to strength training of the speech musculature, there is a definitional hurdle to overcome, namely that if the child has demonstrated weakness of the muscles, that child is by definition dysarthric rather than having a phonological disorder or a dyspraxic disorder (Forrest, 2002). Strength training may indeed be warranted in cases of dysarthria, but there is no reason to undertake strength training for children who have a phonological disorder or DVD without a demonstrated loss of strength.

The findings to date seem counterintuitive until we consider one of the key facts about speech: Speech rides very lightly on the vegetative capabilities of the oral, laryngeal, and respiratory systems. In other words, speech uses little of the capacity of the speech musculature. For example, in respiration, the part of the lung volume used for speech is usually only a small portion of the very large Vital Capacity (although singers and actors can train themselves to use more of that capacity). Similarly, phonation requires very little subglottal pressure compared to the very large pressures that the system is capable of generating. Similarly, the tongue-tip-alveolar pressures used in speaking represent only a fraction of the pressures that can be generated and that might be available for chewing, feeding, and swallowing. Consequently, if the child with a phonological or dyspraxic disorder can handle feeding well, eats typical foods, and is well-nourished, it is highly likely that the oral mechanism has more than enough strength for the production of speech.

With respect to agility, it is difficult to know what is meant by the term when it is applied to structures of the head and neck. Agility generally means the ability to move and respond quickly and efficiently when necessary. Presumably, oral agility means that the oral, pharyngeal, laryngeal, and respiratory structures can respond easily when asked to produce normal speech. Agility must in large part be related to strength, if only because a weak muscle will move an articulator sluggishly, if at all. It appears therefore that if strength is adequate for speech, then agility is also likely to be adequate for speech. Clinical Note 8-1 relates some personal experiences with oral-motor tasks.

---

CLINICAL NOTE 8-1:  How I Learned to Distrust Oral Gymnastics

When I was working on my dissertation study, I had to locate a number of 5-year-old children who had very good articulation to serve as controls for two groups of speech-disordered children. The children in the study had to meet the criterion of having a normal mechanism, and so I did a fairly cursory examination of the oral mechanism, including such oral gymnastics as "Touch your nose with your tongue."

I remember being astonished at the number of these oral non-verbal movements that the super-normal control group could not do, or if they did perform them, it was with groping and hesitancy. Surely, if skill at making such oral movements was related to speaking ability, these children should have serious phonological problems. Yet they had exceptionally good speech. I came to the reluctant conclusion that there was no relationship between ability to carry out oral gymnastics and speaking ability.

Later on, I had a client who was 6 years old and clearly had Developmental Verbal Dyspraxia. He drooled a bit, so we attempted to evaluate oral strength and sensation. Lo and behold, he could not puff out his cheeks, clearly a sign of inadequate strength in the lips! However, the child came to the next session, after a weekend, as proud as could be because he could now puff out his cheeks. His parent said that the child had gone home and figured out how to do this maneuver by trying in out in front of a mirror. To me, this meant that the child did *not* have labial weakness. Rather, he had not figured out the gimmick of sealing both the lips and the tongue in order to trap air in the cheeks.

Instances such as these suggest that oral gymnastics, which are meant to assess the adequacy of the mechanism for speech, in fact assess nothing of the sort. Instead, they probably assess the degree to which a child has experimented with his/her mechanism.

---

There are also problems with claims that oral-motor exercises promote normal oral-facial tactile sensation, increase functional differentiation of the head and face from the rest of the body, build muscle tone, and heighten proprioception, because there is little, if any, evidence that such efforts are related to speech. For example, although proprioception is undoubtedly important during speech, there is little evidence that poor proprioception accounts for phonological or apraxic disorders, nor is there evidence that we can improve oral proprioception, let alone improve speech by improving oral proprioception.

Many of the emphases in these techniques have been borrowed from concepts behind Neurodevelopmental Treatment and/or Sensory Integration in occupational therapy. Unfortunately, research into the efficacy of Neurodevelopmental Treatment with the pediatric population is inconclusive (Brown & Burns, 2001). Sensory Integration is apparently used by 99% of occupational therapists who work with children (Watling, Deitz, Kanny, & McLaughlan, 1999). Nevertheless, there is little empirical evidence that Sensory Integration is effective in occupational therapy in general (Vargas & Camilli, 1999), or for autism (Dawson & Watling, 2000; Gresham, Beebe-Frankenberger, & MacMillan, 1999). Consequently, speech-language pathologists need to be cautious about embracing concepts from Neurodevelopmental Treatment and Sensory Integration therapy.

## Modifying Treatment to Reduce Later Word Retrieval Problems

Several authors have reported that many children with DVD appear to have difficulty with semantics. This difficulty usually shows up as a word retrieval problem, but it is sometimes evident also in word recognition. Very likely this problem stems from the child's hypothesized difficulty in establishing underlying representations for words. In turn, because underlying representations are at best incomplete in these children, the links between stored phonological/phonetic forms and aspects of meaning are likely to be weak. Strengthening all of these links is likely to promote access to vocabulary.

For this reason, it is important when working with children who have DVD to maximize connections between phonological form and meaning. When we present a picture to use in motor drill, we should always say something about it. For example, if the child is working on words with initial /k/, and *cow* is one of the pictures, the SLP could say, "Cow. A cow gives milk. Cow." At the next presentation of the word, the SLP can say something different, such as "Cow. We see cows on farms. Cow."

Equally important is that the child should say the target word many times in response to these stimuli. For example, if the minimal pair *ship* and *tip* are being used to emphasize phonemic differences, the clinician might ask, "Which one is at the end of a pencil?" (Pause for response.) "And which one goes in water?" (Pause.) "And which one carries many people?" (Pause.) "And which one is at the end of your finger?" (Pause.) The child will have produced each word twice in a context that emphasizes the semantic components of these two vocabulary items.

## When Speech-Language Intervention Is Not Enough

There are some children who have DVD who either will not become effective oral communicators, or who will have need of augmentation of their oral speech. The speech-language pathologist should always keep in mind the child's current and future communication needs. If a child who is making slow progress in intervention is having social or academic difficulties due to poor oral communication, then augmentation should be considered. This decision is best taken early rather than late in the child's therapy experience, so that the child's frustration as a communicator does not build to an insurmountable point. One possibility that has been reported in the literature is augmentation with signs, as in Total Communication (e.g., Gibbs, Sherman-Springer, & Cooley, 1990)). We should note, however, that if signing is to be successful, the child should not have a significant limb apraxia. Other possibilities include low-tech or high-tech augmentative or alternative (AAC) devices.

Finally, Hall, Hardy, and LaVelle (1990) reported that certain children with DVD can benefit from using a palatal lift. This intervention may seem extreme in children who do not have a defined motor weakness of the soft palate; nevertheless, in the reported cases, the presence of the lift apparently reduced the motor sequential load on the child's planning of speech messages. These authors reported that improved speech production and intelligibility was the result.

## Efficacy of Treatments for DVD

A number of authors have presented one or more case studies using their recommended forms of intervention for children with DVD. However, there have been few controlled studies, and no group studies. There is one experimental study with one subject which suggests that an MIT-based approach leads to better productions than a touch-cue type of approach (see Clinical Note 8-2), but otherwise there is little evidence that one form of intervention is more effective than another. Despite the lack of comparative research, however, it should be noted that most authorities on DVD rule out traditional treatment on the grounds that it is not appropriate for such children.

CLINICAL NOTE 8-2:  A Head-to-Head Comparison
Between a Touch-Cue Method and an Intonation Method
to Treat Developmental Verbal Dyspraxia

A 1996 Master's thesis by Colleen Wade at Kansas State University was a direct comparison between a touch-cue method and an intonation method. The client was a child, AM, who had just turned three when the study began. She had severe phonological delay with DVD, as diagnosed by a speech-language pathologist and by a pediatric neurologist (see the thesis for details). AM used few consonants (none consistently), and she had many vowel errors. Her word shapes were primarily combinations of CV syllables, although she also used CVC occasionally. She was quite unintelligible except to her family when they knew the context. Typical utterances taken from a conversational sample at the onset of intervention included:

| | |
|---|---|
| "Don't want it here." | [ʌʔwawahʌ] |
| "It's full now." | [əhaha] |
| "It's stuck." | [haʔndʌʔ] |
| "I want that." | [ənʌhə] |
| "It's on my toe." | [ʌbʌdaa:dʌ] |

AM had been in treatment for a year by the time that this study began. The first half of the year was spent in treatment with a focus on improving expressive language and intelligibility; however, there was little change. The second half of that year was focused on articulation and on overcoming tactile defensiveness around the mouth. Progress in articulation was negligible, although the tactile defensiveness decreased considerably.

Colleen Wade chose to compare the two approaches using a single-subject design called alternating treatments (McReynolds & Kearns, 1983). In each session, she did 15 minutes of intervention using one method and then 15 minutes using the other method. The order was alternated each session in order to control for sequence effects. Also, in order to ensure that AM discriminated between the two different treatments, the intonation treatment was always conducted at one table in the room, and the touch-cue treatment at a different table.

The 15 phonemes that girls age 3 are expected to have acquired (Smit, et al., 1990) were divided into three sets based on AM's responses to 10-word imitative probes: five "easy" phonemes (correctly produced eight out of 10 times in baseline), five "difficult" phonemes (never produced in baseline), and five "intermediate" phonemes (produced one to seven of 10 times in baseline). The "easy" and "difficult" phonemes were randomized over the first 10 sessions, and the "intermediate" phonemes were randomly administered over the subsequent five sessions for confirmation of the results.

The two treatment approaches were an adaptation of the Elementary Level of Melodic Intonation Therapy (Helm-Estabrooks, Nicholas, & Morgan, 1989) and an adaptation of the PROMPT system (Chumpelik, 1984). In order to carry out the intonation approach, it was necessary to use two-word stimuli (in order to have an intonation contour) with accompanying pictures. These phrases were spoken with stress on the first syllable. The target phoneme was utterance-initial, as in "foot out" or "cat eat." In order to maintain equality across conditions, the stimuli in the touch-cue

*(continues)*

*(continued)*

session were also two words long. For the intonation cue, the clinician presented a dramatic intonation change between syllables as well as beating the syllables on the table.

Each touch-cue session began with a warm-up—exercises and activities to make the child aware of the targeted articulators for the day. For example, the warm-up for /g/ was for AM to lie on the floor facing up and make gargling sounds while the clinician rubbed the area where chin and neck intersected. Then the clinician pushed the back of AM's tongue upward and backward with a tongue depressor. Stimuli included a model of the target phrase plus a tactile cue similar to those used in the PROMPT system.

In order to make the intonation therapy sessions comparable to the touch-cue sessions, these sessions had a warm-up also, during which time the child and clinician sang three nursery songs. In order to make the two conditions as comparable as possible to each other, the child had the same number of opportunities to respond to the stimulus in each session (15). Correct responses were reinforced the same way in both sessions. The data were the number of correct productions out of 15 productions elicited in each half of the session.

The results were completely straightforward: the intonation approach was unequivocally more effective at eliciting correct productions than was the touch-cue method. For each day's data, the number of correct responses elicited using intonation treatment was greater than or equal to the touch-cue data (nine days greater, six days equal). There were *no* days when more correct responses were elicited using the touch-cue method. This result held for the "easy" sounds, the "difficult" sounds, and the "intermediate" sounds. (It should be noted that during this intervention, AM produced a wide variety of phonemes that were not heard in her spontaneous speech.)

Of course this result cannot be generalized to all children who have DVD—there was a single experimental subject. AM may have been an atypical child because she had residual tendencies toward tactile defensiveness that probably made it difficult for her to use touch cues to shape sound production. On the other hand, many children with DVD have a history of tactile sensitivity. Nevertheless, the findings from this careful research were so clear cut that it becomes important to replicate this study with other children.

Clinical Note 8-2 describes a single-subject experimental study that compared a PROMPT-type intervention with an intervention based on Helfrich-Miller's (1984) adaptation of Melodic Intonation Treatment. It should be noted that the child described here, AM, was very young and had very impaired oral communication when this study was undertaken. Nevertheless, the clinician was able to elicit a wide variety of consonants in two-word phrases from her over the course of the intervention. It was also clear that the MIT-based intervention was more efficacious in eliciting these consonants than was the touch-cue type of intervention.

## *PROCEDURES FOR THE TREATMENT OF DEVELOPMENTAL VERBAL DYSPRAXIA*

### Background

| | |
|---|---|
| **WHO?** | A child of almost any age who shows indicators of Developmental Verbal Dyspraxia (DVD). |
| **WHAT?** | There is no single treatment for DVD. The elements of treatments indicated below are those recommended by several authorities on DVD. Additionally, the treatments for DVD in preschoolers should differ from those for older children. |
| **WHY?** | Most authorities agree that conventional treatments, including traditional articulation training and phonological intervention, are inappropriate (traditional articulation training) or insufficient (phonological intervention) for children with DVD. |
| **WHEN?** | Whenever the speech-language pathologist notes potential dyspraxic elements or suspects DVD. |
| **SUPPORT:** | At this time, there is very little evidence beyond case studies that any of the many treatments proposed for DVD is effective, or that one is more effective than another. |

## PROCEDURES FOR THE TREATMENT OF DEVELOPMENTAL VERBAL DYSPRAXIA

### *Procedures*

The speech-language pathologist will, of course, need to plan treatment specific to the needs of the child and within the parameters that the child sets. A problem-solving approach is most helpful. In addition, preschoolers with DVD have different needs than do school age children.

## ALL CHILDREN

**Principle 1:** *Schedule frequent short treatment sessions.*

The research on motor learning shows that short but frequent practice sessions result in more efficient learning than does massed practice. This principle appears to be especially true for children with DVD. If only a few sessions per week are possible, put part of the motor practice at the beginning and part at the end, with other types of activities in between.

**Principle 2:** *Target functional words and phrases as well as speech sounds.*

Several authorities note that the child with DVD often has no means to communicate important information because she is not understood. Therefore, children with DVD should learn some intelligible, useful words or phrases (e.g., "Leave me alone!") that convey this information.

**Principle 3:**  *As much as possible, work with meaningful material.*

The child with DVD needs to be linking phonological information with semantic information as much as possible. Consequently, the SLP should target words, phrases, and sentences as much as possible. The child should have opportunities to attempt these words in real-life or play situations. In addition, the SLP should provide the label and semantic information about pictures (and objects) used in intervention and should elicit many productions from the child in conjunction with the semantic information.

**Principle 4:**  *Vary targets and materials frequently within the treatment session.*

Materials and targets that are practiced too much lose their meaning, and so varying them should improve learning. In addition, children with DVD may perseverate on one response—that is, may continue to use one word-initial consonant when it is no longer appropriate—zand they need practice in getting out of perseverations.

**Principle 5:**  *Do warm-ups at the beginning of each session.*

In McDonald's (1964a) sensory-motor intervention, each session starts with practice in sequencing syllables that are *within* the child's repertory. For example, the child might repeat [bababa…], first with equal stress on syllables, and later using disyllable rhythms. The emphasis for the child is on how these sequences feel and sound, that is, smooth and easy. Early school-age children may be wary of this task, which involves imitating a model. Fortunately, however, this type of task lends itself to silliness and novel play routines that may appeal to the child.

**Principle 6:**  *Use multiple modalities in providing models, cues, and prompts.*

Virtually every author who writes about DVD notes that children do best with multimodal cues. For example, the clinician might present the /k/ in the word *duck* with a picture of a duck and a written form with the *-ck* underlined, as well as a touch cue to the throat area to indicate the "back-ness" of /k/. Other authors have reported that using exaggerated intonation contours improves the child's performance.

**Principle 7:**  *Let the severity of the DVD be the guide to the number of exemplar words used in a session.*

Strand and Skinder (1999) suggest using fewer exemplar words with more severe children, such as four to five words for children with severe DVD and eight or more for the child with less severe DVD.

**Principle 8:**  *Provide alternative or augmented communication for the child whose speech is not functional for conveying wants, needs, and thoughts.*

Not being understood can have many negative effects for the child with DVD. Consequently, it is important that the child, family, and school personnel understand that the child may need a supplemental means to communicate.

**Principle 9:**  *Include phonological awareness activities in treatment.*

Compared to other children with severe phonological difficulties, children who have DVD are as much at risk, or perhaps more at risk, for problems learning to read. Consequently, children with DVD should also participate in activities that encourage phonological awareness.

## SCHOOL-AGE CHILDREN

**Principle 1:** *Target as many different phonemes and other phonological targets as the child can handle.*

One of the criticisms of using traditional treatment for children with DVD is its one-phoneme-at-a-time approach, which is just too inefficient for children who can produce very few sounds.

**Principle 2:** *Target language forms along with phonetic forms.*

Crary (1993) holds that the difficulty that children with DVD have in planning sequences of phonemes is best addressed by asking them to program linguistic responses. These responses should be meaningful and communicative utterances, such as plurals and possessives.

**Principle 3:** *Provide large amounts of practice.*

It is clear that most authorities believe that large amounts of practice are necessary for children with DVD to progress. This practice should be distributed over the treatment session.

**Principle 4:** *Vary the prosody and perhaps the rate of the desired responses.*

Children with DVD often have prosodic difficulties as part of their communication disability. It is important that they not only learn words and phrases, but also that they learn to vary prosody and rate in order to maximize intelligibility.

**Principle 5:** *Pay attention to facilitating and non-facilitating phonetic contexts.*

Because children with DVD usually have considerable difficulty in sequencing speech sounds with accuracy, it is important to use facilitating phonetic contexts first and non-facilitating contexts later.

## PRESCHOOLERS

**Principle 1:** *Use procedures developed for phonological disorders.*

Like other children with phonological disorders, children with DVD probably have difficulty figuring out the sound system of their language. It makes sense to use procedures that have been developed for phonological disorders, and to augment them with additional motor practice and emphases on functional communication.

**Principle 2:** *Help the child get past difficulties with imitation.*

Children with DVD often have great difficulty in imitation. They may refuse to imitate, may cover the mouth when imitating, or may find ways to deflect requests for imitation. All of these behaviors reflect the child's lack of success when attempting to imitate models. Unfortunately, they *must* learn to imitate in order to progress. The best way to handle this issue is to de-emphasize imitation in the early parts of intervention. For example, the clinician can do auditory bombardment with instructions to the child that he absolutely must *not* say the words he hears. A play-based approach to production is helpful as well. The clinician can provide many models of selected words/structures in play situations and just wait for the child to attempt one. When the child's attempt is not accurate, the clinician simply remodels the word.

**Principle 3:** *The first goal of intervention should be to fill out the consonant and vowel inventory.*

The preschooler with DVD typically has very few consonants and is also missing some vowels. Rather than massive amounts of practice on a few sounds, the preschooler first needs to fill out the consonant inventory, with the targets being those sounds that are expected by the child's age. That is, the child needs to learn three to five words for each of the targeted sounds. This will give the child more options for putting words together, which is important for the large amount of vocabulary learning that takes place in the preschool years. The vowel inventory may not need to be targeted specifically, because vowels often improve during practice with words that contain target consonants.

**Principle 4:** *Focus on consistent and fully correct productions of words.*

The focus of intervention should be on production of words that will be fully correct (and intelligible) when the target sound is said correctly. This means that words should have only sounds that are already in the child's repertory, except for the target sound.

**Principle 5:** *Provide as much motor practice as possible.*

For preschoolers, massive amounts of motor practice should take a back seat to other kinds of goals. However, as much motor practice as possible should be incorporated into treatment.

**Principle 6:** *Reinforce in terms of success at communication.*

Because the preschooler with DVD is so rarely a successful communicator, when the child does produce a word that is correct because he "fixed" the target sound, the clinician should reinforce in terms of successful communication, such as "Wow! I understand that whole word!"

---

## CHILDREN AND ADULTS WHO SPEAK ENGLISH AS A SECOND LANGUAGE

Children who speak English as a second language (or as a third, or a fourth language) are a unique but not homogeneous population. Some of these children may learn to speak English that is unaccented compared to the "school English" predominant in their part of the United States. Other children will speak English with noticeable influence of the first language. In a recent and very comprehensive book on the topic of cultural and linguistic diversity, Goldstein (2000) reviews current thinking on the topic of second language issues for the profession of communication sciences and disorders. Clinical Note 8-3 provides some important ways to think about second language acquisition.

---

**CLINICAL NOTE 8-3: Maxims about Second-Language Learning**

1. The child who has, or has had, difficulty acquiring the first language will also have difficulty acquiring a second language.
2. Children who get a lot of exposure to the second language during childhood will very likely use the type of English that they hear, whether school English or a local variant.

*(continues)*

*(continued)*

3. Children who learn a second language in early childhood typically become fluent in that language for conversational purposes within a year or two, but they may not become academically proficient in that language for another five years (Cummins, 1984). Note however, that the frequency and intensity of the exposure to the second language may influence these times.

Sometimes adults who have learned English as a second language seek speech-language pathology services. These clients may want to reduce the degree to which they sound different from native English speakers, or they may want to improve their intelligibility. In such cases, of course, speech-language pathology services are optional. The majority of adults seeking either type of SLP service did not grow up in an English-speaking country. In our clinic, most of the ESL clients requesting services grew up in Asian countries, they learned English through print, and they had very little exposure to spoken English. They range in intelligibility from perhaps 20% intelligible to 90% intelligible.

## Children Who Speak English as a Second Language

There are two situations concerning second language learning that may come to the attention of the speech-language pathologist who works with children. The first is the child who is having clear difficulty learning the phonology of both the first language and the second language. There is no question that this child requires services, preferably from a clinician who knows both languages. Goldstein (2000) discusses at length our professional obligations in cases where children exhibit disorders in both languages.

The second situation that may come to the attention of the SLP is that of the child who speaks English with an accent or whose intelligibility in English is greatly reduced and whose abilities in the first language are either unknown or marginally within normal limits. The status of the child with respect to the first language may be unknown because of inability to communicate with informants, as in a foster care situation, or because it is difficult to communicate with family members even when they are face to face.

Cases in which the child appears to be at least marginally intelligible in the first language but not in English can arise from a number of sources, including poor teaching of English, little exposure to spoken English, and extensive exposure to speakers of English who themselves are poorly intelligible. This situation may arise as well if the client is of older school age and exhibits potential dyspraxic elements (PDEs). PDEs could have delayed development in the first language somewhat but may not have had a continuing influence on the phonology of the first language. Such PDEs may still influence the acquisition of a second language for a time.

Our professional guidelines appear to suggest that we treat these cases as if the children speak a social dialect such as African-American Vernacular English (American Speech-Language Hearing Association, 1983 and 1985). The idea that underlies the guidelines is that an language or dialect that is used in a community for purposes of communication within that community should not be regarded as inferior or problematic, merely different.

There is apparently a widespread understanding within the profession of speech-language pathology that English spoken with a noticeable accent is not considered to be disordered and therefore intervention is not warranted. This understanding is based on language in public laws relating to education, and within the profession of speech-language pathology on ASHA position statements. The goal of such laws is to prevent discrimination against social dialects because a social dialect is the living language of a community, used by its members to communicate with other members of the community.

The ASHA position papers seem to acknowledge that there may be clients with Limited English Proficiency. However, they then deal with the issue of Limited English Proficiency as if it were a social dialect, that is, the living language of a community. In such cases, any speech-language services would be elective. Although most federal laws relating to public education prohibit using federal funds for such services, school districts may choose to provide such elective services.

However, only a few forms of accented English used in the United States qualify as living languages of a community. These include Spanish-accented English, which is used, along with Spanish, in large, well-established Hispanic communities. The only other form of accented English that is a community language is the dialect of English spoken by natives of India, a variant which is used by Indian speakers who may all have different first languages. When such speakers move away from India, they still use this variant of English to communicate with others from their country.

The second-language learner whose English is difficult to understand is most often from a language/cultural group that does not use this form of accented English for communication within the group; rather, the ambient language is primarily the first language. In other words, the situation is *not* analogous to social dialects. In such cases, I maintain that services should be considered even if the client's first-language skills are reported to be within normal limits. If this client is a child, she is just as much at risk for communicative, social, and academic problems as a child whose *first* language is poorly intelligible.

In fact, I would argue that accented English that is intelligible should *never* be a concern of the SLP unless a client (or her parent) wants accent reduction services and the clinician is in a position to provide them. On the other hand, accented English that is poorly intelligible should *always* be a concern of the SLP. In such cases the therapeutic goal is to help the child become as intelligible as other children her age in her community, even if her English continues to be accented.

Unfortunately, the widespread impression that all second-language accents should be considered as social dialects has in some cases led to a hands-off policy toward ESL learners who have difficulties with communication. Some SLPs seem to believe that even doing an evaluation could be discriminatory. It stands to reason, however, that communication disorders are represented in the second-language-learning population to the same extent as in the first language-learning population. We do not expect to see *fewer* bilingual children with phonological problems than in the monolingual population. Clinical Note 8-4 describes a case in which real problems were never uncovered, apparently because of a hands-off approach to an instance of presumed second-language learning.

---

**CLINICAL NOTE 8-4: A Case of Misdiagnosis**

Lee was a freshman when he first came to the Speech and Hearing Center at his university in a large city in the Midwest. He was a charming, gregarious young man with poorly intelligible speech. He came to the clinic in the middle of his first year. At that time he reported that his scores on a standardized college entrance exam were below the fifth percentile. Lee was also having a very difficult time academically, and he was close to flunking out. Lee reported that he was the youngest of many children in his family, and that he, his parents, and his siblings had immigrated from the

*(continues)*

*(continued)*

Philippines when he was 6 years of age. In the U.S., he had gone through public schools in a small town in a rural area. He reported that he himself spoke and understood primarily English, although he could converse with his parents in their native language. Lee reported that he had participated in speech therapy for a short time in about the eigth grade.

Results of an evaluation of Lee's communication abilities showed that he had many sound deletions and many weak productions of sounds. Some of his speech characteristics were consistent with a mild dysarthria, such as slowed production and weak contacts. During the oral examination he showed considerable muscle weakness along with mild spasticity. He denied problems with chewing and swallowing, nor were any difficulties obvious in the clinical exam. His command of syntax and vocabulary were at the very low end of the normal range. He also walked with an unusual gait and sometimes had hand motions that appeared somewhat athetotic.

School records indicated that Lee had received group language services in the eigth grade and had received resource room services at various times. There was an assessment of articulation revealing many errors that were attributed to second language learning. There was apparently no assessment of oral-motor function, nor any examination of Lee's cognitive status. There was no mention that Lee might have a generalized motor disorder such as a mild cerebral palsy. Instead, there were multiple references to his second-language accent. There was, however, information from a neurologist dated several years previously concerning muscle weakness, suggesting that the clinical picture was not a new one.

As we reflected on Lee's history, it seemed that Lee may not have received appropriate speech-language pathology services, to say nothing of a lack of appropriate physical therapy and occupational therapy services. Although we know nothing about the relationship between his parents and the school system, it appears that Lee's very real communication and related problems might have been swept under the rug of "second-language accent." Ironically, English was Lee's more proficient language.

We often wondered whether more appropriate intervention and guidance services would have steered Lee away from going to college, where the kind of disastrous academic performance that he showed was highly predictable. Before that could happen, however, someone in the school environment had to be willing to say that something besides second language interference was going on with Lee.

## Adults Who Speak English as a Second Language

In our clinic we see a number of adult international graduate students who fit the description of a person who is apparently intelligible in a first language but not in the second (English). Rather, these are adults whose first language is an Asian language and who learned English primarily through texts and written materials. Their reading and writing abilities in English are often very good. They usually indicate that their exposure to spoken English was less than 5% of their formal instruction in English. They do not use English to communicate with their families or friends from the same country. In fact, most of them report that they speak English less than 15 minutes per day. A surprisingly high proportion of these clients (about 25-30%) have other communication difficulties, including voice, fluency, and the presence of potential dyspraxic elements.

It is clear that these adults do not use a social dialect. In fact, they are often referred to our clinic by their professors, who are concerned about the students' intelligibility. Nevertheless, these adults can elect to use or not to use our clinical services.

## How a First Language Influences a Second Language

The ways in which a first language might influence the acquisition of a second language have been debated for years in linguistics. However, from a pragmatic point of view, it appears that features of the first language that are different from features of the second language can set up some expectations for interference. Consequently, languages that are quite similar to English in phonological structure appear to pose fewer problems for intelligibility than languages that are quite dissimilar. Languages can differ in allowable syllable structures, prosody, and consonant and vowel inventories. I will contrast two languages to illustrate this point: namely, Spanish and Mandarin Chinese.

Spanish-accented English is intelligible to most speakers of the "standard" dialect of American English. Spanish phonology shares quite a number of features with English. For example, Spanish has at least a few consonants that can occur in final position. English has many more such consonants, but Spanish speakers learning English are likely to understand that final consonants might be needed. There is also considerable overlap of the consonant repertory between the two languages. Although Spanish appears to be primarily a syllable-timed language, Spanish speakers have little trouble realizing the reduced syllables that characterize English. Spanish also appears to indicate emotion and meaning using utterance-length intonation contours, such as surprise or disbelief, in ways similar to English.

In contrast, Mandarin Chinese is about as different from English as a language can be, differing in syllable structure, prosody, consonant repertory, and vowel repertory. According to Cheng (1991), Mandarin Chinese has few final consonants (only the sonorant /n/ and /ŋ/) and no clusters. Mandarin collapses distinctions between [l] and [r], which becomes very obvious when a Mandarin speaker speaks English, because /r/ is one of the more common consonants in English. Mandarin is also a tone language, which means that the contours of intonation that occur over a vowel are phonemic, and the English distinctions between tense and lax vowels are new to Mandarin speakers. Mandarin is a syllable-timed language, so that the distinctions between stressed and unstressed vowels are not present. Also, English word-level stress patterns and utterance-length intonation contours appear to be quite difficult for native Mandarin speakers.

## Assessment Issues when Intelligibility Is in Question

There are a great many issues related to the assessment of communication in children who are learning more than one language. These are admirably presented in Goldstein's (2000) Resource Guide in this same series. For the specific purposes of evaluating intelligibility and documenting factors that contribute to poor intelligibility, there are a number of procedures to consider.

At the same time, it is well to keep in mind that the United States as a whole is becoming more, rather than less, diverse. In the future, there will probably be increased social and educational tolerance for accents and dialects that differ from so-called Standard English. However, that tolerance will probably not extend to speakers who are perceived not only to have an accent but also to be poorly intelligible.

## *PROCEDURES TO EVALUATE AND DOCUMENT INTELLIGIBILITY IN SECOND LANGUAGE LEARNERS*

### Background

**WHO?** A person of almost any age who is learning English as a second language and who may or may not have difficulties with intelligibility in both English and the first language.

**WHAT?** Assessment procedures designed to document intelligibility and indicate factors that may contribute to reduced intelligibility.

**WHY?** Clients who are learning English as a second language may have some unique contributions to reduced intelligibility.

**WHEN?** This type of assessment is done as part of an evaluation of the communication abilities of persons who are learning or speaking English as a second language when there are concerns about the person's ability to communicate effectively.

**SUPPORT:** This approach is an extension of procedures used to assess monolingual children, with particular attention given (a) to the determination of the social contexts in which the client exhibits limited intelligibility, and (b) to the factors that contribute to reduced intelligibility.

## PROCEDURES TO EVALUATE AND DOCUMENT INTELLIGIBILITY IN SECOND LANGUAGE LEARNERS

### *Procedures*

In addition to the more routine elements of a diagnostic evaluation, such as a screening of hearing and administration of a single-word test of articulation or phonology (if needed), the following are important:

A. Determine which important persons, if any, in the client's environment have difficulty understanding him or her. Note in which language the problem exists.

B. Make a good recording of spontaneous conversation. Gloss and transcribe this recording, being as complete as possible. Based on this transcription, determine the Percent of Consonants Correct (Shriberg & Kwiatkowski, 1982a; see also Section 2). In addition, determine the Percent of Vowels Correct (Shriberg, 1993) from this sample.

C. Using the recording of spontaneous speech, determine the person's intelligibility by having an unfamiliar listener gloss the sample. From this gloss, determine the Percent of Intelligible Words (Shriberg & Kwiatkowski, 1982a; see also Section 2). An alternative or perhaps additional procedure for adults is to administer the *Sentence Intelligibility Test* (Yorkston, Beukelman, & Tice, 2000), which is then transcribed by two persons who are not familiar with the client.

D. List the client's speech-sound errors completely, using a segmental or phonemic inventory form for both consonants and vowels, if necessary (Reproducible Forms 6, 7, and 8).

E. If the client is a child, determine, if at all possible, what speech-sound errors the child makes in the first language. Goldstein (2000) provides considerable information about assessment of bilingual children.

F. Determine the client's speaking rate in English using standard procedures (see Section 1)

G. Assess prosody informally but thoroughly, with attention to both word-level and utterance-level prosody.

   1. *Word-level prosody.* Appendix A contains two-syllable words with differing stress patterns, as well as multisyllabic words with a variety of stress patterns. Adult clients can be asked to read some of these words, or the clinician can say each one for the client to imitate. Of course, if these words are used with children, the clinician should choose words that children are likely to understand. Deviations from the appropriate stress pattern should be noted.

   2. *Utterance-level stress and prosody.* The client can be asked to read or repeat sentences with a variety of stress patterns and prosodic contours. Alternatively, prosody used in the spontaneous speaking sample can be analyzed.

H. Assess the oral mechanism, fluency, and voice characteristics carefully.

I. Develop a comprehensive statement of contributors to poor intelligibility. This statement should guide the goals of intervention. A sample statement might look like this for a teenager of Chinese descent who had recently settled in a small city in a Midwestern state, and who had had about two years of English instruction in his home country prior to emigration:

> *Joe's first language is Cantonese. At the time of evaluation, his conversational speech in English was about 40% intelligible based on percent of glossable words. Joe's facility in Cantonese was not known because he was living temporarily with an English-speaking family. The primary contributors to poorly intelligible English at that time were features predictable from Cantonese (Cheng, 1991), in the rank order judged by the clinician (with 1 being the biggest contributor):*
>
> *1. Final consonant omission*
>
> *2. Misplaced stress in two- and three-syllable words*
>
> *3. Confusions of /l r/*
>
> *4. Separation of clustered consonants by vowels*
>
> *5. Difficulty with lax vowels and /r/-colored vowels*
>
> *6. Inconsistent use of appropriate intonation contours for utterances.*
>
> *None of these difficulties is considered to represent any kind of disability. Furthermore, it is likely that as Joe listens to many different English speakers as part of his immersion into American culture, he will quickly correct some of the previously mentioned difficulties.*

## Intervention for Intelligibility Difficulties

Although intervention for language-learning disabilities in ESL speakers often takes place in the first language, there are occasions when the SLP needs to work on difficulties in intelligibility in the second language due to first-language interference. The extent of intervention will depend not only on the client's needs, but also on the availability of other forms of intervention, such as placement in a class for persons with Limited English Proficiency. There are, however, a few common principles for clinicians to follow if they provide services to improve intelligibility in English.

- We cannot assume that the meaning of each word or phrase that we use for practice is known to the client, and many of our clients are too polite or too shy to tell us if they do not know a word. However, it stands to reason that clients will make better progress with words that they understand and that have utility in the second language.

- Make use of the auditory channel as much as possible. For children, auditory bombardment using objects or pictures, carried out on a daily basis, will help them develop appropriate auditory images of English target sounds. For adults, who may have little experience with spoken English, watching TV may actually be helpful because the context of utterances is usually obvious. In addition, the SLP can ask the client to "hang out" in a shopping mall or coffee shop, observing the rhythms of English.

- Use of multiple modalities is likely to help most clients learn difficult aspects of English. Multiple modalities might include objects, drawings, photographs, and graphemes (if the client can read).

- The clinician should use materials that acknowledge and respect the client's cultural background.

- When working with phonological targets, the clinician should choose stimuli over which the client has reasonably good prosodic control. For example, if the client is working on the [eɪ] vowel, a word like *hazy* may be appropriate but a word like *delay* may be more difficult because of the initial unstressed syllable.

## Choosing Phonological Targets for Bilingual Children

Yavas and Goldstein (1998) have provided recommendations for choosing phonological targets when working with bilingual children. They recommend choosing processes for intervention as follows:

- Highest priority goes to those processes that affect both first and second language at similar rates.

- Second priority goes to processes that affect one language more than the other, assuming that treatment is provided in the affected language.

- Third priority goes to processes that are operative in only one language.

Appendix A contains a number of sets of words that can be used to target vowel and consonant distinctions, as well as words that can be used for practice on word-level prosody and sentences for practice on utterance-length materials.

## Choosing Targets for Teenagers and Adults

For teenage and adult bilingual persons, the prosodic aspects of spoken English are often equal in importance to the other phonological aspects. There are a number of published programs and/or software to assist with assessing and remediating prosodic difficulties, including *SPEECHWORKS* (Version 3.15, Blackmer & Ferrier, 2002) and an excellent print resource by Edwards and Strattman (1996). There is also a proprietary program called the *Compton P-ESL Program*™ (Compton, n.d.) managed by the Institute of Language and Phonology, which trains SLPs to evaluate and remediate phonology and prosody for ESL speakers. Clinicians must be trained and certified to use the *P-ESL*™ materials, which appear to be very comprehensive.

When the SLP works with teenagers and adults to improve intelligibility, the goals should reflect the statement about the relative contribution of various factors to reduced intelligibility. For example, for Joe, the teenager mentioned earlier, production of final consonants is an important goal. The clinician can draw on approaches used in both phonological intervention and traditional intervention to remediate final consonants. Both minimal pairs and articulation drills may be useful.

When treating prosodic differences, such as word-level stress patterns, the clinician can use some of the materials found in Appendix A relating to word-level stress. For utterance-level stress, materials available in Edwards and Strattman (1996), as well as in the other commercially available programs can be very useful.

Some ESL clients who want services for intelligibility actually have little experience with spoken English. For these clients, it may be helpful to record materials for them, or use materials available from Dialect Accent Specialists, Inc., which include recorded speech that clients can listen to at home. In addition, some communities and universities sponsor Communication Partners, in which an ESL client is paired with a native English speaker. The partners get together weekly for an hour or so of conversation in English. These conversations also help the ESL client to understand American culture.

## Efficacy of Interventions to Improve Intelligibility in ESL Speakers

As is the case with many other interventions offered by speech-language-pathologists, intervention procedures to improve intelligibility are buttressed primarily by case studies. The *SPEECH-WORKS* manual does include some reports of efficacy and time to completion of the program. As always, the SLP needs to document that the chosen procedures are producing the desired changes in the speech of individual clients, whether or not controlled efficacy studies exist.

## CHILDREN WITH DEVELOPMENTAL DELAY

Many children who have moderate to severe developmental delay also have difficulty acquiring the sound system of English. In many such cases a component of the difficulty is that the child also exhibits potential dyspraxic elements to some degree. Nevertheless, a minimum level of cognitive capacity appears to be a prerequisite for adequate acquisition of a sound system. It is not entirely clear which aspects of cognitive delay contribute to difficulties in acquiring sounds. However, at least three capacities must be involved, namely the ability to synthesize, the ability to generate hypotheses, and the ability to generalize.

We need to consider the ability to synthesize and to hypothesize in order to understand what children with cognitive delays do or do not do with input from the ambient language. It appears that typically developing children begin to see patterns in the input, for example, that words in English often have a closing consonant. From this pattern, the child can then generate a hypothesis about her own output, and she can also test the hypothesis by trying out a new form consistent with the pattern to see what response it elicits.

There appears to be relatively little work on how phonology develops in children with developmental delays, except for a few descriptive studies of children with Down Syndrome. However, we might guess that many children with developmental delay do a certain amount of synthesis and hypothesis testing, if only because their phonologies do, in fact, develop. This cognitive work may not be as efficient as it is in typically developing children, but it does seem to occur.

The greatest hindrance to full development of the phonological system in children with cognitive delay is likely in the area of generalization. A number of persons who have written about phonological treatment when there is developmental delay have suggested that neither traditional nor phonological approaches are particularly effective with these populations. It appears that the difficulty is most evident in the lack of generalization to untrained word positions, and secondarily to untrained partners and untrained locales. Those authors who have made recommendations for direct work on phonology in this population (e.g., McLean, 1970) tend to stress heavy-duty behavioral training, that is, presenting many trials and many exemplars. We can interpret such recommendations as attempts to achieve by "brute force" what the child has difficulty doing spontaneously, that is, generalize what she has learned.

There is one subset of children with developmental delay, namely Down Syndrome children, who appear to have phonological difficulties that exceed their deficits in other cognitive areas. For example, Das (2002) has hypothesized that in Down Syndrome, the most salient deficits are in phonological memory and articulation. Other authors have found that children with Down Syndrome have impairment of short-term memory for verbal information, but no impairment of short-term memory for visual or spatial information (Jarrold, Baddeley, & Phillips, 1999). These writers have suggested that a verbal short-term memory deficit would show up as "difficulties in subvocal rehearsal and phonological storage" (p. 61). Such a deficit would clearly impair the ability to learn the phonology of the ambient language.

## Assessment of Phonology When There Is Cognitive Delay

In planning the assessment process, the SLP may wish to use tests and materials appropriate for children at the client's approximate mental age. Beyond that, all of the procedures appropriate for evaluation are very similar to those used for other children. We should be particularly aware that disfluencies more often characterize children with developmental delays than their typically developing peers.

## Intervention When There Is Cognitive Delay

Based on the foregoing observations, it appears that the prognosis for phonological improvement is uncertain, at best, if conventional intervention is used. As a result, speech-language pathologists may wish to consider alternative strategies to improve the communication of children with cognitive delays. One intervention that is widely used is Total Communication, which is usually conceptualized as simultaneous sign and speech. There are also suggestions in the literature that Down Syndrome children may be uniquely receptive to Total Communication because of their relatively good visual skills.

Given the current state of knowledge about intervention for phonology in children with developmental delays, the approach recommended here is to emphasize functional communication over phonologically accurate communication. Table 8-3 shows some ways to achieve this emphasis in terms of setting priorities.

**TABLE 8-3.** Strategies for improving speech-sound aspects of communication in children who have cognitive delays.

---

1. The top priority should be to teach the child intelligible versions of words that are highly functional for him or her, such as names of family members and significant others, names of pets, important actions such as eat, *drink*, *sleep*, and *go to bathroom*, as well as names of important objects. These lists can be generated with the help of the child's family and teachers.

*(continues)*

**TABLE 8-3.** *(continued)*

2. Then, if the child appears to be capable of doing a certain amount of generalization, intervention can be instituted for specific targets. The phonological targets would be chosen based on developmental ages of acquisition and also on the child's readiness to move on as evidenced by stimulability testing. The SLP will likely need to maintain a very high rate of correct responding in order for the child to generalize a newfound skill or sound.

3. If the child has very poor oral communication and if it appears that intervention will take a long time before oral communication is functional for the child, the clinician should consider an augmentative communication device or Total Communication as a bridge to improved oral communication later on.

4. If the child is learning to read functional materials, incorporate the written words into treatment and even objects such as stop signs as stimuli.

---

If the SLP considers work on individual phonemes or even on phonological processes to be important, it is likely that many exemplars will need to be introduced. That is, use of many exemplars appears to promote generalization. Additionally, considerable drill will likely be needed for every target that is chosen. McLean (1970) developed the stimulus shift system specifically for children with developmental delays. In this system, models of the desired production and pictures of the object being named (held close to the mouth) and a mirror are used in various combinations as cues while the child progresses from words to phrases and sentences. These cues may be reintroduced and then faded in successive steps of the program.

### Efficacy of Interventions to Improve Phonology in Children with Developmental Delay

McLean reported that several children with mental retardation were able to complete the first five steps of his 10-step stimulus shift program, while only one child was not able to do so. With respect to the use of Total Communication, there are several small-scale studies (most lacking controls) and case studies to support this program. A relatively extensive exploration of Total Communication used with Down syndrome children was carried out by Matheson (1987), who studied 22 Down Syndrome children. She found that use of Total Communication increased the children's use of several types of expressive behaviors, although she did not specifically assess phonology.

There appear to be very few, if any, studies of the effectiveness of an emphasis on functional communication, although many classrooms for children with developmental delays emphasize the kind of skills and vocabulary that help children get along in the world. A functional approach also appears to correspond rather well to current emphases in special education on developmentally appropriate practices.

It is clear that a great deal more research is needed on the nature and causes of phonological disorders in developmentally delayed children. Ideally, this research will then lead to specifically targeted interventions that would result in the maximum possible progress in phonology for these children.

## SUMMARY

The goal of this section has been to show how assessment and treatment should be adapted for particular diagnostic groups. Treatment for a child with DVD, an adult ESL client, and a client with developmental delay can look very different because of the unique cognitive and linguistic capabilities of each type of client. These differences challenge the SLP to provide the best and most appropriate forms of assessment and treatment.

# SECTION

# CASE STUDIES

●●●●●●●●●●●●●●●●●●●●●●●●●●●●●●●●●●●●●●●

### CASE I: CHOOSING AN EVALUATION FOCUS—
### AN EARLY SCHOOL-AGE CHILD

**Client:**        Lucy
**Age:**           5;1
**Referral:**     Lucy's pediatrician, at the request of Lucy's mother, referred Lucy for evaluation because very few people outside the immediate family could understand her.

**Background:**  Lucy was the second of three children in a middle-class family. She was enrolled in kindergarten, where she was one of the youngest children in the class. Her mother reported that Lucy "leaves out sounds."

## Issues to Be Considered in the Evaluation:

1. Assessment of phonological processes is appropriate because of the complaint about Lucy's poor intelligibility and the comment that she leaves out sounds. If the assessment instrument does not include many words that are two syllables in length or longer, the clinician may wish to supplement the analysis. In addition, both quantitative and indirect measures of intelligibility will be important, as well as a severity measure such as Percent of Consonants Correct.

2. Assessment of both receptive and expressive language will be important because of the close ties between phonology and language at Lucy's age.

3. The SLP may plan a classroom visit to observe Lucy's communicative interactions with her peers.

4. As with all evaluations, abnormalities in hearing and in the oral mechanism need to be ruled out as contributing factors, and voice, fluency, and cognition need to be assessed formally or informally.

## CASE II: CHOOSING AN EVALUATION FOCUS—
## AN ELEMENTARY SCHOOL-AGE CHILD

**Client:**       Ricardo

**Age:**          7;9

**Referral:**     The classroom teacher (third grade) made the referral, commenting that Ricardo had some problems with the "r" sound, although she rarely misunderstood him.

**Background:**   Ricardo had recently moved into the district (in mid-year). His school records suggested that although some Spanish was spoken in the home, especially with his elderly grandfather, Ricardo had spoken primarily English since he began talking. He had received intervention for several years for phonological processes, and his reading scores were about two years behind those of his peers. At the time of his most recent IEP, two years previously, Ricardo's scores on language test instruments in English were in the low normal range.

## Issues to Be Considered in the Evaluation:

1. Ricardo's exposure to a second language in the home may not be a significant factor in his current academic performance, but the SLP should verify with his parents that the primary language in the home is still English.

2. Very likely Ricardo is now demonstrating residual errors that are motoric or phonetic in nature. For this reason, and because intelligibility is not seriously compromised, a standard inventory test is appropriate. This should be followed by assessment of stimulability for error sounds, especially for /r/.

3. Poor phonological awareness may be one aspect of Ricardo's reading difficulties; consequently, assessment using a standardized test of phonological awareness will be appropriate.

# CASE III: RESULTS OF EVALUATION OF A CHILD WITH A PHONOLOGICAL DISORDER

| | |
|---|---|
| **Client:** | Ben |
| **Age:** | 3;5 |
| **Referral:** | Ben's parents, who were concerned about his poor intelligibility to others, referred him to a university clinic. |
| **Background:** | Ben was an only child, and his parents were both teachers. He had started walking at about 11 months, but did not start talking until 15 months. He was in a home daycare setting with children of a variety of ages. |

## Assessments:

1. The *Smit-Hand Articulation and Phonology Evaluation* (Smit & Hand, 1997) was administered, and its optional phonological process analysis was performed. Ben used the following processes:

   - Stopping of fricatives in all word positions (100%). Not stimulable
   - Fronting (50%).
   - Cluster reduction, initial clusters with /s/ (100%). Not stimulable
   - Cluster reduction, initial clusters with /r l w/ (60%). Note: Some clusters with /w l/ were fully correct.

   •Gliding of /r/ (100%). Note: Syllable-initial /l/ was produced correctly.

   •Vocalization of /r l/ (100%). Not stimulable

2. *Intelligibility*

   Ben's intelligibility as measured using Percent of Intelligible Words was 86%. His mother said that the family understood Ben about 80% of the time, but that "outsiders" understood him less than half the time.

3. *Severity*

   The Percent of Consonants Correct (Shriberg & Kwiatkowski, 1982a) was 62%.

4. *Language*

   Ben's receptive language was in the high normal range. His expressive language was good in terms of content, use, and word order, but his morphology was affected by his tendency to reduce all word-final clusters.

5. *Cognition*

   Because of his good receptive language skills, and because of his general responsiveness during the evaluation, Ben's cognitive level was estimated to be well within normal limits.

6. *Other Assessments*

   Ben's hearing was within normal limits, and there was no history of otitis media. Vocal register, voice quality, fluency, and prosody were within normal limits, and there were no readily apparent dyspraxic elements. There were no concerns in the psychosocial domain.

7. *Recommendation*

The recommendation was to enroll Ben for phonological intervention, largely on the basis of his poor intelligibility to persons outside the family. A second consideration was Ben's lack of stimulability to change a process (Stopping) that was no longer developmentally appropriate and that had a large influence on intelligibility. Treatment based on either a Cycles approach (Hodson and Paden, 1991) or a Pressure Points approach (discussed in Section 6) was recommended. The recommended first targets were the processes of Stopping and Fronting.

8. *Prognosis*

With respect to improvement with intervention, most of the possible prognostic factors were positive except for stimulability.

## CASE IV: DOCUMENTING PROGRESS IN
## PHONOLOGICAL INTERVENTION

**Client:**          James (Jamie)

**Age:**             3;0

**Referral:**        Another speech-language pathologist who had worked with Jamie for 6 months referred him to a university clinic because of his lack of progress. The referring SLP considered his phonological disorder to be very severe and wanted someone else to try to make some headway.

**Background:**      At the onset of this course of intervention, Jamie used every deletion process at high levels except initial consonant deletion, which he only used occasionally. He had an extremely limited phonetic inventory—some, but not all members in the classes of glides, nasals, and stops. He used no final consonants, and he produced only three words that contained intervocalic consonants (*Mommy*, *Daddy*, and *baby*). He also had numerous vowel errors. He exhibited a number of possible dyspraxic elements, although there was no groping of the articulators.

**Intervention:**    A play-based variant of Pressure Points intervention was used with Jamie. The first goal was to expand the repertory of phonemes that he could use in initial and final position of words. The second goal was to expand the number of phonemes that he could use in intervocalic position of disyllabic words with first-syllable stress, such as *Mommy*. In every case, the goal was to elicit acceptable target sounds in three to five words for each phoneme.

**Methods:**         At the beginning of each session, the clinician provided auditory bombardment of the sound or sounds chosen for the day's intervention. The child's mother continued auditory bombardment at home. In addition the clinic room was "seeded" with toys and objects that could be named and used in play. The clinician used focused stimulation (Fey, 1991) to model words with selected targets for Jamie. A second person kept data on Jamie's productions, noting acceptable and incorrect attempts. The second person also noted whether the attempt was a direct imitation (I), a delayed imitation (D), or spontaneous (S).

## Results of Intervention:

1. Because the goal of intervention was to fill out the repertory of phonemes used in meaningful words, the form Reproducible Form 6: Segmental Inventory—Consonants was used to track progress. Figure 9-1 shows Jamie's consonant inventory at the time of the first session, and Figure 9-2 shows his inventory at the time of the last session, his 19th. The inventories also show a coding to indicate the status of each sound, whether stimulable, emerging, or stabilizing. Uncoded items are considered to be stable.

## REPRODUCIBLE FORM 6: SEGMENTAL INVENTORY—CONSONANTS

Name: Jamie      Age: 3; 4      Date: ———————

Use this form to record the child's version(s) of each English target consonant. Tally the number of productions of that type next to each symbol.

| Place/Manner | Initial | | Intervocalic | | Final | |
|---|---|---|---|---|---|---|
| **Glides** | | | | | | |
| Labiovelar | /w/ w | | /w/ | | | |
| Palatal | /j/ [j] | | /j/ | | ▓▓▓ | |
| Glottal | /h/ h | | /h/ | | ▓▓▓ | |
| | | | | | ▓▓▓ | |
| **Nasals** | | | | | | |
| Labial | /m/ m | | /m/ (m) | | /m/ | |
| Alveolar | /n/ n | | /n/ | | /n/ | |
| Velar | ▓▓▓ | | /ŋ/ | | /ŋ/ | |
| | | | | | | |
| | *Voiceless* | *Voiced* | *Voiceless* | *Voiced* | *Voiceless* | *Voiced* |
| **Stops** | | | | | | |
| Labial | /p/ b | /b/ b | /p/ t | /b/ [b] | /p/ | /b/ |
| Alveolar | /t/ | /d/ d | /t/ | /d/ (d) | /t/ | /d/ |
| Velar | /k/ | /g/ [g] | /k/ | /g/ | /k/ | /g/ |
| | | | | | | |
| **Fricatives** | | | | | | |
| Labial | /f/ | /v/ | /f/ | /v/ | /f/ | /v/ |
| Dental | /θ/ | /ð/ | /θ/ | /ð/ | /θ/ | /ð/ |
| Alveolar | /s/ | /z/ | /s/ | /z/ | /s/ | /z/ |
| Palatal | /ʃ/ | /ʒ/ rare | /ʃ/ | /ʒ/ | /ʃ/ | /ʒ/ |
| | | | | | | |
| **Affricates** | | | | | | |
| Palatal | /ʧ/ | /ʤ/ | /ʧ/ | /ʤ/ | /ʧ/ | /ʤ/ |
| | | | | | | |
| **Liquids** | | | | | | |
| Alveolar | /l/ | | /l/ | | /l/ | |
| Palatal | /r/ | | /r/ | | /r/ or /ɚ/ | |

◯ = stimulable — can be elicited in at least one word      ☐ = emerging — can be readily elicited in five or more words

__ = stabilizing — used correctly most of the time

Blanks represent sounds that were rarely attempted and then always deleted.

**Figure 9-1**    Reproducible Form 6: Segmental Inventory—Consonants

# REPRODUCIBLE FORM 6: SEGMENTAL INVENTORY—CONSONANTS

**Name:** Jamie          **Age:** 3; 8          **Date:** ___—___

Use this form to record the child's version(s) of each English target consonant. Tally the number of productions of that type next to each symbol.

| Place/Manner | Initial | | Intervocalic | | Final | |
|---|---|---|---|---|---|---|
| **Glides** | | | | | | |
| Labiovelar | /w/ w | | /w/ | | | |
| Palatal | /j/ ☐j | | /j/ | | ▓▓▓ | ▓▓▓ |
| Glottal | /h/ h | | /h/ | | ▓▓▓ | ▓▓▓ |
| | | | | | ▓▓▓ | ▓▓▓ |
| **Nasals** | | | | | | |
| Labial | /m/ m | | /m/ m | | /m/ m | |
| Alveolar | /n/ n | | /n/ ⃝n | | /n/ ⃝n | |
| Velar | ▓▓▓ | | /ŋ/ | | /ŋ/ | |
| | | | | | | |

| | Voiceless | Voiced | Voiceless | Voiced | Voiceless | Voiced |
|---|---|---|---|---|---|---|
| **Stops** | | | | | | |
| Labial | /p/ ☐p b | /b/ b | /p/ p | /b/ b | /p/ p | /b/ |
| Alveolar | /t/ ☐t d | /d/ d | /t/ | /d/ d | /t/ t | /d/ |
| Velar | /k/ ⃝k gd | /g/ g | /k/ | /g/ | /k/ ⃝k | /g/ |
| | | | | | | |
| **Fricatives** | | | | | | |
| Labial | /f/ | /v/ | /f/ | /v/ | /f/ | /v/ |
| Dental | /θ/ | /ð/ | /θ/ | /ð/ | /θ/ | /ð/ |
| Alveolar | /s/ | /z/ | /s/ | /z/ | /s/ ☐s | /z/ |
| Palatal | /ʃ/ | /ʒ/ rare | /ʃ/ | /ʒ/ | /ʃ/ | /ʒ/ |
| | | | | | | |
| **Affricates** | | | | | | |
| Palatal | /tʃ/ | /dʒ/ | /tʃ/ | /dʒ/ | /tʃ/ ☐ʧ | /dʒ/ |
| | | | | | | |

| Place/Manner | Initial | Intervocalic | Final |
|---|---|---|---|
| **Liquids** | | | |
| Alveolar | /l/ ⃝1 | /l/ ⃝1 | /l/ |
| Palatal | /r/ w | /r/ | /r/ or /ɚ/ |
| | | | |

⃝ = stimulable — can be elicited in at least one word          ☐ = emerging — can be readily elicited in five or more words
__ = stabilizing — used correctly most of the time

Blanks represent sounds that were rarely attempted and then always deleted.

**Figure 9-2**  Reproducible Form 6: Segmental Inventory—Consonants

During this period, Jamie stabilized voiced stops at three places of articulation and in both initial and intervocalic positions. The voiced-voiceless distinction is beginning to appear in initial stops. The /m/ has stabilized, and the /n/ has become stimulable. Jamie now produces sounds from each class, that is, not only stops, nasals, and glides, but also fricatives, affricates, and liquids.

2. Jamie's vowel inventory was not a specific target of intervention. However, his vowel productions improved markedly in the words targeted for production. No doubt, this positive result came about because of the intensive auditory input achieved through the use of auditory bombardment and through focused stimulation.

## CASE V: AN ARTICULATION DIFFICULTY
## WITH AN UNUSUAL EFFECT ON PROSODY

| | |
|---|---|
| **Client:** | Sean (Sean is one of the children discussed in Clinical Note 4-1) |
| **Age:** | 11;7 |
| **Referral:** | Sean had been in articulation therapy for many years. His grandfather brought Sean to our clinic for a second opinion. |
| **Evaluation:** | Sean's articulation errors included lateral distortions of /ʃ tʃ dʒ/ and inconsistent distortions of consonantal /r/. He had a mild hearing loss in the right ear. The most unusual aspect of Sean's speaking patterns was that he was acutely aware of the location of his target fricatives and affricates, and he greatly softened the syllables containing them in connected speech. The effect was that there would be sudden drops in his vocal intensity, giving his speech a somewhat unusual quality, and perceived deviance was relatively high. Sean was stimulable for improved productions, but only when he expended considerably more effort than was heard for these targets in connected speech. He was very stimulable for correct /r/ and he labeled his /r/ errors as "careless." As a result of the evaluation, we recommended treatment in our clinic. |

## Intervention:

1. From the beginning, Sean's productions of /ʃ tʃ dʒ/ had to meet two criteria to be considered acceptable. The criteria were:
   A. Central airflow
   B. Loud enough
2. Also, in the early stages of intervention, Sean did a great deal of self-evaluation, using non-verbal means, such as thumbs up/thumbs down. That is, he indicated whether each of his productions met each of the two criteria.

## Results:

Sean made rapid progress not only on the targeted fricatives and affricates, but also in the perceived naturalness of his speech. He was dismissed after one semester.

## CASE VI: WHEN INTERVENTION DOES NOT SEEM TO WORK

| | |
|---|---|
| **Client:** | Danny (Danny is the child mentioned in Clinical Note 7-2) |
| **Age:** | 14;9 |
| **Referral:** | Danny's mother referred her son to a private practitioner for a second opinion on whether he should continue in treatment in the school setting. |
| **Background:** | Danny's mother indicated that Danny had received speech-language services for articulation for many years, and that he had been working on his unilateral distortions of sounds like /s/ and /ʃ/ for over two years. He was discouraged about his lack of progress, and he wanted to quit therapy. However, when we explained how we planned to tackle his difficulty with him as an active participant, he agreed to give it a try. |

### Results of Re-Evaluation:

Danny's production of /s z ʃ ʧ ʤ / was both acoustically and visually distracting to the listener. He lateralized these productions by sliding the jaw to the right. His attempts at correct production involved a small rightward jaw slide that nevertheless resulted in an acceptable production. However, he was unable to generalize the acceptable productions even to phrases without reverting to his unilateral distortion. Intervention at the speech and hearing center was recommended, and Danny agreed to participate for one semester.

### Intervention and Methods:

1. It was important to enlist Danny as an active partner in remediation. We explained the reason for every procedure in depth to him, and we encouraged him to think about additional ways that he could help himself to solidify the new versions of his old sounds.

2. The initial goal of treatment was nonverbal. Danny was to concentrate on what he felt when he moved the jaw up and down in the midline rather than letting it slide. He used a mirror and kinesthetic cues (a finger on the chin) to help himself. He then progressed to silent mouthing of other tongue-tip sounds like /t d n/, and eventually he was producing syllable trains containing these phonemes with a variety of vowels. The focus throughout remained on the visual and kinesthetic cues associated with midline movements of the jaw.

3. A new criterion for acceptability of productions of the error sounds was introduced. In order for a sound to be acceptable, the production had to meet three criteria:

    A. It was produced with the jaw moving only in the midline.

    B. It was produced with central air flow.

    C. It was sharp enough (Danny was easily trained to the clinician's standard for "sharp enough").

   These criteria were written on three cards that the clinician used when providing feedback and that Danny used when he was asked to evaluate his own productions.

4. Danny was taken all the way back to isolated productions at the start of the treatment period. He was disappointed about this, but we assured him that he would not stay there long and would likely pass through the single-word and subsequent stages quite quickly because he was already keenly aware of where his sounds occurred. In the initial stages, a mirror was used extensively, but its use was discontinued relatively quickly because we wanted Danny to rely on the kinesthetics of the movement.

5. Danny had to achieve 90-95% acceptability over two sessions before he could pass from each level to the next, such as from isolation to words.

6. Self-monitoring was introduced from the beginning, and it was carried out silently. When Danny produced a target sound, the clinician then pointed to each criterion card in turn and Danny gave a thumbs-up or a thumbs-down.

7. Even at the early stages, syllable trains containing the target sound were incorporated into production practice.

8. Near the end of the semester, Danny indicated that he wanted to learn a soliloquy from Shakespeare's *Hamlet*. He thought he should practice it with a mirror first, so that he could be sure that he looked acceptable during the speech. Then he practiced the speech slowly, frequently checking that his jaw was moving in the midline, based on kinesthetic feedback. Only then did he gradually increase the rate and expressiveness of his performance.

## Results:

1. Danny moved rapidly through the stages until he came to answering questions with a sentence response. He faltered a bit at that level, but with review of where he had been and with some concentrated effort, he returned to previous acceptability levels. However, the criterion for passing to the next stage was increased to 95% acceptability in at least 30 productions for a total of four sessions.

2. Danny was able to be dismissed from treatment at the end of the semester, although he returned for monthly follow-ups for two months after dismissal. He was very pleased about his progress, especially when he performed Hamlet's soliloquy for his theater club.

## CASE VII: A CASE OF DEVELOPMENTAL VERBAL DYSPRAXIA

| | |
|---|---|
| **Client:** | Carter |
| **Age:** | 6;0 |
| **Referral:** | Carter's mother referred him for evaluation because Carter seldom used consonants. In addition, his mother thought that his difficulty with speech sounds would interfere with learning to read. Carter had had no previous evaluations or treatment for speech. |
| **Background:** | Carter had been held back from school by his parents because of his poor speech. The family history was positive for dyslexia and for speech problems. Carter had no history of otitis media. He reportedly was reluctant to talk directly with people other than family members, but he was willing to have a family member serve as an intermediary. |

## Initial Evaluation:

1. The *Smit-Hand Articulation and Phonology Evaluation* (Smit & Hand, 1997) was administered to Carter, and the optional phonological process analysis was performed. Based on the sample and on another wordlist elicited 2 weeks previously, several additional analyses were undertaken. These included the following Reproducible Forms:

   3: Phonetic Inventory—Consonants (Figure 9-3)

   5: Syllable and Word–Shape Inventory and Sequential Constraints (Figure 9-4)

   6: Segmental Inventory—Consonants (Figure 9-5)

   7: Segmental Inventory—Word-Initial Clusters (Figure 9-6)

   8: Segmental Inventory—Vowels (Figure 9-7)

# REPRODUCIBLE FORM 3: PHONETIC INVENTORY—CONSONANTS

Name: __Carter_____ Age: __5; 9____ Date: ____—_____

Use this form to record the types of consonants that the client produces, without regard to the English target consonant. Tally the number of productions of that type next to each symbol. *(Based on SHAPE and another wordlist elicited 3 weeks previously.)*

| Place/Manner | Initial | Intervocalic | Final |
|---|---|---|---|
| **Glides** | | | |
| Labiovelar | w ⷌⷌ ⷌⷌ ⏐⏐⏐ w⏐ | w ⏐⏐ | |
| Palatal | j ⏐⏐⏐ | j ⏐ | |
| Glottal | | | |
| | | | |
| **Nasals** | | | |
| Labial | m ⏐⏐⏐ | m ⏐⏐ | m ⷌⷌ mᵊ⏐ |
| Alveolar | n ⏐ | | ŋ ⷌⷌ ⏐⏐⏐ nᵊ⏐⏐ |
| Velar | | ŋ ⏐⏐⏐⏐ | |
| | | | |

| | Voiceless | Voiced | Voiceless | Voiced | Voiceless | Voiced |
|---|---|---|---|---|---|---|
| **Stops** | | | | | | |
| Labial | p ⏐⏐⏐ | b ⷌⷌ ⏐⏐⏐⏐ | p ⏐⏐⏐ p͜b⏐ | | pʰ ⏐⏐⏐ p⏐ | b⏐ bᵊ⏐ |
| Alveolar | | d ⷌⷌ⏐⏐ d̪⏐ | t ⏐ | d ⏐ | tʰ ⏐⏐⏐ t⏐⏐ | d⏐⏐ dᵊ⏐ |
| Velar | k̠ʔ⏐ | g ⏐ | k ⏐ | | kʰ ⏐⏐⏐ k⏐⏐ | gᵊ⏐ |
| Glottal | ʔ ⷌⷌ ⷌⷌ | | | | ʔ ⏐⏐ | |
| | | | | | | |
| **Fricatives** | | | | | | |
| Labial | f̠ʔ⏐ f⏐ | | f ⏐⏐⏐ | v ⏐ | p͜f⏐ f⏐⏐⏐ | v ⏐ |
| Dental | | | | | | |
| Alveolar | | | | z⏐ | ʔts⏐ | z⏐⏐ |
| Palatal | ʃʔ | | ʃ⏐ | | ʃ⏐ | ʒ⏐ |
| | | | | | | |
| **Affricates** | | | | | | |
| Palatal | tʃʔ⏐⏐ | dʒ:⏐⏐⏐ | | | tʃ⏐ tʃ:⏐ | dʒ⏐⏐ dʒᵊ⏐ |
| | | | | | | |
| **Liquids** | | | | | | |
| Alveolar | | | | | l⏐ | |
| Palatal | | | | | ɚ ⏐⏐ | |
| | | | | | | |
| **Clusters** | gw   sʔn | | | | | |

**Figure 9-3**   Reproducible Form 3: Phonetic Inventory – Consonants

## REPRODUCIBLE FORM 5:  SYLLABLE AND WORD-SHAPE INVENTORY AND SEQUENTIAL CONSTRAINTS

Name: __Carter_____ Age: __5; 9____ Date: ___—_____

Shown below are syllable and word shapes commonly used by young children. The C stands for a consonant and the V for a vowel. Parentheses indicate that the C or V within the parenthesis is optional, for example, (C)CV means that the child uses both CV and CCV syllables. Tally the number of syllable/word shapes of each type.  There is space in each section to add additional shapes that the child may use.

Be sure to note what the child actually does rather than comparing to the adult form. For example, if the child's utterance is [fwɪdweto] for *refrigerator*, this form would be listed under Trisyllables even though the adult version has five syllables. Also, for some children who make heavy use of one sound, for example, the only C used in front of vowels is [h], you may want to tally [hV] syllables separately.

Note: Not tallied

### *Shapes of Monosyllables*

( V )                                ( CCV )   extremely rare

( CV )        often [ʔV]            CCCV(C)

( VC )                              (C)VCC

( CVC )       often [ʔVC]

### *Shapes of Disyllables*

( VCV )       often [VʔC]           CCVCV

( CVCV )      often [ʔVʔC]

( VCVC )      often [VʔVC]

CVCVC

### *Shapes of Trisyllables*

VCVCV

CVCVCV

### *Sequential Constraints*

Indicate any limitations on what types of segments cannot be adjacent to each other.

① Few consonant clusters.

② Many initial and intervocalic consonants are glotal stops—a preference for [ʔ].

③ There are are a few initial voiceless fricatives, but they are followed immediately by a glotal stop: [pʔæk] for p<u>ack</u>.

**Figure 9-4**   Reproducible Form 5: Syllable and Word-Shape Inventory

## REPRODUCIBLE FORM 6: SEGMENTAL INVENTORY—CONSONANTS

Name: Carter                              Age: 5; 9      Date: ⎯

Use this form to record the child's version(s) of each English target consonant. Tally the number of productions of that type next to each symbol. (*Not tallied, but most frequent production listed first.*)

| Place/Manner | Initial | | Intervocalic | | Final | |
|---|---|---|---|---|---|---|
| **Glides** | | | | | | |
| Labiovelar | /w/  w m | | /w/ | | | |
| Palatal | /j/  j | | /j/ | | ▓▓▓ | |
| Glottal | /h/  ʔ ∅ | | /h/ | | ▓▓▓ | |
| | | | | | ▓▓▓ | |
| **Nasals** | | | | | | |
| Labial | /m/  m | | /m/  m | | /m/  m mᵊ | |
| Alveolar | /n/  n | | /n/ | | /n/  n ŋ ∅ | |
| Velar | ▓▓▓ | | /ŋ/ | | /ŋ/  n nᵊ ŋ | |

| | Voiceless | Voiced | Voiceless | Voiced | Voiceless | Voiced |
|---|---|---|---|---|---|---|
| **Stops** | | | | | | |
| Labial | /p/  p | /b/  b | /p/  p | /b/  p͟b | /p/  p pʰ | /b/  b bᵊ |
| Alveolar | /t/  k̲ʔ ∅ | /d/  d ḓ | /t/ | /d/ | /t/  t tʰ | /d/  d dᵊ |
| Velar | /k/  ʔ ∅ g | /g/  d | /k/  k | /g/  d | /k/  kʰ k | /g/  gᵊ k d |
| **Fricatives** | | | | | | |
| Labial | /f/  ∅ f̲ʔ | /v/  w | /f/  f | /v/  v | /f/  f p͟f | /v/  ʔ |
| Dental | /θ/  f̲ʔ ʔ ∅ | /ð/  ʔ ∅ | /θ/ | /ð/  ∅ | /θ/  f | /ð/ |
| Alveolar | /s/  ∅ ʧ ʃ | /z/  w | /s/ | /z/  z | /s/  ∅ ʃ ʧ | /z/  ʒ z ʤ |
| Palatal | /ʃ/  ∅ ʃ̲ʔ | /ʒ/  rare | /ʃ/  f | /ʒ/ | /ʃ/  f ʔ͟ts | /ʒ/ |
| **Affricates** | | | | | | |
| Palatal | /ʧ/  ∅ ʧ̲ʔ | /ʤ/  ∅ ʤ | /ʧ/ | /ʤ/  ∅ | /ʧ/  ʧ ʧ: | /ʤ/  ʤ ʤᵊ |

| Place/Manner | Initial | | Intervocalic | | Final | |
|---|---|---|---|---|---|---|
| **Liquids** | | | | | | |
| Alveolar | /l/  w | | /l/  j w | | /l/  v l | |
| Palatal /r/ | /r/  w | | /r/  w | | /r/ or /ɚ/  ∅ ə ɚ V:  ɪ ə ɚ ∅ | |

**Figure 9-5**  Reproducible Form 6: Segmental Inventory – Consonants

## REPRODUCIBLE FORM 7: SEGMENTAL INVENTORY— WORD-INITIAL CLUSTERS

Name: Carter _____ Age: 5; 9 _____ Date: __—__

Use this form to record the child's version(s) of each English target cluster. Tally the number of productions of that type next to each symbol. (*Not tallied*)

| Two-Element Clusters | Voiceless Initial C | Voiced Initial C | | Two-Element Clusters with /s/ | |
|---|---|---|---|---|---|
| With /w/ | /tw/   ʔØ | | | /sm/   Øm | |
| | /kw/   k̲ʔØ | | | /sn/   sʔn | |
| | /sw/   ʤØ | | | | |
| | | | | /sp/   Øb | |
| With /l/ | /pl/   bØ   pØ | /bl/   bØ | | /st/   Øʤ | |
| | /kl/   ʔØ   gw | /gl/   gᵘ | | /sk/   Øʔ | |
| | /fl/   ØØ | | | | |
| | /sl/   ØØ | | | **Three-Element Clusters with /s/** | |
| With /r/ | /pr/   bØ | /br/   bØ | | /skw/   ØØØ   Øgᵘ | |
| | /tr/   Ø   ʧØ | /dr/   ØØ   ʤ:Ø | | /spl/   ØbØ | |
| | /kr/   gᵘ   ØØ | /gr/   gØ | | /spr/   ØbØ | |
| | /fr/   ʔØ | | | /str/   ØʔØ | |
| | /Ør/   ʤØ | | | /skr/   Øʧʔ | |
| Rare Clusters | /sf/ | /dw/ | | | |
| | /ʃl/ | /gw/ | | | |
| | /ʃr/ | /vr/ | | | |
| | /hj/ | /mj/ | | | |
| | /pj/ | /bj/ | | | |
| | /gj/ | /kj/ | | | |

*Note:* We may have here a philosophical difference in the use of the Ø (null) symbol. I prefer to make it explicit.

**Figure 9-6**   Reproducible Form 7: Segmental Inventory – Word-Initial Clusters

## REPRODUCIBLE FORM 8: SEGMENTAL INVENTORY—VOWELS

Name: _Carter_____ Age: __5; 9___ Date: ____—_____

Use this form to determine the vowels the child uses for each English target. Enter the symbol for the vowel used on a line in the relevant category. Use tally marks to indicate the number of tokens containing this vowel. (*Not tallied, but most common varient listed first.*)

| | | | | | |
|---|---|---|---|---|---|
| High front – | /i/ | i | ɪ | | |
| | /ɪ/ | ɪ | | | |
| | /e/ | e | ɪ | | |
| Mid-low front – | /ɛ/ | ʌ | | | |
| | /ɚ/ | ɑ | ʌ | | |
| High back, rounded – | /u/ | u | | | |
| | /ʊ/ | ʊ | | | |
| Mid back, rounded – | /o/ | o | | | |
| | /ɔ/ | ɑ | | | |
| Low Back – | /ɑ/ | ɑ | (OK for this dialect) | | |
| Central – | /ə/ | ʌ | | | |
| | /ʌ/ | ʌ | | | |
| [r]-colored – | /ɝ/ | 3 | | | |
| | /ɚ/ | ɚ | ə | | |
| | /ɪr/ | ʌ | | | |
| | /ɛr/ | ʌ | | | |
| | /ʊr/ | ʌ | | | |
| | /ɔr/ | ʌ | | | |
| | /ɑr/ | ʌ | | | |
| Diphthongs – | /aɪ/ | ɪ | | | |
| | /aʊ/ | aʊ | ʌ | | |
| | /ɔɪ/ | ɔə | | | |

**Figure 9-7**   Reproducible Form 8: Segmental Inventory – Vowels

2. Perusal of these analyses showed some rather unusual findings:

   A. Carter used few of the typical phonological processes other than gliding of liquids. However, that does not mean that he used target structures correctly.

   B. The phonetic inventory for consonants showed that Carter used a wide variety of speech sounds. However, the segmental inventory for consonants indicated that Carter rarely used these sounds in the correct places. For example, his [w] could be used for /w/, /l/, /r/, and—surprisingly—for word-initial /v/ and /z/. He also had other unusual errors. He used glottal stops to replace some initial consonants and clusters, and he broke many syllables using glottal stops. For example, his production of *shoe* was [ʃʔu].

   C. Carter used a variety of one- and two-syllable word shapes, excepting those that involved clusters. However, many of those shapes could be counted only because he used a glottal stop, for example, for some word-initial C and most intervocalic C.

   D. Carter used single consonants, glottal stops, and outright deletions for word-initial clusters.

   E. Carter also had several vowel errors, as seen in the segmental inventory for vowels.

   F. Carter exhibited unusual assimilations and metatheses, although they were not frequent. For example, *window* was said as [mɪndo], and *fishing* was said as [ɪfɪŋ] (although *fish* was said as [fʔɪʔts]).

3. Carter was completely unintelligible to the clinician. Because of his relatively slow speaking rate, it was easy to transcribe syllables, but the problem was that transcription did not help in understanding what they meant.

4. Receptive vocabulary was at the 97th percentile on the Peabody Picture Vocabulary Test (Dunn, 1965), but his expressive language could not be evaluated due to poor intelligibility. Cognitive function was estimated to be well within normal limits.

5. With respect to prosody, Carter's connected speech sounded like strings of stressed syllables and as mentioned earlier, his speech was slow enough that we could easily transcribe individual syllables. Hearing status and voice quality were within normal limits. It was not possible to evaluate fluency because many of Carter's syllables sounded the same, and they might or might not have been repetitions.

6. In several different evaluations of the oral mechanism and its function, Carter's responses were often within the normal range, but for some of the tasks he demonstrated slowness, weakness of closures, and groping. Alternating motion rates (diadochokinesis) were slow. It is worth noting that the minor deficiencies in the oral mechanism did not adequately account for Carter's errors. For example, he could not keep his lips together with enough force to prevent the clinician from gently pulling a tongue blade from between his closed lips. Nevertheless, his production of bilabials was adequate.

7. A diagnosis of Developmental Verbal Dyspraxia was made on the basis of the preponderance of the evidence as shown in Reproducible Form 12: Checklist for Characteristics of Developmental Verbal Dyspraxia (Figure 9-8).

## REPRODUCIBLE FORM 12: CHECKLIST FOR CHARACTERISTICS OF DEVELOPMENTAL VERBAL DYSPRAXIA

Name:_____Carter_____ Age: _5; 9_____ Date: ____—_____

This checklist can help the SLP determine from the preponderance of the evidence if a child has Developmental Verbal Dyspraxia.

### Speech and Oral Behaviors

✓    1. Significant disturbances in intelligibility or naturalness* (Poor intelligibility is a common characteristic in young children who have DVD. Some older children who have undergone treatment have speech that is mostly intelligible, but slow and deliberate.)

✓    2. Severely limited consonant repertory, with many omission errors*

✓    3. Reduced syllable shape inventory*

✓    4. Assimilation and metathetic (transposition) errors*

✓    5. Vowel errors*

✓    6. Presence of an oral, non-verbal apraxia*

✓    7. Groping for articulatory contacts*

✓    8. Inconsistency in production, especially within the same word*

✓    9. Increase in errors when word length increases or when word complexity increases*

✓    10. Errors in prosody* (Little alternating stress because of few unstressed syllables)

    11. Increase in errors in connected speech compared to single words

    12. Occasional well-articulated word that is not heard again*

✓    13. Other (specify)

### History

✓    1. Poor feeding in infancy and/or persistent drooling after an age when most children reduce drooling

    2. Sensory aversions such as tactile defensiveness in infancy and early childhood—that is, unwillingness to put certain textures or tastes in the mouth or to encounter certain textures on the skin

    3. Relative silence during infancy

    4. Generalized clumsiness

    5. Slow progress in treatment*

    6. Other (specify)

*(continues)*

**Figure 9-8**    Reproducible Form 12: Characteristics of Developmental Verbal Dyspraxia

## Checklist for Characteristics of Developmental Verbal Dyspraxia *(continued)*

### *Non-Speech Indicators of Difficulty in Speaking*

      1. Unwillingness or refusal to imitate modeled words

      2. Well-developed gesture system to supplement speech*

✓    3. Avoidance of speaking situations

✓    4. Reliance on parent or older sibling as a translator

      5. Other (specify)

### *Concomitant Characteristics*

✓    1. Expressive language depressed in comparison to receptive language

      2. Specific difficulty with vocabulary, especially word-finding

✓    3. Signs typically associated with central neuromotor disorders: perseveration, difficulty inhibiting gestures or behaviors that interfere with production attempts, and evidence of fatigue relatively early in a task

      4. Other (specify)

*Note: Characteristics which have widespread support, and which some authorities consider to be strong indicators of DVD if they are present, are indicated with an asterisk. It is well to note that Marquardt and Sussman (1991) consider the severity of reported DVD behaviors to be as diagnostic as their presence.*

**Figure 9-8** *(continued)*

## Initial Steps in Intervention:

1. We recommended that the parents try to provide some peer group experiences for Carter, which they did after they found some other home-schooled children in the area. By that time Carter was already more intelligible and willing to participate.

2. Except for some initial work in isolation for newly targeted sounds, only real words were used in treatment with Carter, and they had to be words that would be fully acceptable when he "fixed" the target. We also used graphemes extensively with him. The requirement for using real, meaningful words with Carter was difficult to meet because of his limited sound inventory. In the early stages, we sometimes made up words, which he found to be fun.

3. Because the need for correct use of a variety of speech sounds was so important for Carter, we targeted specific phonemes only until he could readily produce them in five or six words, then chose a new target.

4. Because it was clear that Carter had difficulty sequencing oral sounds, we incorporated considerable drill, which was necessary to achieve the five or six words mentioned above.

5. Because Carter used many glottal stops in word-initial position, we targeted that structure first, beginning with the consonant /h/ (which requires that the vocal folds be open rather than closed as for a glottal stop but which also requires no oral articulation). Carter was taught to make a smooth transition into a vowel. Words used were *hi, hoe, who, he, hay* and *hey*, and *How!* (stereotypical Native American greeting).

6. We then went to initial /k/, because it has a long Voice Onset Time, during which the aspiration sounds a lot like an /h/. So we introduced the /k/ as being similar to /h/.

## Results:

1. After a year of intervention, Carter's family moved away. However, by that time Carter had filled out the complete segmental inventory, including /r/, except for the frequent substitution of [ʃ] for /s/. He had corrected most but not all of the vowel errors. Interestingly, no change was noted in the vowel errors until they became direct targets of intervention.

2. Carter's prosody did not become completely natural during this period. He continued to use a fairly slow rate of speech, and he did not make as great a distinction between stressed and unstressed syllables as other English speakers. However, he was able to include all sounds in all syllables, which for him was probably the more important result.

## CASE VIII: A CASE OF DEVELOPMENTAL DELAY
## AND PHONOLOGICAL PROBLEMS

**Client:**        Sunday

**Age:**           8;7

**Referral:**      Sunday was in a multicategorical class in a small rural school in a small rural school district. The teacher referred her to the school's speech-language pathologist because she wanted to know if Sunday could become more verbal and more intelligible.

**Background:**    Sunday was the youngest child of five in a family that farmed on rented land. Although her parents readily gave consent for evaluation and treatment, they made it clear that such activities would be part of school and not part of home. The family had kept Sunday at home without the knowledge of the school district, sending her to kindergarten at age 8;5 when they "thought it was time for her to go to school." Consequently, Sunday's communication and academic skills had never before been evaluated.

## Evaluation:

1. Sunday was quite cooperative despite a short attention span. It took five half-hour sessions to complete a brief assessment of language using the *Preschool Language Scale-3* (Zimmerman, Steiner, & Pond, 1991), using the norms for Sunday's estimated mental age, the *Khan-Lewis Phonological Analysis* (Khan & Lewis, 1986), and a conversational sample.

2. Results showed that Sunday had receptive language and phonology scores consistent with a child of about age 4, while expressive language was consistent with an age of about 3;8. Her utterances usually were short and often somewhat repetitive, for example, "Me like this teddy bear. You like this teddy bear?"

3. A psychometric evaluation completed when Sunday was entering kindergarten suggested that her IQ on the WISC-R was about 60.

4. Sunday used a variety of typical phonological processes, unstressed syllable deletion, gliding and vocalization of /r/ but not /l/, and fronting of palatals. Her speech was characterized by considerable variability that included the occasional correct production for such typical error sounds as /s ʃ tʃ dʒ l r/.

5. The recommendation was that the SLP work closely with the classroom teacher to help Sunday become as intelligible as possible with curricular materials. For example, the class was working on being able to communicate their full name and address to others in a way that could be understood, and the SLP elicited intelligible productions of *Sunday* and of the words in her home address, which the classroom teacher also reinforced.

# CASE IX: A CASE OF "TERMINAL /R/"
# AND INTELLIGIBILITY PROBLEMS

| | |
|---|---|
| **Client:** | Jill (Jill is one of the children discussed in Clinical Note 4-1) |
| **Age:** | 9;3 |
| **Referral:** | Jill's school speech-language pathologist suggested that Jill's parents consider a summer program for Jill at a speech camp in a different state. They applied, and Jill was accepted along with other children with speech and language problems. |
| **Background:** | Jill was in third grade, having been held back after her first year in kindergarten. She had received school SLP services for language and articulation for four years. The school SLP reported that Jill had corrected most sounds that were in error except for the /r/, which she had worked on for about 18 months. |

## Results of Evaluation:

1. In a probe for /r/ and /l/, Jill used vowel substitutions for post-vocalic /l/ and /r/ 100% of the time. She used a derhotacized consonantal /r/ 78% of the time and a [w] for /r/ substitution the rest of the time. She was stimulable for /-l/ and also for the /tr-/ cluster, but only in the words *tree* and *treat*, and not *true* or *troll*.

2. Jill's receptive language scores were at about the 7;6-year-old level and expressive scores at about 7;0. She did not have difficulty with morphology at the one-word level. Her reading skills were at the early second grade level.

3. Jill's connected speech was characterized by "islands of unintelligibility." These islands appeared to result from dropped unstressed syllables and word endings, as well as her /r/-errors.

4. Jill was very talkative and would happily hold the floor whenever possible. She did not repair misunderstandings of her speech except to repeat what she had just said, without modification.

## Intervention:

1. Early in the intervention period, it became apparent that Jill did not hear differences between her own error productions of /r/ and the clinician's correct productions; however, she could detect differences between other children's versions of /r/ and the clinician's. She could also detect differences between her own productions and the correct productions of /r/ by peers. Consequently, Jill was grouped with several children who had acceptable /r/, but who were working on sounds that Jill was able to produce. Thus the children could act as providers of models to each other.

2. By the end of 10 hours of intensive intervention, Jill had a tenuous /r/ in isolation. At that point the goal was for that /r/ to become very stable and easily produced, which took another three hours of intensive drill. After that, once Jill had the /r/ in /rV/ syllables, she began to practice syllable chains with /r/, varying the vowels and the stress patterns of the syllables.

3. In parallel with Jill's work on /r/, she worked on improving intelligibility. She learned about the cues that indicated that listeners had not understood her, progressing from noting a listener's raised hand to noting "squeezing" of the eyebrows to being aware

of inappropriate responses by listeners to what she had said. Her utterances in structured conversation were evaluated on a sentence-by-sentence basis for the answer to the question "Did Jill say all the sounds?" and later "Did Jill talk clearly?"

## Results:

1. After her initial slow beginning with /r/, Jill moved relatively quickly through word, phrase, and sentence levels by the end of the summer session. Her school SLP continued to see progress when Jill returned to school in the fall.

2. In the area of clear speech, Jill was able to maintain clear speech through conversations in sessions with her peers and the clinicians, but unfortunately, little carryover to other situations was noted.

# CASE X: A CASE OF DEVELOPMENTAL DELAY IN A CHILD WITH SECOND LANGUAGE ISSUES

**Client:** Sheila

**Age:** 3;7

**Referral:** Sheila's parents brought her for evaluation and treatment on the recommendation of an internationally known neurological institute.

**Background:** Sheila was the fourth child of highly educated parents from India. Her father was an international consulting geologist, and the family had lived for periods of one to two years in several different countries. The parents reported that all other members of the family were fluent in both Gujarati (one of the languages of India) and English, and that the older children attended English-language schools wherever the family lived. Sheila had been hypotonic when she was born, and her development was markedly delayed. At the time of the evaluation, she was also beginning physical therapy and occupational therapy services. Feeding and nutrition had been ruled out as concerns.

## Evaluation and Recommendations:

1. Parental report and clinician observation confirmed that Sheila's vocalizations were primarily vowels, although an occasional [m] could be heard in her jargon. She used pointing gestures and hand-closing ("give me") gestures to indicate her wants.

2. In communication development, Sheila appeared to be at about an 18-month level. Using the *MacArthur Communicative Development Inventory: Words and Gestures* (Fenson, et al., 1993), her parents reported that she understood about 70 words and phrases in either English or Gujarati. They said that she attempted both English and Gujarati words at home.

3. One of Sheila's strengths was that she was interactive and responsive, even with the clinician, whom she did not know.

4. Between the time of the neurological evaluation and their coming to the clinic, the parents had researched the effects of exposure to two languages on development in both languages. They had concluded that the whole family should speak only English with Sheila at home. Their rationale was that Sheila was clearly going to have trouble learning to communicate, and she did not need any other factor that could further delay language development. Moreover, they anticipated that any schooling she received would be in English-language environments. They had come to the conclusion that Sheila should receive treatment in English.

5. The clinician recommended that SLP treatment concentrate on functional vocabulary for Sheila, initially words typical in a young child's vocabulary and also distinctive names for family members, which she did not yet have. Consequently, the focus in the phonological aspects of intervention would be on early-developing sounds—stops, nasals, and glides, as well as CV and reduplicated CV syllables that Sheila could use functionally. The clinician also recommended that not only the clinician but also one or both of the parents participate in the sessions to provide stimuli and reinforcement to Sheila and to carry on the work at home.

   *Note:* If the family had made the decision that Sheila should learn Gujarati first, and English later, the clinician (who was not a speaker of Gujarati) and the parents would have developed the vocabulary to be taught. In addition, a parent would probably need to administer the treatment with the clinician's coaching, because it would be very difficult to find other speakers of Gujarati in the vicinity, let alone a Gujarati-speaking SLP.

## CASE XI: EVALUATION OF A COMPLICATED CASE INCLUDING ENGLISH AS A SECOND LANGUAGE

**Client:** Lee (Lee is the subject of Clinical Note 8-4.)
**Age:** 20
**Referral:** The campus advising office for undecided majors referred Lee because of problems understanding his speech.
**Background:** See information in Clinical Note 8-4.

## Evaluation:

Speech sound production was assessed in connected speech from conversation and from reading Reproducible Form 10: The Rainbow Passage (Client's Copy) and transcribing it onto Reproducible Form 11: The Rainbow Passage (Clinician's Copy), shown in Figure 9-9. In addition, an examination of the oral mechanism with special attention to neuromotor aspects was performed. Language assessment included the Oral Directions Subtest and the Story Construction Subtest of the *Detroit Tests of Learning Aptitude-2* (Hammill, 1985).

---

### REPRODUCIBLE FORM 11: THE RAINBOW PASSAGE (CLINICIAN'S COPY)
*Reproduced with permission from Fairbanks (1960).*

Name:_____ Age: _____ Date: _____

Phonemes correct except as noted.

---

Figure 9-9  Reproducible Form 11: The Rainbow Passage (Clinician's Copy)

and    its    two    ends    apparently    beyond    the    horizon.

(æ)n̦(d)  ɪ t s  tu  ɛ n(d) z  ə pɛr ən ʔlɪ  bɪ j ɑ n(d)  ð ə  h ɔ r aɪ z n̦

There    is,    according    to    legend,    a    boiling    pot    of

ð ə r  ɪ z  ə k ɔ r d n̦  t ə  lɛ ʤ n̦ d  ə  b ɔɪ l n̦  p ɑ t  ə v

gold    at    one    end.    People    look,    but    no    one    ever

g o l d  æ ʔ  w ʌ n  ɛ n d  p i p l  l ʊ k  b ə ʔ  n oʊ  w ʌ n  ɛ v ɚ

finds    it.    When    a    man    looks    for    something

f aɪ n(d) z  ɪ ʔ  w ɛ n  ə  m æ n  l ʊ k s  f ɔ r  s ʌ m θ ɪ ŋ

beyond    his    reach,    his    friends    say    he    is    looking

b ɪ j ɑ n d  h ɪ z  r i ʧ  h ɪ z  f r ɛ n(d) z  s eɪ  h i·  ɪ z  l ʊ k n̦

for    the    pot    of    gold    at    the    end    of    the    rainbow

f ɔ r  ð ə  p ɑ t  ə v  g o l d  æ ʔ  ð ɪ  ɛ n d  ə v  ð ə  r eɪ n b oʊ.

**Figure 9-9** *(continued)*

## Results:

1. The Rainbow Passage was difficult for Lee to read out loud, so the clinician read it a sentence at a time and Lee repeated it while looking at the text. We then filled out Reproducible Forms 6 and 7 (shown in Figure 9-10 and 9-11), the segmental inventories for consonants and clusters, respectively. Based on these analyses, Lee exhibited frequent deletion of syllable-final consonants and consonant clusters, especially involving nasals, simplification of initial clusters, and substitutions for interdental consonants.

2. The results of the examination of the oral mechanism were that Lee exhibited motor weakness and incoordination in virtually all oral systems. He also experienced "overflow" activity when attempting some of the oral motor tasks, for example, his head turned to the side. Diadochokinetic tasks resulted in slow, weak, arrhythmic productions.

# REPRODUCIBLE FORM 6: SEGMENTAL INVENTORY—CONSONANTS

Name: __Lee__ Age: __20__ Date: __—__

Use this form to record the child's version(s) of each English target consonant. Tally the number of productions of that type next to each symbol.

| Place/Manner | Initial | Intervocalic | Final |
|---|---|---|---|
| **Glides** | | | |
| Labiovelar | /w/   w ‖‖ | /w/ | |
| Palatal | /j/   j | | /j/   j | | |
| Glottal | /h/   h ‖‖ Ø | | /h/ | |
| | | | |
| **Nasals** | | | |
| Labial | /m/   m | | /m/ | /m/   Ṽ Ø ‖ |
| Alveolar | /n/   n | | /n/   n | | /n/   Ṽ Ø ⅏ ⅏ | |
| Velar | | /ŋ/ | /ŋ/   ŋ| n| ‖ |

| Place/Manner | Voiceless | Voiced | Voiceless | Voiced | Voiceless | Voiced |
|---|---|---|---|---|---|---|
| **Stops** | | | | | | |
| Labial | /p/   p ‖‖ | /b/   b ⅏ | | /p/   p | | /b/   b | | /p/   β | | /b/ |
| Alveolar | /t/   t ‖‖ | /d/ | /t/   ɾ| | /d/ | /t/ ø ⅏ ɾ| ʔ ‖| | /d/   d | |
| Velar | /k/   k | | /g/ | /k/   k ‖ | /g/ | /k/   k ‖| Ø | | /g/ |
| | | | | | | |
| **Fricatives** | | | | | | |
| Labial | /f/   f ‖ | /v/ | /f/ | /v/   f ‖ | /f/ | /v/ θ ‖| f ‖ ʔ| |
| Dental | /θ/   ɾ| | /ð/ d ⅏| ⅏ | /θ/ | /ð/ | /θ/   θ ‖ | /ð/ |
| Alveolar | /s/   s | | /z/ | /s/ | /z/ | /s/ | /z/ s ⅏ d| Ø | |
| Palatal | /ʃ/   s | | /ʒ/ rare | /ʃ/ | /ʒ/ | /ʃ/ | /ʒ/   Ø | |
| | | | | | | |
| **Affricates** | | | | | | |
| Palatal | /tʃ/ | /dʒ/ | /tʃ/ | /dʒ/   d| | /tʃ/   tʃ ‖| | /dʒ/ |
| | | | | | | |
| **Liquids** | | | | | | |
| Alveolar | /l/   l ⅏ ‖ | /l/   l ‖ | /l/   ɔ ‖ | | | |
| Palatal | /r/   r ⅏ w| | /r/   r ‖ | /r/ or /ɚ/   ə ‖ | | | |

**Figure 9-10**   Reproducible Form 6: Segmental Inventory – Consonants

## REPRODUCIBLE FORM 7:
## SEGMENTAL INVENTORY—WORD-INITIAL CLUSTERS

Name: __Lee_____ Age: __20____ Date: ___—_____

Use this form to record the child's version(s) of each English target cluster. Tally the number of productions of that type next to each symbol. *(Not tallied)*

| Two-Element Clusters | Voiceless Initial C | Voiced Initial C | | Two-Element Clusters with /s/ |
|---|---|---|---|---|
| With /w/ | /tw/ | | | /sm/ |
| | /kw/ | | | /sn/ |
| | /sw/ | | | |
| | | | | /sp/ |
| With /l/ | /pl/ | /bl/ | | /st/ |
| | /kl/ | /gl/ | | /sk/ |
| | /fl/ | | | |
| | /sl/ | | | **Three-Element Clusters with /s/** |
| With /r/ | /pr/   pØ \| | /br/ | | /skw/ |
| | /tr/ | /dr/   dr \| | | /spl/ |
| | /kr/ | /gr/ | | /spr/ |
| | /fr/   fw \| | | | /str/   str \| |
| | /Ør/ | | | /skr/ |
| Rare Clusters | /sf/ | /dw/ | | |
| | /ʃl/ | /gw/ | | |
| | /ʃr/ | /vr/ | | |
| | /hj/ | /mj/ | | |
| | /pj/ | /bj/ b Ø \| | | |
| | /gj/ | /kj/ | | |
| Final Clusters | -ks   [kØ] \|\| | | | |
| | -ps   [ØØ] | | | |
| | -ts   [ØØ] \|\| | | | |
| | -vnd   [v̄ØØ] 卌 | -n̥d   [n̥Ø] \|\| | | |
| | -vn(d)₂   [v̄ØØØ] \|\|\| | -ld   [Ød] \|\| | | |
| | -nt   [v̄ØØ] | | | |

**Figure 9-11**   Reproducible Form 7: Segmental Inventory – Word-Initial Clusters

3. The language testing revealed that story construction was adequate, but the comprehension task of following oral directions resulted in a score at the ninth percentile for persons of age 18, the oldest age covered by the test norms.

4. As was indicated in Clinical Note 8-4, Lee considered his "best" language to be English.

## Recommendations:

1. We recommended that Lee receive speech intervention to improve intelligibility.

2. We communicated with the advising center (with Lee's permission) and referred Lee to a neurologist and then to Vocational Rehabilitation Services.

# APPENDIX

# EVALUATING SUCCESS

● ● ● ● ● ● ● ● ● ● ● ● ● ● ● ● ● ● ● ● ● ● ● ● ● ● ● ● ● ● ● ● ● ● ● ● ●

This appendix includes reproducible forms that can be used as part of a complete assessment of articulation and phonology. They include:

Reproducible Form 1: Checklist for the Diagnostic Evaluation of a Client with Phonological or Articulatory Disorder

Reproducible Form 2: Voice-Prosody and Register Checklists (Adapted from Shriberg, 1993)

Reproducible Form 3: Phonetic Inventory—Consonants

Reproducible Form 4: Phonetic Inventory—Vowels

Reproducible Form 5: Syllable and Word-Shape Inventory and Sequential Constraints

Reproducible Form 6: Segmental Inventory—Consonants

Reproducible Form 7: Segmental Inventory—Word-Initial Clusters

Reproducible Form 8: Segmental Inventory—Vowels

Reproducible Form 9: A Checklist of Listener Responses to Client's Speech

Reproducible Form 10: The Rainbow Passage (Client's Copy)

Reproducible Form 11: The Rainbow Passage (Clinician's Copy)

Reproducible Form 12: Checklist for Characteristics of Developmental Verbal Dyspraxia

Reproducible Form 13: Speech-Language Pathologist's Self-Evaluation

# REPRODUCIBLE FORM 1: CHECKLIST FOR THE DIAGNOSTIC EVALUATION OF A CLIENT WITH PHONOLOGICAL OR ARTICULATORY DISORDER

Name:_____ Age: _____ Date: _____

## Case History

____ Caregiver concerns

____ Perinatal history

____ Developmental history

____ Medical history

____ Social history

____ Current communication status

____ Current communication interactions

____ **Hearing Screening, Hearing History**

____ **Assessment of Speech**

____ Test of phonological processes or articulation (specify)

____ Connected speech sample

   ____ Percent of Intelligible Words

   ____ Intelligibility ratings

   ____ Percent of Consonants Correct or Articulation Competence Index

____ Inventory (Phonetic/Segmental: C, CC, V)

## Possible Related Variables

____ Register

____ Voice    ____ Loudness

             ____ Pitch

____ Voice Quality

             ____ Laryngeal

             ____ Nasal

____ Prosody    ____ Phrasing

             ____ Rate

             ____ Stress

____ Phonological awareness assessment

____ Possible Dyspraxic Elements (list):

*(continues)*

## Diagnostic Checklist *(continued)*

___ **Assessment of language**
(Specify any formal tests used, and measures such as MLU)

   ___ Comprehension

      ___ Content

      ___ Form

      ___ Use  (Pragmatics)

   ___ Expression

      ___ Content

      ___ Form

      ___ Use (Pragmatics)

___ **Estimate of cognitive level**
May be based on:

   ___ Behavior that is alert, responsive, interactive, and appropriate for age

   ___ Results of comprehension testing

   ___ Assessment of stage of play (Westby, 2000)

**Psychosocial Inputs and Concerns (list):**

**Psychosocial Behaviors and Concerns (list):**

## REPRODUCIBLE FORM 2:  VOICE-PROSODY AND REGISTER CHECKLISTS
*(Adapted from Shriberg, 1993)*

Name:_____ Age: _____ Date: _____

### Instructions
1. Describe the speech sample with respect to context, number of usable utterances and participants.
2. Check all that apply. If desired, the following scale can be used:

1 = Occasional      2 = Frequent      3 = Always

| VOICE | | |
|---|---|---|
| **REGISTER** | **LOUDNESS** | **PITCH** |
| ___ Character register, such as cartoon character | ___ Appropriate | ___ Appropriate |
| ___ Narrative register | ___ Soft | ___ Low pitch/glottal fry |
| ___ Negative register, such as whining | ___ Loud | ___ Low pitch |
| ___ Sound effects | | ___ High pitch/falsetto |
| ___ Whisper | | ___ High pitch |

| VOICE QUALITY | |
|---|---|
| **LARYNGEAL FEATURES** | **RESONANCE FEATURES** |
| ___ Appropriate | ___ Appropriate |
| ___ Breathy | ___ Hypernasal |
| ___ Rough | ___ Denasal |
| ___ Strained | ___ Nasopharyngeal |
| ___ Break/shift/tremulous | |
| ___ Register break | |
| ___ Diplophonia | |
| ___ Multiple laryngeal features | |

*(continues)*

## Voice-Prosody and Register Checklists *(continued)*

| PROSODY | | |
|---|---|---|
| **PHRASING AND FLUENCY** | **RATE** | **STRESS** |
| ___ Appropriate | ___ Appropriate | ___ Appropriate |
| ___ Sound/syllable repetition | ___ Slow rate not due to pause time | ___ Incorrect multisyllabic word stress |
| ___ Word repetition | ___ Slow rate due to pause time | ___ Reduced/equal stress |
| ___ Sound/syllable *and* word repetition | ___ Slow articulation rate | ___ Excessive/equal/ misplaced stress |
| ___ Repetition of more than one word, such as phrase | ___ Fast rate | ___ Multiple stress features |
| ___ One-word revision | ___ Fast rate with acceleration | |
| ___ Revision of more than one word, such as phrase | | |
| ___ *Failure to mark end of clause/sentence with pitch declination or pause | | |
| ___ *Failure to use appropriate question intonation | | |
| *Added by Smit | | |

## REPRODUCIBLE FORM 3: PHONETIC INVENTORY—CONSONANTS

Name:_____ Age: _____ Date: _____

Use this form to record the types of consonants that the client produces, without regard to the English target consonant. Tally the number of productions of that type next to each symbol.

| Place/Manner | Initial | Intervocalic | Final |
|---|---|---|---|
|  |  |  |  |
| **Glides** |  |  |  |
| Labiovelar |  |  |  |
| Palatal |  |  |  |
| Glottal |  |  |  |
|  |  |  |  |
| **Nasals** |  |  |  |
| Labial |  |  |  |
| Alveolar |  |  |  |
| Velar |  |  |  |
|  |  |  |  |

|  | Voiceless | Voiced | Voiceless | Voiced | Voiceless | Voiced |
|---|---|---|---|---|---|---|
| **Stops** |  |  |  |  |  |  |
| Labial |  |  |  |  |  |  |
| Alveolar |  |  |  |  |  |  |
| Velar |  |  |  |  |  |  |
| Glottal |  |  |  |  |  |  |
|  |  |  |  |  |  |  |
| **Fricatives** |  |  |  |  |  |  |
| Labial |  |  |  |  |  |  |
| Dental |  |  |  |  |  |  |
| Alveolar |  |  |  |  |  |  |
| Palatal |  |  |  |  |  |  |
|  |  |  |  |  |  |  |
| **Affricates** |  |  |  |  |  |  |
| Palatal |  |  |  |  |  |  |
|  |  |  |  |  |  |  |
|  |  |  |  |  |  |  |
| **Liquids** |  |  |  |  |  |  |
| Alveolar |  |  |  |  |  |  |
| Palatal |  |  |  |  |  |  |
|  |  |  |  |  |  |  |
| **Clusters** |  |  |  |  |  |  |

## REPRODUCIBLE FORM 4:  PHONETIC INVENTORY—VOWELS

**Name:**_____ **Age:** _____ **Date:** _____

Use this form to determine which types of vowels the client uses, regardless of the English target. Enter the symbol for the vowel used on a line in the relevant category. Use tally marks to indicate the number of tokens containing this vowel. Include diphthongized tense vowels in the category in which the tense vowel falls. The English tense vowels are [i e u o ɑ].

*Note:* Some features that children may manipulate include rounding, nasalization, lengthening/shortening, and degree of jaw opening.

High front (English uses [i ɪ e])          _____   _____   _____   _____

Mid-low front (English uses [ɛ æ])        _____   _____   _____   _____

High back, rounded (English uses [u ʊ])    _____   _____   _____   _____

Mid back, rounded (English uses [o ɔ])     _____   _____   _____   _____

Low back (English uses [ɑ])               _____   _____   _____   _____

Central (English uses [ə ʌ])              _____   _____   _____   _____

Central [r]-colored V (English uses [ɚ ɝ])  _____   _____   _____   _____

Other [r]-colored V
    (English uses [ ɪr ɛr ʊr ɔr ar])       _____   _____   _____   _____

Diphthongs (English uses [aɪ aʊ ɔɪ]       _____   _____   _____   _____

## REPRODUCIBLE FORM 5: SYLLABLE AND WORD-SHAPE INVENTORY AND SEQUENTIAL CONSTRAINTS

Name:_____ Age: _____ Date: _____

Shown below are syllable and word shapes commonly used by young children. The C stands for a consonant and the V for a vowel. Parentheses indicate that the C or V within the parenthesis is optional, for example, (C)CV means that the child uses both CV and CCV syllables. Tally the number of syllable/word shapes of each type. There is space in each section to add additional shapes that the child may use.

Be sure to note what the child actually does rather than comparing to the adult form. For example, if the child's utterance is [fwɪdweto] for *refrigerator*, this form would be listed under Trisyllables even though the adult version has five syllables. Also, for some children who make heavy use of one sound, for example, the only C used in front of vowels is [h], you may want to tally [hV] syllables separately.

---

### *Shapes of Monosyllables*

---

| | |
|---|---|
| V | CCV(C) |
| CV | CCCV(C) |
| VC | (C)VCC |
| CVC | |

---

### *Shapes of Disyllables*

---

| | |
|---|---|
| VCV | CCVCV |
| CVCV | |
| VCVC | |
| CVCVC | |

---

### *Shapes of Trisyllables*

---

VCVCV
CVCVCV

---

### *Sequential Constraints*

---

Indicate any limitations on what types of segments cannot be adjacent to each other.

# REPRODUCIBLE FORM 6: SEGMENTAL INVENTORY—CONSONANTS

Name:_____ Age: _____ Date: _____

Use this form to record the child's version(s) of each English target consonant. Tally the number of productions of that type next to each symbol.

| Place/Manner | Initial | | Intervocalic | | Final | |
|---|---|---|---|---|---|---|
| | | | | | | |
| **Glides** | | | | | | |
| Labiovelar | /w/ | | /w/ | | | |
| Palatal | /j/ | | /j/ | | | |
| Glottal | /h/ | | /h/ | | | |
| | | | | | | |
| **Nasals** | | | | | | |
| Labial | /m/ | | /m/ | | /m/ | |
| Alveolar | /n/ | | /n/ | | /n/ | |
| Velar | | | /ŋ/ | | /ŋ/ | |
| | | | | | | |
| | Voiceless | Voiced | Voiceless | Voiced | Voiceless | Voiced |
| **Stops** | | | | | | |
| Labial | /p/ | /b/ | /p/ | /b/ | /p/ | /b/ |
| Alveolar | /t/ | /d/ | /t/ | /d/ | /t/ | /d/ |
| Velar | /k/ | /g/ | /k/ | /g/ | /k/ | /g/ |
| | | | | | | |
| **Fricatives** | | | | | | |
| Labial | /f/ | /v/ | /f/ | /v/ | /f/ | /v/ |
| Dental | /θ/ | /ð/ | /θ/ | /ð/ | /θ/ | /ð/ |
| Alveolar | /s/ | /z/ | /s/ | /z/ | /s/ | /z/ |
| Palatal | /ʃ/ | /ʒ/ rare | /ʃ/ | /ʒ/ | /ʃ/ | /ʒ/ |
| | | | | | | |
| **Affricates** | | | | | | |
| Palatal | /ʧ/ | /ʤ/ | /ʧ/ | /ʤ/ | /ʧ/ | /ʤ/ |
| | | | | | | |
| **Liquids** | | | | | | |
| Alveolar | /l/ | | /l/ | | /l/ | |
| Palatal | /r/ | | /r/ | | /r/ or /ɚ/ | |

## REPRODUCIBLE FORM 7: SEGMENTAL INVENTORY—
## WORD-INITIAL CLUSTERS

Name:_____ Age: _____ Date: _____

Use this form to indicate how the child produces each English target cluster. Tally the number of productions of that type next to each symbol.

| Two-Element Clusters | | | | Two-Element Clusters with /s/ |
|---|---|---|---|---|
| | Voiceless Initial C | Voiced Initial C | | |
| With /w/ | /tw/ | | | /sm/ |
| | /kw/ | | | /sn/ |
| | /sw/ | | | |
| | | | | /sp/ |
| With /l/ | /pl/ | /bl/ | | /st/ |
| | /kl/ | /gl/ | | /sk/ |
| | /fl/ | | | |
| | /sl/ | | | **Three-Element Clusters with /s/** |
| | | | | |
| With /r/ | /pr/ | /br/ | | /skw/ |
| | /tr/ | /dr/ | | /spl/ |
| | /kr/ | /gr/ | | /spr/ |
| | /fr/ | | | /str/ |
| | /θr/ | | | /skr/ |
| | | | | |
| **Rare Clusters** | /sf/ | /dw/ | | |
| | /ʃl/ | /gw/ | | |
| | /ʃr/ | /vr/ | | |
| | /hj/ | /mj/ | | |
| | /pj/ | /bj/ | | |
| | /gj/ | /kj/ | | |

# REPRODUCIBLE FORM 8: SEGMENTAL INVENTORY—VOWELS

Name:_____ Age: _____ Date: _____

Use this form to determine the vowels the child uses for each English target. Enter the symbol for the vowel used on a line in the relevant category. Use tally marks to indicate the number of tokens containing this vowel.

| High front | /i/ | _____ | _____ | _____ | _____ |
| | /ɪ/ | _____ | _____ | _____ | _____ |
| | /e/ | _____ | _____ | _____ | _____ |
| Mid-low front | /ɛ/ | _____ | _____ | _____ | _____ |
| | /æ/ | _____ | _____ | _____ | _____ |
| High back, rounded | /u/ | _____ | _____ | _____ | _____ |
| | /ʊ/ | _____ | _____ | _____ | _____ |
| Mid back, rounded | /o/ | _____ | _____ | _____ | _____ |
| | /ɔ/ | _____ | _____ | _____ | _____ |
| Low back | /ɑ/ | _____ | _____ | _____ | _____ |
| Central | /ə/ | _____ | _____ | _____ | _____ |
| | /ʌ/ | _____ | _____ | _____ | _____ |
| [r]-colored | /ɝ/ | _____ | _____ | _____ | _____ |
| | /ɚ/ | _____ | _____ | _____ | _____ |
| | /ɪr/ | _____ | _____ | _____ | _____ |
| | /ɛr/ | _____ | _____ | _____ | _____ |
| | /ʊr/ | _____ | _____ | _____ | _____ |
| | /ɔr/ | _____ | _____ | _____ | _____ |
| | /ar/ | _____ | _____ | _____ | _____ |
| Diphthongs | /aɪ/ | _____ | _____ | _____ | _____ |
| | /aʊ/ | _____ | _____ | _____ | _____ |
| | /ɔɪ/ | _____ | _____ | _____ | _____ |

## REPRODUCIBLE FORM 9:  A CHECKLIST OF LISTENER RESPONSES TO CLIENT'S SPEECH

Date: _____

Dear _____ ,

Please respond to the following scales concerning the speech of _____ .
On each scale, please check the item that most closely describes your opinion.

### SCALE 1: HOW THE SPEECH PATTERN SOUNDS TO ME

_____ I generally pay attention only to what this child says, not how it is said.

_____ I notice the child's speaking pattern, but I easily concentrate on the content.

_____ I am distracted by the speaking pattern, and I work to concentrate on the content.

_____ I am so distracted by the speaking pattern that I miss some of the content.

_____ Because of the speaking pattern, I have difficulty paying attention to content.

**COMMENTS:** _____

_____

_____

_____

### SCALE 2: HOW THIS CHILD REACTS TO HIS OR HER OWN SPEECH

_____ The child seems unaware of any speaking differences.

_____ The child occasionally seems to be aware that the speaking pattern is somewhat different.

_____ The child is mildly frustrated by his/her speaking pattern, for example, avoids talking, ordering on the phone.

_____ The child is very frustrated and perhaps discouraged by the speaking pattern.

**COMMENTS:** _____

_____

_____

_____

## REPRODUCIBLE FORM 10:  THE RAINBOW PASSAGE (CLIENT'S COPY)
*Reproduced with permission from Fairbanks (1960).*

Name:_____ Age: _____ Date: _____

Instructions: Please read the following out loud at your normal reading rate.

When the sunlight strikes raindrops in the air, they act like a prism and form a
rainbow. The rainbow is a division of white light into many beautiful colors. These
take the shape of a long round arch, with its path high above, and its two ends
apparently beyond the horizon. There is, according to legend, a boiling pot of gold
at one end. People look, but no one ever finds it. When a man looks for something
beyond his reach, his friends say he is looking for the pot of gold at the end of
the rainbow.

# REPRODUCIBLE FORM 11: THE RAINBOW PASSAGE (CLINICIAN'S COPY)
*Reproduced with permission from Fairbanks (1960).*

**Name:**_____ **Age:** _____ **Date:** _____

| When | the | sunlight | strikes | raindrops | in | the | air, |
|---|---|---|---|---|---|---|---|
| wɛn | ðə | sʌnlaɪt | straɪks | reɪndrɑps | ɪn | ðɪ | ɛr |

| they | act | like | a | prism | and | form | a | rainbow. |
|---|---|---|---|---|---|---|---|---|
| ðeɪ | æk(t) | laɪk | ə | prɪzm | n̩(d) | fɔrm | ə | reɪnboʊ |

| The | rainbow | is | a | division | of | white | light | into |
|---|---|---|---|---|---|---|---|---|
| ðə | reɪnboʊ | ɪz | ə | dɪvɪʒn̩ | əv | waɪt | laɪt | ɪntu |

| many | beautiful | colors. | These | take | the | shape | of |
|---|---|---|---|---|---|---|---|
| mɛnɪ | bjutɪfl̩ | kʌlɚz | ðiz | teɪk | ðə | ʃeɪp | əv |

| a | long | round | arch, | with | its | path | high | above, |
|---|---|---|---|---|---|---|---|---|
| ə | lɑŋ | raʊnd | arʧ | wɪθ | ɪts | pæθ | haɪ | əbʌv |

| and | its | two | ends | apparently | beyond | the | horizon. |
|---|---|---|---|---|---|---|---|
| (æ)n(d) | ɪts | tu | ɛn(d)z | əpɛrənʔlɪ | bɪjɑn(d) | ðə | hɔraɪzn̩ |

| There | is, | according | to | legend, | a | boiling | pot | of |
|---|---|---|---|---|---|---|---|---|
| ðər | ɪz | əkɔrdn̩ | tə | lɛʤn̩d | ə | bɔɪln̩ | pɑt | əv |

| gold | at | one | end. | People | look, | but | no | one | ever |
|---|---|---|---|---|---|---|---|---|---|
| gold | æʔ | wʌn | ɛnd | pipl | lʊk | bəʔ | noʊ | wʌn | ɛvɚ |

| finds | it. | When | a | man | looks | for | something |
|---|---|---|---|---|---|---|---|
| faɪn(d)z | ɪʔ | wɛn | ə | mæn | lʊks | fɔr | sʌmθɪŋ |

| beyond | his | reach, | his | friends | say | he | is | looking |
|---|---|---|---|---|---|---|---|---|
| bɪjɑnd | hɪz | riʧ | hɪz | frɛn(d)z | seɪ | hi | ɪz | lʊkŋ̩ |

| for | the | pot | of | gold | at | the | end | of | the | rainbow |
|---|---|---|---|---|---|---|---|---|---|---|
| fɔr | ðə | pɑt | əv | gold | æʔ | ðɪ | ɛnd | əv | ðə | reɪnboʊ. |

## REPRODUCIBLE FORM 12: CHECKLIST FOR CHARACTERISTICS OF DEVELOPMENTAL VERBAL DYSPRAXIA

Name:_____ Age: _____ Date: _____

This checklist can help the SLP determine from the preponderance of the evidence if a child has Developmental Verbal Dyspraxia.

### *Speech and Oral Behaviors*

_____ 1. Significant disturbances in intelligibility or naturalness* (Poor intelligibility is a common characteristic in young children who have DVD. Some older children who have undergone treatment have speech that is mostly intelligible, but slow and deliberate.)

_____ 2. Severely limited consonant repertory, with many omission errors*

_____ 3. Reduced syllable shape inventory*

_____ 4. Assimilation and metathetic (transposition) errors*

_____ 5. Vowel errors*

_____ 6. Presence of an oral, non-verbal apraxia*

_____ 7. Groping for articulatory contacts*

_____ 8. Inconsistency in production, especially within the same word*

_____ 9. Increase in errors when word length increases or when word complexity increases*

_____ 10. Errors in prosody*

_____ 11. Increase in errors in connected speech compared to single words

_____ 12. Occasional well-articulated word that is not heard again*

_____ 13. Other (specify)

### *History*

_____ 1. Poor feeding in infancy and/or persistent drooling after an age when most children reduce drooling

_____ 2. Sensory aversions such as tactile defensiveness in infancy and early childhood—that is, unwillingness to put certain textures or tastes in the mouth or to encounter certain textures on the skin

_____ 3. Relative silence during infancy

_____ 4. Generalized clumsiness

_____ 5. Slow progress in treatment*

_____ 6. Other (specify)                                                                *(continues)*

# Checklist for Characteristics of Developmental Verbal Dyspraxia *(continued)*

---

## *Non-Speech Indicators of Difficulty in Speaking*

---

_____ 1. Unwillingness or refusal to imitate modeled words

_____ 2. Well-developed gesture system to supplement speech*

_____ 3. Avoidance of speaking situations

_____ 4. Reliance on parent or older sibling as a translator

_____ 5. Other (specify)

---

## *Concomitant Characteristics*

---

_____ 1. Expressive language depressed in comparison to receptive language

_____ 2. Specific difficulty with vocabulary, especially word-finding

_____ 3. Signs typically associated with central neuromotor disorders: perseveration, difficulty inhibiting gestures or behaviors that interfere with production attempts, and evidence of fatigue relatively early in a task

_____ 4. Other (specify)

---

*Note: Characteristics which have widespread support, and which some authorities consider to be strong indicators of DVD if they are present, are indicated with an asterisk. It is well to note that Marquardt and Sussman (1991) consider the severity of reported DVD behaviors to be as diagnostic as their presence.*

**Reproducible Form 13:**

# SPEECH-LANGUAGE PATHOLOGIST'S SELF-EVALUATION

| QUESTION (Do I...) | YES | NO |
|---|---|---|
| 1. Understand the difference between "residual or phonetic" errors and "phonological" errors? | | |
| 2. Know when phonological and articulatory assessment is needed? | | |
| 3. Measure intelligibility directly and indirectly, as needed for a given client? | | |
| 4. Use prosody and register checklists as needed for a given client? | | |
| 5. Understand the importance of phonological awareness and assess it when appropriate for a given client? | | |
| 6. Understand the reasons for and the elements of "independent" analyses? | | |
| 7. Understand the reasons for and the elements of "relational" analyses? | | |
| 8. Understand the various types of phonological processes and evaluate a child's use of phonological processes when appropriate? | | |
| 9. Understand the role that knowledge hierarchies may play in diagnostics and intervention? | | |
| 10. Know the basic principles underlying non-linear phonology and use them in planning evaluations and treatment? | | |
| 11. Know how to determine possible dyspraxic elements and use them in planning intervention? | | |
| 12. Understand the role that intelligibility, severity, and perceived deviance play in the evaluation of the speech of the school-aged child, and how to assess them? | | |
| 13. Know what the important prognostic variables are for children with articulation difficulties? | | |
| 14. Use the intervention principles that will help fine-tune treatment to improve outcomes? | | |
| 15. Distinguish between "training broad" and "training deep" and know when each is appropriate? | | |

*(continues)*

## Speech-Language Pathologist's Self-Evaluation *(continued)*

| QUESTION (Do I...) | YES | NO |
|---|---|---|
| 16. Know what kinds of auditory training are appropriate in phonological approaches ("training broad")? | | |
| 17. Know what principles are involved in choosing processes and exemplars in phonological treatments? | | |
| 18. Understand the strengths of the various phonological approaches? | | |
| 19. Know what methods promote rapid change in the three phases of traditional intervention—<br>• Elicitation?<br>• Transfer?<br>• Maintenance? | | |
| 20. Use the key elements of each of the treatment approaches for DVD? | | |
| 21. Know what appropriate speech sound goals are for children whose first language is not English? | | |
| 22. Understand what appropriate speech sound goals are for children with cognitive delays? | | |

# APPENDIX

# MATERIALS USEFUL FOR OLDER SCHOOL-AGE CLIENTS AND FOR ADULTS WHO SPEAK ENGLISH AS A SECOND LANGUAGE

• • • • • • • • • • • • • • • • • • • • • • • • • • • • • • • • • • • •

Part I: Consonants
Part II: Vowels
Part III: Word-Level Stress Patterns

The materials included in this appendix cover those aspects of English phonology that are frequently problematic for speakers of English as a second language (ESL). Wherever possible, alternate spellings are provided for homophones, e.g. *right* and *write*.

These materials can be used in a number of ways:

- Wordlists for each phoneme target or for each word-level stress pattern can be used for both auditory bombardment and production practice.

- Minimal contrasts can be used for both auditory bombardment and production practice.

- In some cases, sentences are provided to increase task complexity. These can be modelled and practiced with or with out the text visible.

It is important that the client know the meaning of each word presented. For less-advanced ESL speakers, words should be selected that the client is likely to know.

## PART I: CONSONANTS

### Syllable-Final Consonant—Voiceless

| | | |
|---|---|---|
| 1. cup | 15. wash | 29. bathtub |
| 2. chip | 16. dish | 30. ruthless |
| 3. cat | 17. cash | 31. baseball |
| 4. hat | 18. watch | 32. faster |
| 5. bite | 19. catch | 33. restaurant |
| 6. back | 20. reach | 34. dish cloth |
| 7. duck | 21. cupcake | 35. washtub |
| 8. laugh | 22. update | 36. wishbone |
| 9. half | 23. bat wing | 37. mushroom |
| 10. bath | 24. eight thirty | 38. beach ball |
| 11. faith | 25. acting | 39. watchman |
| 12. boss | 26. actor | 40. switchback |
| 13. race | 27. laughter | |
| 14. base | 28. half-baked | |

*Note:* Final /t/ is often produced as [ʔ] in American English

### Syllable-Final Consonants—Nasals

| | | |
|---|---|---|
| 1. home | 8. sun/son | 15. main/Maine/mane |
| 2. come | 9. fun | 16. rain/reign |
| 3. comb | 10. can | 17. tune |
| 4. ham | 11. run | 18. mean |
| 5. sum/some | 12. bean | 19. sing |
| 6. rim | 13. bone | 20. wing |
| 7. hum | 14. one/won | 21. sang |

## Syllable-Final Consonants—Nasals *(continued)*

22. rang
23. king
24. song
25. comeback
26. hamster
27. hamburger
28. homebound
29. Kansas
30. under
31. winter
32. wonder
33. enroll
34. handy
35. fancy
36. hundred
37. engine
38. England
39. monkey
40. banker
41. anger
42. thank you

## Syllable-Final Consonants—Voiced

1. tub
2. lab
3. mob
4. robe
5. mad
6. ride
7. could
8. bread
9. big
10. bag
11. dog
12. drug
13. have
14. five
15. live
16. drive
17. bathe
18. smooth
19. soothe
20. breathe
21. lose
22. noise
23. cheese
24. breeze
25. days
26. does
27. has
28. boys
29. rage
30. edge
31. age
32. gauge
33. absent
34. abstain
35. obstruct
36. observe
37. substitute
38. advertise
39. goldfish
40. headline
41. seedless
42. ignore
43. ragweed
44. hogwash
45. exact
46. exam
47. cheesecake
48. wisecrack
49. business
50. dismal
51. doesn't
52. husband
53. judgment
54. ageless

## Consonants /r/ and /l/

Minimal Pairs, /r/ and /l/

1. ray       lay
2. race      lace
3. rack      lack
4. rake      lake
5. ram       lamb
6. ramp      lamp
7. rap       lap
8. rash      lash

*(continues)*

## Consonants /r/ and /l/ *(continued)*

### Minimal Pairs, /r/ and /l/

| | | | | | |
|---|---|---|---|---|---|
| 9. | rate | late | 19. | rip | lip |
| 10. | raw | law | 20. | road | load |
| 11. | reach | leach/leech | 21. | rock | lock |
| 12. | read | lead | 22. | wrong | long |
| 13. | reef | leaf | 23. | room | loom |
| 14. | red | led | 24. | racing | lacing |
| 15. | rice | lice | 25. | rater | later |
| 16. | right/write | light/"lite" | 26. | reader | leader |
| 17. | rim | limb | 27. | river | liver |
| 18. | rhyme | lime | | | |

### Consonant Clusters with Minimal Pairs

| | | | | | |
|---|---|---|---|---|---|
| 1. | brand | bland | 12. | grow | glow |
| 2. | breed | bleed | 13. | cram | clam |
| 3. | breast | blest/blessed | 14. | crime | climb |
| 4. | broom | bloom | 15. | crowd | cloud |
| 5. | brush | blush | 16. | pray | play |
| 6. | frame | flame | 17. | frame | flame |
| 7. | fresh | flesh | 18. | Fred | fled |
| 8. | free | flea/flee | 19. | freeze | fleas |
| 9. | fright | flight | 20. | fresh | flesh |
| 10. | fry | fly | 21. | fruit | flute |
| 11. | grass | glass | 22. | fry | fly |

## Consonants /n/ and /l/

### Minimal Contrasts

| | | | | | |
|---|---|---|---|---|---|
| 1. | night | light | 10. | nook | look |
| 2. | net | let | 11. | nab | lab |
| 3. | node | load | 12. | news | lose |
| 4. | name | lame | 13. | snap | slap |
| 5. | nap | lap | 14. | snow | slow |
| 6. | knack | lack | 15. | snip | slip |
| 7. | know | low | 16. | snack | slacks |
| 8. | nine | line | 17. | snug | slug |
| 9. | nuke | Luke | | | |

## Consonants /s ʃ tʃ/

Minimal Contrasts

| *Syllable-Initial* | | |
|---|---|---|
| 1. save | shave | |
| 2. sigh | shy | chai |
| 3. sew | show | |
| 4. sip | ship | chip |
| 5. saw | Shaw | |
| 6. see | she | |
| 7. sear | sheer/shear | cheer |
| 8. sake | shake | |
| 9. Sam | sham | |
| 10. same | shame | |
| 11. seep | sheep | cheap |
| 12. seen | sheen | |
| 13. said | shed | |
| 14. sin | shin | chin |
| 15. sue | shoe | chew |
| 16. seat | sheet | cheat |
| 17. | share | chair |
| 18. sap | | chap |

| *Syllable-Final* | | |
|---|---|---|
| 1. Cass | cash | catch |
| 2. bass | bash | batch |
| 3. mass | mash | match |
| 4. lass | lash | latch |
| 5. | hash | hatch |
| 6. | wish | witch |
| 7. muss | mush | much |
| 8. fasten | fashion | |

## Consonants /z dz dʒ/

Minimal Contrasts

| 1. zip | jip | |
|---|---|---|
| 2. zany | Janie | |
| 3. zoo | Jew | |
| 4. Zach | Jack | |
| 5. raise | raids | rage |
| 6. pays | | page |

| 7. ways | wades | wage |
|---|---|---|
| 8. buzz | buds | budge |
| 9. | weds | wedge |
| 10. bins | | binge |
| 11. | rids | ridge |

## Consonant /v/

### /v-/

| | | | |
|---|---|---|---|
| 1. vain/vein | 7. vend | 13. view | 19. valley |
| 2. van | 8. vent | 14. voice | 20. value |
| 3. vague | 9. verb | 15. volt | 21. victim |
| 4. vase | 10. vet | 16. vacant | 22. vapor |
| 5. vast | 11. vest | 17. vaccine | 23. visa |
| 6. vault | 12. vice | 18. valid | 24. visit |

### /-v/

| | | | |
|---|---|---|---|
| 1. five | 7. groove | 13. of | 19. believe |
| 2. cave | 8. have | 14. wave | 20. captive |
| 3. brave | 9. leave | 15. above | 21. derive |
| 4. dive | 10. live | 16. alive | 22. improve |
| 5. give | 11. love | 17. approve | 23. native |
| 6. gave | 12. prove | 18. behave | 24. remove |

## Consonant /θ/

### /θ-/

| | | | |
|---|---|---|---|
| 1. thank | 6. thigh | 11. thorn | 16. thickness |
| 2. thaw | 7. thin | 12. thumb | 17. thirty |
| 3. thief | 8. think | 13. thug | 18. thunder |
| 4. theme | 9. thing | 14. thermos | |
| 5. thick | 10. third | 15. thesis | |

### /-θ/

| | | | |
|---|---|---|---|
| 1. bath | 7. faith | 13. teeth | 19. Zenith |
| 2. booth | 8. fifth | 14. truth | 20. twentieth |
| 3. both | 9. math | 15. youth | 21. thirtieth |
| 4. breath | 10. mouth | 16. beneath | |
| 5. cloth | 11. path | 17. mammoth | |
| 6. death | 12. south | 18. warpath | |

## Phrases with /θ/

1. a concern about ethics
2. How thoughtful!
3. hurt your thumb
4. Thursday is the big day
5. we are thankful
6. please be thorough
7. through the door
8. a great athlete
9. an ethnic conflict
10. clean the bathroom
11. Don't drink methyl alcohol
12. in fifth grade (Note: "fith" is OK)
13. a lethal dose
14. the fourth item
15. a southwest wind
16. a ruthless person
17. a militant atheist
18. How pathetic!
19. in the depths of despair
20. we question authority
21. the sixth day
22. a love of mathematics
23. a new threat
24. What a heart throb!
25. a filthy room

## Phrases with /ð/

1. now and then
2. That rascal!
3. What about those?
4. all by themselves
5. 50 points or thereabouts
6. although it is snowing
7. Still breathing?
8. my younger brother
9. a feather in your cap
10. it ran smoothly
11. a real featherbrain
12. a southern exposure
13. the baby is teething
14. work up a lather
15. neither Jack nor Jill
16. awful weather
17. a motherless child
18. a gathering of scholars
19. Americans like togetherness
20. worthy of honor
21. bathe the sore limb
22. the Northern Lights (aurora borealis)
23. the farthest place
24. other than that
25. either will do

## Syllable-Final Clusters with Nasals

| | | |
|---|---|---|
| 1. want | 19. bunk | 37. amount |
| 2. wants | 20. honk | 38. invent |
| 3. bend | 21. dance | 39. advance |
| 4. bond | 22. once | 40. announce |
| 5. fund | 23. chance | 41. defense |
| 6. find | 24. fence | 42. distance |
| 7. bump | 25. ounce | 43. finance |
| 8. lump | 26. prince | 44. nonsense |
| 9. dump | 27. sense | 45. patience |
| 10. damp | 28. tense | 46. pronounce |
| 11. lamp | 29. attend | 47. assumes |
| 12. can't | 30. husband | 48. bedrooms |
| 13. won't | 31. expand | 49. blue jeans |
| 14. dent | 32. extend | 50. complains |
| 15. wink | 33. behind | 51. remains |
| 16. blink | 34. command | 52. Wednesday |
| 17. sink | 35. accent | |
| 18. junk | 36. absent | |

## Consonants—Vocalic and Post-Vocalic /r/

Minimal Contrasts with /-r/

| | | | | | | | |
|---|---|---|---|---|---|---|---|
| 1. pair | peer | per | poor | pore | par | pyre | power |
| 2. wear | we're | whir | | wore | | wire | |
| 3. fair | fear | fur | | four | far | fire | |
| 4. air | | ear | | or | are | ire | hour |
| 5. dare | dear | | doer | door | | dire | dour |
| 6. share | sheer | sure | | shore | | | shower |
| 7. mare | mere | myrrh | Moor | more | mar | mire | |
| 8. hair | hear | her | who're | whore | | hire | how're |
| 9. snare | sneer | | | snore | | | |
| 10. stair | steer | stir | | store | star | | |
| 11. care | | cur | Coor(s)/ cure | core | car | | cower |
| 12. spare | spear | spur | spoor | spore | spar | spire | |

## Disyllables with Final and Embedded /-r/

| | | | |
|---|---|---|---|
| 1. before | 12. barber | 23. urgent | 34. surplus |
| 2. acquire | 13. urban | 24. gorgeous | 35. partial |
| 3. affair | 14. carbon | 25. workbook | 36. portion |
| 4. bizarre | 15. purchase | 26. charcoal | 37. cartoon |
| 5. cashier | 16. fortune | 27. nearly | 38. forty |
| 6. conspire | 17. order | 28. early | 39. birthday |
| 7. detour | 18. harden | 29. army | 40. northern |
| 8. devour | 19. careful | 30. German | 41. harvest |
| 9. guitar | 20. perfect | 31. journal | 42. perverse |
| 10. somewhere | 21. argue | 32. morning | 43. doorway |
| 11. occur | 22. jargon | 33. airport | 44. firewood |

## Minimal Contrasts with /-l/

| | | | | | | | | | | |
|---|---|---|---|---|---|---|---|---|---|---|
| 1. fell | fail | fill | feel | fall | full | fool | foal | file | foul | foil |
| 2. Pell | pail | pill | peel | Paul | pull | pool | pole | pile | Powell | |
| 3. sell | sale | sill | seal | Saul | | Sue'll | soul | | | soil |
| 4. L | ail | ill | eel | all | | | | aisle | owl | oil |
| 5. Mel | mail | mill | meal | mall | | mule | mole | mile | | |
| 6. | kale | kill | keel | call | | cool | coal | Kyle | cowl | coil |
| 7. spell | | spill | spiel | | | spool | | | | spoil |
| 8. well | whale | will | wheel | wall | wool | | | while | | |
| 9. tell | tail | till | teal | tall | | tool | toll | tile | towel | toil |
| 10. bell | bail | bill | | ball | bull | Boole | bowl | bile | bowel | boil |

## Disyllables with Final, Embedded, and Syllabic /-l/

| | | | |
|---|---|---|---|
| 1. distill | 15. album | 29. film | 43. camel |
| 2. cancel | 16. elbow | 30. calm | 44. little |
| 3. baseball | 17. builder | 31. elk | 45. bottle |
| 4. cruel | 18. children | 32. balk | 46. channel |
| 5. install | 19. selfish | 33. held | 47. funnel |
| 6. Brazil | 20. sulfa | 34. spoiled | 48. careful |
| 7. airmail | 21. Elgar | 35. bulge | 49. cheerful |
| 8. exile | 22. welcome | 36. overwhelm | 50. awful |
| 9. conceal | 23. bulky | 37. help | 51. angle |
| 10. fragile | 24. ailment | 38. nailed | 52. uncle |
| 11. jewel | 25. Walmart | 39. old | 53. pickle |
| 12. rainfall | 26. walnut | 40. smelled | 54. normal |
| 13. vowel | 27. helper | 41. bald | 55. apple |
| 14. royal | 28. alter | 42. calm | 56. castle |

## Sentences with Word-Final Clusters and Morphological Endings

1. The chemist titrated the solution.
2. David swims two miles every day.
3. Once that rocket has been launched, nothing can stop it.
4. When Bob was in army basic training, he missed his wife.
5. In Manhattan, it seems like everyone drives everywhere.
6. In Hawaii, life is very relaxed (according to the ads).
7. The "good Samaritan" acted quickly to save the woman's baby.
8. That kid never asks before he takes something of mine!
9. When one jumps over a fence, one should look first.
10. We went to an arts and crafts fair.
11. He thinks that salt dissolves faster than sugar.
12. The settlers warmed themselves by the fire and toasted their bread.
13. The teacher's son confessed that he had carried out the prank.
14. We walked to Food for Less and staggered home with our bags.
15. If Jackie doesn't call, we won't know if she arrived.
16. That professor has published many papers with his (her) students.
17. One gets used to flying in airplanes, but there is still something unnatural about the experience.
18. In some labs, everything is computerized.
19. The defendants explained their position once more.
20. Politics is only for those with strong hearts and iron stomachs.
21. Mr. Brown hasn't felt well enough to respond to your questions.

## PART II: VOWELS

If a vowel can be spelled in a number of different ways, all relevant spellings have been included. The vowels /ə/, /ʌ/, /ɔ/, and /ɑ/ have not been included because they are rarely in error. The /r/-colored vowels are included under the Consonant section of the Appendix because of the analogies with syllable-final /l/.

### High Front Vowels

| /ɪ/ | /ɪ/ | /i/ | /i/ |
|---|---|---|---|
| 1. bridge | 9. liquid | 1. dream | 9. repeat |
| 2. fist | 10. equip | 2. free | 10. antique |
| 3. cling | 11. him | 3. clean | 11. he |
| 4. brick | 12. his | 4. breeze | 12. she |
| 5. kick | 13. kiss | 5. team | 13. hero |
| 6. fix | 14. flip | 6. keep | 14. flee/flea |
| 7. finger | | 7. Lee | 15. Z (letter) |
| 8. script | | 8. screen | 16. key |

### Minimal Pairs

| /ɪ/ | /i/ | /ɪ/ | /i/ |
|---|---|---|---|
| 1. bit | beat | 10. mitt | meat/meet |
| 2. bid | bead | 11. lid | lead |
| 3. lip | leap | 12. sit | seat |
| 4. hip | heap | 13. fill | feel |
| 5. hit | heat | 14. will | wheel |
| 6. rim | ream | 15. pick | peak |
| 7. shin | sheen | 16. fit | feet |
| 8. pit | peat/Pete | 17. rid | read/reed |
| 9. sin | seen/scene | 18. ship | sheep |

### Phrases with /ɪ/ and /i/

1. make a bid
2. buy a bead
3. kick the ball
4. on the team
5. pick some fruit
6. take a peek
7. do sit down
8. have a seat
9. over the bridge
10. make a fist
11. clean the peaches
12. he said "No"
13. she said "No"
14. shoes fit your feet

*(continues)*

## High Front Vowels *(continued)*

### Phrases with /ɪ/ and /i/

15. a ship full of sheep
16. use the key
17. please repeat that
18. fix the door
19. a liquid diet
20. a nice breeze
21. what a scene
22. time to flee the city
23. read the fine print
24. wearing jeans
25. easy does it

## Mid-Front Vowels

| /ɛ/ | /ɛ/ | /e/ | /e/ |
|---|---|---|---|
| 1. F (letter) | 11. pest | 1. A (letter) | 11. pay |
| 2. M (letter) | 12. plenty | 2. H (letter) | 12. paper |
| 3. X | 13. leather | 3. J | 13. replace |
| 4. N | 14. expect | 4. K | 14. straight |
| 5. S | 15. Texas | 5. may | 15. radiate |
| 6. left | 16. bed | 6. eight | 16. gate |
| 7. step | 17. leg | 7. steak/stake | 17. rain |
| 8. spend | 18. head | 8. snake | 18. neighbor |
| 9. guest/guessed | 19. said | 9. clay | 19. weight/wait |
| 10. sense | 20. catch | 10. vein/vain | 20. Hey! |
|  | (some dialects) |  |  |

### Minimal Pairs

| /ɛ/ | /e/ | /ɛ/ | /e/ |
|---|---|---|---|
| 1. red | raid | 9. west | waist/waste |
| 2. let | late | 10. rest | raced |
| 3. wet | wait | 11. mess | Mace |
| 4. men | main/mane | 12. shed | shade |
| 5. sex | sakes | 13. pest | paste |
| 6. well | wail/whale | 14. get | gate |
| 7. fed | fade | 15. pen | pain |
| 8. bread | braid | 16. wet | wait/weight |

## Phrases with /ɛ/ and /e/

1. they met today
2. the pets ate today
3. a step away
4. for her sake
5. waste of motion
6. spend too much
7. place mat
8. go straight ahead
9. leather shoe
10. replace the plate
11. eat bread too
12. braid the yarn
13. snakes bite
14. plenty of money
15. write a paper
16. the guest house
17. what to expect
18. table for eight
19. the month of May
20. in that vein
21. rest at home
22. radiation alert
23. did not pay attention
24. in left field
25. wait for me

## Low Front Vowel /æ/

1. wrap
2. cap
3. nap
4. hat
5. cat
6. mat
7. bad
8. Dad
9. had
10. back
11. sack
12. rack
13. lack
14. man
15. can
16. hand
17. band
18. ran
19. fan
20. sad
21. ram
22. Sam
23. jam
24. bang
25. hang
26. rang
27. fast
28. cash
29. ash
30. trash
31. crash
32. mash
33. class
34. laugh
35. faster
36. classic
37. ashes
38. camera
39. hammer
40. attack
41. abstract
42. hanger
43. happy
44. attic
45. drastic
46. apple
47. aptitude
48. handle
49. manage

Minimal Pairs

| | /ɛ/ | /æ/ | | | /ɛ/ | /æ/ |
|---|---|---|---|---|---|---|
| 1. | bed | bad | | 11. | fed | fad |
| 2. | head | had | | 12. | met | mat |
| 3. | pest | past | | 13. | dead | Dad |
| 4. | leg | lag | | 14. | men | man |
| 5. | hem | ham | | 15. | bend | band |
| 6. | X | ax | | 16. | Esther | aster |
| 7. | M | am | | 17. | wren | ran |
| 8. | mess | mass | | 18. | said | sad |
| 9. | ten | tan | | 19. | gem | jam |
| 10. | mesh | mash | | | | |

## High Back Vowels

/u/

(See also the "hidden vowel" words)

| | | | | | |
|---|---|---|---|---|---|
| 1. two/to/too | 12. blue | 23. goose |
| 2. new | 13. doom | 24. rude |
| 3. chew | 14. true | 25. crude |
| 4. shoe | 15. crude | 26. nuclear |
| 5. clue | 16. flu/flew | 27. kangaroo |
| 6. room | 17. school | 28. tourist |
| 7. boom | 18. tool | 29. Jupiter |
| 8. noon | 19. cool | 30. lukewarm |
| 9. moon | 20. do/dew | 31. lagoon |
| 10. June | 21. woo | |
| 11. rude | 22. Jewish | |

/ʊ/

| | | | | | |
|---|---|---|---|---|---|
| 1. put | 6. shook | 11. would/wood |
| 2. nook | 7. hook | 12. should |
| 3. look | 8. foot | 13. roof (some dialects) |
| 4. took | 9. root | 14. tush (some dialects) |
| 5. book | 10. could | |

## Mid-Back Vowel

### /o/

1. boat
2. coat
3. bone
4. node
5. code
6. goat
7. note
8. flow
9. grow
10. sew/so
11. no/know
12. slow
13. coal
14. row
15. bowl
16. Coke
17. dome
18. home
19. comb
20. vote
21. coast
22. toast
23. roast
24. boast
25. post
26. lower
27. compose
28. over
29. October
30. component
31. amino-
32. Post Office
33. Kodak

## Diphthongs

### /aʊ/

1. out
2. house
3. mouse
4. shout
5. town
6. clown
7. frown
8. down
9. pound
10. mound
11. ground
12. sound
13. found
14. round
15. loud
16. proud
17. cloud
18. spout
19. about
20. around
21. downpour

### /ɔɪ/

1. boy
2. joy
3. boil
4. noise
5. coil
6. coin
7. toy
8. soy
9. join
10. rejoice
11. royal
12. soy sauce

### /aɪ/

1. time
2. bike
3. fight
4. right/write
5. I
6. sight/site
7. shine
8. rhyme
9. hide
10. side
11. hike
12. type
13. ice
14. five
15. rise
16. my
17. item
18. wider
19. pilot
20. dynamite

"Hidden /ɪ/"

| | | |
|---|---|---|
| 1. pure | 11. muse | 21. confuse |
| 2. cure | 12. music | 22. manuscript |
| 3. cube | 13. use | 23. regular |
| 4. cute | 14. beauty | 24. uniform |
| 5. fume | 15. unite | 25. obscure |
| 6. fuse | 16. beautiful | 26. peculiar |
| 7. fuel | 17. university | 27. Bermuda |
| 8. huge | 18. vacuum | 28. humid |
| 9. few | 19. future | |
| 10. mute | 20. computer | |

# PART III: STRESS PATTERNS AT THE WORD LEVEL

## Two-Syllable Words (Disyllables)

Most two-syllable words have stress on the first syllable. However, disyllables that contain a Latinate prefix, such as *in-*, *re-*, and *de-*, have primary stress on the second syllable.

When two-syllable base words add suffixes at the end, the primary stress usually stays with the syllable that would be stressed without the suffix.

## Three-Syllable Words (Trisyllables)

Trisyllables vary quite a bit in stress pattern. Generally, however, if the word includes a Latinate prefix, that prefix is almost always unstressed.

### Stress Patterns in Disyllables

#### Trochaic Stress Pattern

1-3 or 1-2

| | | | |
|---|---|---|---|
| 1. butter | 6. Kansas | 11. anger | 16. chapter |
| 2. better | 7. captain | 12. better | 17. beaker |
| 3. language | 8. thankful | 13. likely | |
| 4. maybe | 9. grateful | 14. exit | |
| 5. China | 10. accent | 15. diesel | |

Sentences

1. We are learning English.
2. The people are happy.
3. I am reading the story now.
4. Send a letter to your mother.
5. That is a pretty picture.
6. What a tiny office!
7. We are in Parker Hall.
8. They study in the evenings.
9. If you open the door, be careful.

### Stress Patterns in Disyllables

#### Iambic Stress Pattern

3-1 or 2-1

| | | | |
|---|---|---|---|
| 1. about | 8. attract | 15. decide | 22. describe |
| 2. ahead | 9. abstain | 16. remind | 23. machine |
| 3. around | 10. advise | 17. refine | 24. enroll |
| 4. alike | 11. assign | 18. remain | 25. connect |
| 5. behind | 12. define | 19. reply | |
| 6. between | 13. defend | 20. protect | |
| 7. beside | 14. delight | 21. provide | |

Sentences

1. He likes all food, except eggs.
2. Beware the black bears.
3. Please respond at once.
4. She complained about the rooms.
5. Germs can infect our cells.
6. What does this box contain?
7. Children can't behave all the time.
8. What does this report imply?
9. That hotel is too fancy for me.

## Stress Patterns in Three-Syllable Words (Trisyllables)

Stress Pattern

1-3-2

| | | | |
|---|---|---|---|
| 1. unity | 13. isolate | 25. criminal | 37. delicate |
| 2. unify | 14. parasite | 26. motorbike | 38. educate |
| 3. margarine | 15. parachute | 27. ecstasy | 39. applicant |
| 4. marginal | 16. penetrate | 28. vaccinate | 40. medicate |
| 5. parallel | 17. dominate | 29. taxpayer | 41. handicap |
| 6. chemistry | 18. satellite | 30. flexible | 42. algebra |
| 7. isotherm | 19. separate | 31. maximum | 43. logical |
| 8. algorithm | 20. tolerate | 32. Mexico | 44. register |
| 9. copyright | 21. manuscript | 33. oxygen | 45. teenager |
| 10. kilowatt | 22. strategy | 34. broccoli | 46. afterward |
| 11. estimate | 23. afterthought | 35. chocolate | 47. atmosphere |
| 12. opposite | 24. versatile | 36. coconut | 48. Saturday |

Sentences

1. Ride the motorbike.
2. We have to be flexible.
3. The oxygen is almost gone.
4. At last the traveler reached his goal.
5. Broccoli is good for you.
6. The design is based on triangles.
7. The answer to this question is not trivial.
8. We will have to compromise.
9. Please do it as a personal favor.

Center-stress, for example, 3-1-2, 2-1-3, 3-1-3

| | | | |
|---|---|---|---|
| 1. attraction | 8. Manhattan | 15. official | 22. united |
| 2. unhappy | 9. September | 16. creation | 23. professor |
| 3. unlucky | 10. October | 17. elastic | 24. computer |
| 4. remainder | 11. November | 18. tobacco | 25. condition |
| 5. reminder | 12. December | 19. Korea | |
| 6. retainer | 13. assignment | 20. Bermuda | |
| 7. linguistic | 14. assistant | 21. delightful | |

Final stress, for example, 2-3-1

1. engineer
2. Chevrolet
3. Taiwanese
4. reinforce
5. recommend
6. trampoline
7. Vaseline
8. disregard
9. disrespect (n.)
10. Japanese
11. supersede
12. intercede
13. redirect

## Addition of Morphological Endings—Effects on Word-Level Stress Patterns

Most two-syllable base words with primary stress on the second syllable retain primary stress on that syllable when endings are added. However, some endings signal a special stress pattern.

1. attract    attraction    attracting
2. remain    remainder    remaining
3. retain    retention    retaining
4. arouse    arousal    arousing
5. rely    reliance    relying    reliable
6. delight    delightful
7. profess    professor    profession    professional
8. provide    provision    providing    provisional
9. enroll    enrollment    enrolling
10. respond    responsive    responding    responsiveness
11. refine        refining    refinery
12. allow    allowance    allowing    allowable
13. explode    explosion    exploding
14. supply    supplier    supplying
15. complex            complexity
16. erase    eraser    erasing    erasure
17. exhaust    exhaustion    exhausting

*Words that end in *-ition* or *-ation* always have primary stress on the second-to-last syllable.

1. compute    computer    computing    computation*
2. explore    explorer        exploration*
3. repeat        repeating    repetition*
4. restore        restoring    restoration*

Other examples are as follows:

1. separation
2. position
3. dissertation
4. administration
5. arbitration
6. definition
7. abolition
8. conglomeration
9. inhibition
10. distribution
11. accreditation
12. communication

Some words that end in *-ence* or *-ent* have primary stress on the third syllable from the end, but not all such words have this.

| | | | |
|---|---|---|---|
| 1. excel | | excelling | excellence |
| 2. refer | referral | referring | reference |
| 3. neglect | | neglecting | negligent |
| 4. confide | | confiding | confidence |
| 5. confer | | conferring | conference |

Words ending in *-ology* always have the primary stress on the third to the last syllable, such as the following:

1. psychology
2. biology
3. pathology
4. immunology
5. sociology
6. anthropology
7. geology
8. ideology

Words with primary stress on the penultimate (second to last) syllable:
Stress pattern 2-3-1-2 or 2-3-1-3

1. independence
2. supercilious
3. developmental
4. incidental
5. accidental
6. governmental

# GLOSSARY

● ● ● ● ● ● ● ● ● ● ● ● ● ● ● ● ● ● ● ● ● ● ● ● ● ● ● ● ● ● ● ● ● ● ● ● ●

**4-exemplar rule:** A child cannot be said to use a phonological process productively unless there are at least four exemplars of that process in the speech sample.

**40% rule:** A child uses a phonological process productively if she uses it in 40% or more of the opportunities to use that process.

**50-word point:** The point at which the child uses 50 different words, usually at about 18 months. It is at this point that children typically begin using two-word utterances. In addition, they also begin to "phonologize" their speech sound system, that is, they begin to differentiate words into the phonemes that make up the words.

**Affricate:** A sound made up of a stop component followed by a fricative component, for example, /ʧ/

**Age of acquisition for a phoneme:** The earliest age at which 75% or 90% of children produce that phoneme correctly

**Allophone:** An articulatory or acoustic variant of a phoneme that is still considered to represent that phoneme

**Alveolar:** Relating to articulatory placement on the alveolar ridge, most often the upper alveolar ridge. In English, /n t d s z l/ are alveolar sounds.

**Alveolar assimilation:** A phonological process in which a velar target early in the word changes to an alveolar in the presence of an alveolar later in the word, for example, [dot] for *goat*

**Approximant:** A shorthand way of referring to liquids and glides, that is, to non-nasal consonants with a strong resonance structure

**Antecedent event:** An event that precedes the client's attempt to produce the desired response. Such events may include models, cues, and other devices to assist the client.

**Articulation:** The motoric, phonetic, and acoustic aspects of speech production

**Articulation Competence Index (ACI):** A measure of severity developed by Shriberg (1993) for children whose errors are primarily distortions

**Assessment:** Administration of a procedure intended to determine performance in a given area of function

**Assimilation process:** A phonological process that involves changing a consonant to make it similar to a consonant elsewhere in the word

**Auditory bombardment:** A procedure developed by Hodson and Paden (1991) in which a child hears a number of words that contain a particular phonological structure, for example, initial /r/-consonants. May be provided using amplification.

**Backing:** A phonological process involving substitution of a velar for an alveolar, for example, [gɪr] for *deer*

**Bizarreness:** The degree to which the child's error pattern draws attention to the speech

**Bracket:** The symbol used to indicate that one is referring to a particular production or type of production, such as [eɪ]

**Breath group:** The group of syllables spoken on one breath

**C:** Abbreviation for a consonant

**Capability:** The linguistic characteristics and risk factors affecting a client's ability to learn phonology

**Carryover:** Generalization to situations, locations, or conversational partners other than the situation in which the treatment for speech sound problems is provided (usually a clinical room with a speech-language pathologist)

**Case history:** The body of information obtained from the client or from a person who is knowledgeable about the client concerning aspects of the client's history, onset of communication difficulties, and current function

**Causal-correlates:** Variables that have been identified in the past as related to the presence of a speech sound disorder, and also variables that are plausibly related on the basis of phonological theories

**Citation form:** A word spoken as a single word in an isolated utterance

**Clear speech:** The connected-speech equivalent of citation forms, usually spoken rather slowly and with emphasis on acoustic distinctions

**Cluster reduction:** A phonological process resulting in deletion of one or more elements of a consonant cluster

**Coarticulation:** The overlapping of articulatory gestures for neighboring speech sounds

**Coda:** In a syllable, all of the consonants at the end of the syllable

**Cognitive phonology:** A theory of phonological acquisition that focuses on the child's active processing of phonological information

**Colloquial speech:** The everyday conversational form of speech, which typically includes many deletions and assimilations

**Confidence interval:** In statistics, a range on either side of a score obtained on a test such that one can have a certain level of assurance that the true score lies in that range. Confidence intervals are usually determined by taking the obtained score plus or minus one standard deviation for the 65% confidence interval or plus or minus two standard deviations for the 95% confidence interval.

**Consequent event:** An event that occurs after the client has attempted the desired response. Such events include positive reinforcement and feedback.

**Consistency:** The degree to which performance stays the same from exemplar to exemplar

**Consonant cluster:** A sequence of two or more consonants within a syllable, also called a "blend"

**Context-related shortening of a segment:** Regular changes to the duration of a segment such as a phoneme or syllable that are due to the context in which the segment is produced. For example, the duration of the segment *speed* is much shorter in the word *speedily* than it is when *speed* is said in citation form.

**Contextual variation:** The degree to which production of a phoneme varies with the phonetic content of the phonemes surrounding it

**Continuum of treatment:** A way to conceptualize the phases involved in the treatment process

**Contrastive speech:** A production in which the differences between two words are emphasized

**Cross-sectional design:** A research design that involves studying groups of children at successive age levels, usually contrasted with "longitudinal design"

**Cutoff for the lowest 10%:** In formal tests of articulation and phonology, the scores that fall at or below the 10th percentile of the norming population. Children with these scores usually qualify for further assessment and/or intervention. This criterion is in common use.

**Cutpoint at two standard deviations below the mean:** In formal tests of articulation and phonology, the scores that fall at or below the point that represents two standard deviations below the mean, or approximately 2.5% of the population. This is an extremely conservative criterion.

**Depalatalization:** A phonological process that involves substitution of an alveolar for a palatal consonant, for example, [sip] or [tip] or [dip] for *chip*

**Developmental Verbal Dyspraxia (DVD):** A condition of speech impairment characterized by a presumed difficulty in sequencing speech movements, also called **Developmental Verbal Apraxia (DVA)** and **Developmental Apraxia of Speech (DAS or DAOS)**

**Diacritics:** Symbols that can be placed adjacent to a phoneme symbol to represent a particular characteristic of the production

**Diagnostic evaluation:** A formal evaluation, usually comprehensive, done to determine the dimensions of the communication difficulties, the factors that may be related to the problem, the need for further referrals, and the likely outcomes with and without intervention

**Dialects:** Distinctive but mutually intelligible varieties of a language that are spoken by large groups of people

**Diphthong:** A single vowel phoneme that involves the successive articulation of two different vowel qualities. English phonemic diphthongs include /aɪ aʊ ɔɪ/.

**Diphthongized vowel:** A tense vowel that has an off-glide similar to a different vowel, such as [eɪ] for /e/

**Discrimination training:** See **Perceptual training.**

**Disfluencies:** Repetitions, hesitations, prolongations, blocks, and intrusive sounds that interrupt the flow of speech

**Distinctive feature:** The smallest characteristic that can make a difference between two phonemes

**Duration of speech sounds:** The length of a segment or segments as measured in milliseconds or portions of a second. There are a number of different computerized systems for measuring the durations of speech sounds.

**Dynamic assessment:** Assessment that takes account of the child's performance in a social environment. Dynamic assessment involves searching for ways to assist the child to move forward. In phonology, this means looking for points at which the child appears ready to change.

**Dyspraxia:** Difficulty in sequencing volitional movements. The adjective form is **dyspraxic.**

**Ear training:** See **Perceptual training.**

**Epenthesis:** The addition of a sound or a syllable to a word

**ESL:** Abbreviation for English as a Second Language

**Establishment (elicitation) phase:** The early part of the continuum of treatment. The goal during this phase is stable, accurate production of the target sound or syllable in at least one phonetic context, for example, isolation or syllable.

**Etiology:** The origin or cause of a phenomenon. In speech language-pathology, etiology is used most often in reference to a type of communication disorder.

**Exaggerated speech:** Speech in which certain words are emphasized in a dramatic way

**Exemplar:** A phoneme or a word in which a given phonological process has an opportunity to occur

**Facilitating context:** The context in which the target phoneme is uttered contains other speech sounds that appear to make the phoneme easier to say. For example, if /r/ is the target, then the word *grow* might represent a facilitating context because both the /g/ and the /o/ are made in the back of the mouth, as is /r/.

**Favorite sound:** An idiosyncratic phonological process whereby the child chooses to say words that contain a particular sound, and also uses this sound to substitute for a variety of other consonants, such as [t], as in [ti] for *see*, [tɪp] for *ship*, [tin] for *green*, and [bɛt] for *best*

**Final:** Occupying the last position in a word or syllable, that is, the coda

**Final consonant deletion:** A phonological process in which final consonants are deleted, resulting in open syllables

**Final declination:** The decrease in both pitch and intensity that occurs at the end of a typical breath group, if the utterance is declarative

**Fluency:** The degree to which speech is forward-moving, smooth, and rhythmic

**Focus:** Client-based factors affecting phonological learning, including ability to attend, recognition of need to change, and effort applied in learning

**Foot:** In poetry and in some types of speech analysis, the basic unit of rhythm. In English, the foot is one stressed syllable with one or two adjacent unstressed syllables.

**Formal speech:** The type of speech used in giving presentations, speaking to a person worthy of respect, and engaging in professional interactions

**Frame-and-content theory:** A theory of phonological acquisition that has a focus on the child's differentiation of consonants and vowels

**Fricative:** A speech sound made with a continuous airstream forced past an obstruction, for example, /s/

**Fronting:** A phonological process that involves substitution of an alveolar for a velar consonant, such as [tʌm] for *come*

**Frozen form:** Versions of words that a child produced at a much younger age and that the child continues to produce in the same way despite advances in the phonological system

**Function words (functors):** The set of words that includes copular verbs, auxiliary verbs, modal verbs, prepositions, pronouns, relative pronouns, and certain adverbs (those not formed by adding -*ly* to adjectives). These words are all members of classes of words that do not admit new members, and they are mostly unstressed in connected speech.

**Functionality:** A measure of how useful the child's speech is for activities of daily communication

**Generalization phase:** A part of the continuum of treatment during which the client learns to use the target in a variety of linguistic contexts and a number of speaking situations

**Generative phonology:** A theory of phonology that has a focus on the nature of the child's implicit knowledge about the speech sound system

**Gliding:** A phonological process that involves substitution of a glide for a liquid in initial or intervocalic position, for example, [waɪt] for *light*

**Gloss:** The listener's interpretation of the words that he understands the speaker to say

**Glottal:** Referring to characteristics of sounds made at the glottis. In English, the two glottal sounds are the glottal stop /ʔ/ and the /h/.

**Glottal Replacement:** An idiosyncratic process in which some or all consonants are replaced with glottal stops, such as [ʔɪʔ] for *fish*

**Iamb:** A foot that has two syllables with the stress pattern weak-strong, as in the word *beside*. The related adjective is *iambic*.

**Idiosyncratic processes:** Regularities in a given child's phonology that are unique to the child, that is, are uncommon among typically developing children. An example might be the process called Initial Glottal Replacement, in which the child substitutes a glottal stop for the first consonant in a word such as *shoe*.

**Inconsistency:** A tendency to vary the production of a given phoneme or phonological structure

**Inconsistency with hits:** Variable productions that include one or more in which the target segment is correct

**Independent analyses:** Procedures for describing a child's sound system without reference to the adult system

**Inflectional morphemes:** Elements of meaning that are added to a content word, for example, the plural marker -*s*, the past tense marker -*ed*, and so forth

**Initial:** Occupying the first position in a syllable or word, that is, the onset

**Intelligibility:** A measure of how understandable the child's conversational speech is to others

**Interdental:** Made with the tongue between the teeth. In English, the interdentals include /θ ð/.

**International Phonetic Alphabet (IPA):** The standard transcription system used in linguistics and speech-language pathology

**Intervocalic:** Occurring between two vowels

**Intonation contour:** A schematic of the perceived change in vocal intonation over the entire utterance

**Knowledge hierarchies:** A listing of a child's relative knowledge of phonological structures from most to least

**Lax vowels:** Vowels produced with relatively little effort or muscle tension, including /ɪ ɛ æ ʊ ə/. Lax vowels cannot occur in open syllables in English.

**Liquid:** A type of non-nasal consonant characterized by its resonance structure. Liquids include /l/ and /r/.

**Longitudinal design:** A research design that involves following the same children over time, usually contrasted with "cross-sectional design"

**Loudness contour:** A schematic of the perceived change in vocal loudness over the entire utterance

**Maintenance phase:** A part of the continuum of treatment in which the clinician gradually transfers responsibility for carryover into other speaking situations and contexts to the client

**Mean:** In statistics, the average of a set of numbers. In practice, the mean test score is the most typical score for a group of children of a particular age.

**Medial:** A position within a word that is anywhere between the first phoneme and last phoneme. This term was used frequently in the early years of the profession; however, currently this term is not often used because of its imprecision.

**Metaphonology:** The ability to reflect on one's own speech productions

**Metathesis:** A phonological process in which one phoneme-sized unit is shifted from one position to another, for example, [nupɪs] for *Snoopy*

**Morphology:** The study of units of meaning in a language. Also, systematic changes to words that change the meaning of those words in a specific way. For example, in English, inflectional morphemes are often added to the beginning or end of content words, such as, adding *s* to the word *cat* to make the plural *cats*.

**Nasal:** A speech sound made with an oral obstruction and nasal opening so that there is a characteristic nasal resonance structure. English nasals include /m n ŋ/.

**Natural phonology:** A theory of phonology that is oriented toward discovering the common features of languages and especially the common aspects shown by children acquiring the sound system of their native language

**Natural processes:** Phonological processes that appear to be a result of every child's biological predisposition because they are very commonly used by young children learning a variety of languages

**Neurodevelopmental Treatment (NDT):** A method of treating motor dysfunction in children, developed by Bobath (1980). NDT has a focus on inhibiting abnormal tone and reflexes and on normalizing movement, balance, and equilibrium. Although NDT was originally developed for children with cerebral palsy, it is used with other populations as well.

**Nonlinear phonology:** A theory of phonological acquisition and performance that has a focus on hierarchical relationships that exist within words and phrases

**Norms:** Levels of typical performance on a given measure at specific chronological ages in the population sampled

**Nucleus:** The part of a syllable that is either a vowel or a syllabic consonant. The nucleus comes between the onset, if any, and the coda, if any.

**Obstruent:** A non-nasal speech sound made with an obstruction in the oral cavity such that pressure builds up behind the obstruction. In English, the obstruents include the stops, fricatives, and affricates.

**Onset:** All the consonants at the beginning of a syllable

**Oral-motor treatments:** Methods of treating speech sound disorders that have as their goal increasing the strength and agility of the articulators. A broader definition would include treatments that also emphasize sensory and reflexive aspects of the articulators.

**Open syllable:** A syllable with no ending consonant, such as V or CV

**Palatal:** A speech sound made with an approximation to the hard palate. In English, /j/ is a palatal glide and /ʃ ʒ tʃ dʒ/ are palatal obstruents.

**Percentage of Consonants Correct (PCC):** A metric for determining severity of a phonological disorder

**Percentage of Intelligible Words (PIW):** A metric for determining how intelligible (understandable) a person is

**Percentile rank**: In statistics, a way of showing where in a population a particular score lies. For example, a score at the 25th percentile is at the point where 25% of the population have scores below that level and 75% have scores above that level.

**Perceptual training**: Teaching the child to identify sounds in isolation and in the stream of speech and to perceive differences among sounds

**Phonetic error**: An error that appears to be due to failure to move an articulator appropriately

**Phonetic inventory**: An independent analysis system that is an organized list of the types of speech sounds the child uses. This can be done for both consonants and vowels.

**Phonological awareness**: The capacity to see relationships among phonemes, syllables, and words, and also to manipulate these structures

**Phonological idiom**: A word produced in a surprisingly advanced form compared to the rest of the child's phonology

**Phonological process**: A description of a regularly occurring pattern in the child's production, stated in terms of the adult system

**Phonology**: (1) The sound system of a language, (2) an individual child's sound system, or (3) the study of speech sound systems

**Positive reinforcement**: A consequent event that increases the probability of an acceptable response in the future

**Potential dyspraxic element (PDE)**: A characteristic or behavior that would be considered a marker for Developmental Verbal Dyspraxia if that characteristic or behavior were accompanied by several others that are typically associated with DVD

**Pragmatics**: The way that language and speech are used. For example, if a speaker is going to change the topic, she usually indicates that to the listener, perhaps saying, "I want to tell you about something else."

**Praxis**: As defined by Velleman and Strand (1994), "praxis is the ability to select, organize, and initiate the motor pattern (for a particular action)" (p 110).

**Prevalence**: The proportion affected in the population at any one point in time

**Probe**: A mini-assessment intended to capture any changes that are taking place in a system

**Productive Use**: Refers to a phonological structure or a phonological process. The child uses the structure or process frequently enough that the use is not random. See **40% rule**.

**Prognosis**: An educated forecast about the client's future with respect to a speech sound disorder

**Prosody**: The rhythm, intonation contour, loudness contour, rate, and perceived stress in an utterance

**Reduplication**: A phonological process that results in the repetition of a syllable in whole or in part, resulting in a CVCV or a VCVC form. In full reduplication, the two CVs are the same, for example, [baba] for *blanket*, while in partial reduplication either the two Cs or the two Vs may differ, for example, [babo] for *bottle*.

**Register**: A mode of talking that can affect phonology, prosody, level of fundamental frequency, variations in laryngeal tone, and word choice. Examples are whispering, baby talk, and formal speech.

**Relational analyses**: Procedures for describing a child's phonological system with reference to the adult system

**Reliability:** In statistical terms, the degree to which a given result may vary between two administrations of the same test instrument, or among different persons administering the same instrument, or between a small group of subjects and an expanded group of subjects

**Residual errors**: Errors on individual phonemes past the age of acquisition for that phoneme

**Response definition:** A statement of the criteria for considering a response to be acceptable

**Rime:** The part of a syllable that comes after the onset. It consists of a nucleus (usually a vowel or a syllabic consonant) and a coda.

**Schedule of positive reinforcement:** The plan for positive reinforcement that determines how frequently and when a correct response will be reinforced

**Screening:** A type of quick but representative test, often informal, to indicate if further evaluation is necessary

**Segmental (phonemic) inventory:** An organized list of adult phoneme targets and the child's corresponding productions that can be carried out for both consonants and vowels

**Self-evaluation:** The client evaluates his or her own productions with respect to accuracy.

**Sensory aversion:** A condition in which the client does not want to encounter particular textures or tastes in the mouth or particular textures on the body

**Sensory Integration (SI) Therapy:** A system of therapy developed by Ayres (1972) for children who appear to have difficulties in integrating tactile, kinesthetic, and other sensory input to interact with their environment. Although not developed specifically for autism, SI therapy is often used with this population.

**Sentence-level stress:** The location of emphasized words in an utterance

**Sequential constraints:** An independent analysis that indicates what kinds of speech sounds can follow each other. For example, the child may have no word-initial consonant clusters, that is, no words in which one consonant directly follows another in the same syllable.

**Severity:** A measure of how disordered or deviant the child's speech is in terms of its deviation from some standard

**Singleton consonant**: A consonant not preceded or followed by another consonant in a syllable

**Slash:** The symbol used to indicate that one is referring to a particular phoneme, such as /e/

**Sound Production Task (SPT):** A probe in which a target phoneme is placed in a variety of contexts from isolation to sentences

**Speaking rate:** The rate at which a person talks, usually measured in words per minute or syllables per minute. Pauses longer than two seconds are usually excised.

**Special-purpose test:** In phonology, a test designed for a specific purpose other than comparing the child's performance to norms

**Speech-language pathologist:** A person who provides professional services to persons with speech and language disorders and who holds either the Certificate of Clinical Competence from the American Speech-Language-Hearing Association, or state licensure, or both

**Speech sound discrimination:** The ability to hear the difference between different productions of a target phoneme or segment, most importantly the difference between correct and incorrect productions. Also called speech sound perception.

**Speech sounds:** All types of oral production of sounds intended for communication

**Standard deviation:** In statistics, a mathematical way to describe the variability of a set of numbers (scores) based on the distance of each score from the mean

**Standard scores:** A transformation of the mean and standard deviation of a set of scores to a frequently used scale, such as one with a mean of 50 or 100 and a standard deviation of 10

**Standardized test:** A test that is developed so as to be representative of a large population. A standardized test usually provides some form of norms to the user.

**Stimulability:** The ability to imitate correctly an errored sound under specified conditions

**Stopping:** A phonological process that involves the substitution of a stop for a fricative or an affricate, such as [du] for *zoo*

**Stress-timed languages:** Languages in which the basic unit of rhythm is the foot, and the feet tend to come at equal intervals. (A foot is one stressed syllable and zero, one, or two adjacent unstressed syllables.)

**Strident:** A feature of some speech sounds that have high-frequency noise as a component. In English, the strident phonemes include /f v s z ʃ ʒ ʧ ʤ/.

**Substitution process:** A phonological process that involves the substitution of one phoneme-sized unit for another

**Suprasegmentals:** Characteristics of an utterance that transcend the segments, including intonation pattern, intensity variations, and duration (rate)

**Syllabic consonant:** A consonant that can function as a syllable. Examples in English include /l/, /r/, /m/, /n/, and /ŋ/.

**Syllable and word shape inventory:** An independent analysis that is a listing of the types of syllable shapes and word shapes the child uses

**Syllable coalescence:** Two or more syllables are said as one syllable, but aspects of the two original syllables are preserved

**Syllable shape:** An indication of the order of consonants and vowels in the syllable using C for any consonant and V for any vowel

**Syllable Structure Processes:** Phonological processes that affect syllable and word shapes

**Syllable-final:** The position of a segment at the end of a syllable

**Syllable-initial:** The position of a segment at the beginning of a syllable

**Syllable-timed languages:** Languages in which the basic unit of rhythm is the syllable, and the syllables tend to come at equal intervals

**TALK:** A procedure for sampling a client's productions of a target phoneme in a three-minute sample of conversation

**Tactile defensiveness:** A child's unwillingness to be touched in particular places, such as around the mouth, or to encounter particular textures on the skin or in the mouth

**Tangible reinforcer:** A reinforcer that can be handled, such as a token, an object, or a food item

**Team:** The group of persons involved in providing services to a client, usually including a variety of professionals as well as family members

**Tense vowels:** Vowels produced with a relatively large amount of effort. Tense vowels can be diphthongized. In English, only tense vowels can occur in open syllables. The tense vowels include /i e ʌ u o ɔ ɑ/.

**Token economy:** A system of tangible rewards that the client can accumulate and exchange later for a desired object

**Total Communication:** A method of intervention for speech and language problems in children with developmental disorders that involves signing plus speech

**Training broad:** Remediation directed to several exemplars of one phonological process and/or to several processes at the same time, with no expectation of bringing the child to a high level of correct production through training alone

**Training deep:** Remediation directed to just one or two sounds, taking them from the establishment phase through the maintenance phase

**Transcription, broad or systematic**: Use of the traditional consonant and vowel symbols to indicate the phoneme class and identity of the speech sound that was produced

**Transcription, narrow or phonetic**: Use of diacritics and/or words to capture additional details about the way the sound was produced

**Trochee:** A foot that has two syllables with the stress pattern strong-weak, as in the word *baby*. The related adjective is *trochaic*.

**Underlying representation (UR):** A hypothesized stored form for a word or a phoneme that serves as an internal reference. There may be separate URs for perception and production. It is sometimes called underlying form.

**Utterance-final lengthening:** The strong tendency for the last word or the last syllable in an utterance to be longer than it would be if embedded within the utterance

**V:** Abbreviation for a vowel

**Velar:** A speech sound made with an obstruction at the velum. English velars include /k g ŋ/.

**Velar Assimilation:** A phonological process that involves an alveolar target early in the word changing to a velar in the presence of a velar later in the word, for example, [gagɪ] for *doggie*

**Vernacular:** Colloquial speech

**Vocalization:** (1) Any sound made using voice, including grunts, squeals, and cries, or (2) the phonological process of changing a consonant segment into a vowel. For example, when /l/ or /r/ is syllabic and the child substitutes a vowel such as the schwa instead, that is called the process of Vocalization.

**Vowel quadrilateral:** A four-sided figure that is a schematic representation of the vowels of English in terms of the tongue's height and the tongue's position from front to back of the mouth

**Vowel reduction**: The use of a more central vowel for a vowel target that is less central, usually occurring in unstressed syllables

**Weak Syllable Deletion:** The phonological process of deleting unstressed syllables, for example, saying *remember* as [mɛmbɚ]

**Word recipes:** A type of idiosyncratic process in which words of a given type are produced in a similar way, such as *bunny* said as [bʌji], *tummy* said as [tʌji], *monkey* said as [mʌji], and *baby* said as [beji]

**Word shape:** An indication of the order of consonants and vowels in the word using C for any consonant and V for any vowel

**Word-final:** The position of a segment at the end of a word

**Word-initial:** The position of a segment at the beginning of a word

**Word-level stress:** A description of the relative prominence of syllables in a word

# REFERENCES

●●●●●●●●●●●●●●●●●●●●●●●●●●●●●●●●●●●●●

Aase, D., Hovre, C., Krause, K., Schelfhout, S., Smith, J., & Carpenter, L. (2000). *Contextual Test of Articulation*. Eau Claire, WI: Thinking Publications.

American Psychiatric Association. (2000). *Diagnostic and statistical manual of mental disorders, text revision (DSM-IV-TR)*. Washington, DC: Author.

American Speech-Language Hearing Association. (1983). Social dialects. *Asha, 25*(9), 23–24.

American Speech-Language Hearing Association. (1985). Clinical management of communicatively handicapped minority language populations. *Asha, 27*(6), 29–32.

Andrews, G., & Ingham, R. (1971). Stuttering: Considerations in the evaluation of treatment. *British Journal of Communication Disorders, 6*, 129–138.

Aram, D. (1984). Preface to the issue of *Seminars in Speech and Language, 5*(2), devoted to Developmental Verbal Apraxia, unnumbered pages.

*ASHA Leader*. (2001, May 1). SLPs face average monthly caseload of 53, pp. 3, 29. Rockville, MD: American Speech-Language Hearing Association.

Ayres, A. J. (1972). *Sensory integration and learning disorders*. Los Angeles, CA: Western Psychological Services.

Bain, B. A. (1994). A framework for dynamic assessment in phonology: Stimulability revisited. *Clinics in Communication Disorders, 4*, 12–22.

Baker, R. D., & Ryan, B. P. (1971). *Programmed conditioning for articulation*. Monterey, CA: Monterey Learning Systems.

Bankson, N. W. , & Bernthal, J. E. (1990). *Bankson-Bernthal Test of Phonology (BBTOP)*. Austin, TX: Pro-Ed.

Bankson, N. W., & Byrne, M. C. (1972). The effect of a timed correct sound production task on carryover. *Journal of Speech and Hearing Research, 15*, 160–168.

Bashir, A., Grahamjones, F., & Bostwick, R. (1984). The touch-cue method of therapy for Developmental Verbal Apraxia. *Seminars in Speech and Language, 5*, 127–137.

Bauman-Waengler, J. (2000). *Articulatory and phonological impairments: A clinical focus*. Boston: Allyn & Bacon.

Bernhardt, B., & Stemberger, J. P. (1998). *Handbook of phonological development: From the perspective of constraint-based nonlinear phonology*. San Diego, CA: Academic Press.

Bernhardt, B., & Stemberger, J. P. (2000). *Workbook in nonlinear phonology for clinical application*. Austin, TX: Pro-Ed.

Bernhardt, B., & Stoel-Gammon, C. (1994). Nonlinear phonology: Introduction and clinical application. *Journal of Speech and Hearing Research, 37*, 123–143.

Bernthal, J., & Bankson, N. (1998). *Articulation and phonological disorders* (4th ed). Boston: Allyn & Bacon.

Blache, S. (1982). Minimal word pairs and distinctive feature training. In M. Crary (Ed.), *Phonological Intervention: Concepts and Procedures* (pp. 61–96). San Diego, CA: College-Hill Press.

Blackmer, E. R., & Ferrier, L. (2002). *SPEECHWORKS, 3.15*. Plymouth, NH: Trinity Software.

Blakely, R. (1980). *Screening Test for Developmental Apraxia of Speech*. Tigand, OR: C. C. Publications.

Bleile, K. (1995). *Manual of articulation and phonological disorders*. San Diego, CA: Singular Publishing Group.

Bobath, K. (1980). A neurophysiological basis for the treatment of cerebral palsy. Cambridge, UK: Cambridge University Press.

Boshart, C. (1998). *Oral motor analysis and remediation techniques*. Temecula, CA: Speech Dynamics, Inc.

Bradford, A., & Dodd, B. (1996). Do all speech-disordered children have motor deficits? *Clinical Linguistics and Phonetics, 10,* 77–101.

Bridgeman, E., & Snowling, M. (1988). The perception of phoneme sequence: A comparison of dyspraxic and normal children. *British Journal of Disorders of Communication, 23,* 245–252.

Broen, P.A., & Westman, M.J. (1990). Project Parent: A preschool speech program implemented through parents. *Journal of Speech and Hearing Disorders, 55,* 495-502.

Brown, G. T., & Burns, S. A. (2001). The efficacy of neurodevelopmental treatment in paediatrics: A systematic review. *British Journal of Occupational Therapy, 64,* 235–244.

Camarata, S. (1993). The application of naturalistic conversation training to speech production in children with speech disabilities. *Journal of Applied Behavior Analysis, 26,* 173–182.

Carter, E., & Buck, M. (1958). Prognostic testing for functional articulation disorders among children in the first grade. *Journal of Speech and Hearing Disorders, 23,* 124–133.

Caruso, A., & Strand, E. (Eds.). (1999). *Clinical management of motor speech disorders in children*. New York: Thieme.

Charles-Luce, J., Luce, P., & Vitevich, M. (2000, November 16). *Models of the lexicon*. Paper presented at the Annual Convention of the American Speech-Language-Hearing Association, Washington, DC.

Cheng, L. R. L. (1991). *Assessing Asian language performance: Guidelines for evaluating Limited-English-Proficient students*. Oceanside, CA: Academic Communication Associates.

Chomsky, N., & Halle, M. (1968). *The sound pattern of English*. New York: Harper & Row.

Chumpelik, D. (1984). The PROMPT system of therapy: Theoretical framework and applications for Developmental Apraxia of Speech. *Seminars in Speech and Language, 5,* 139–156.

Compton, A. (n.d.). *Compton P-ESL program*. San Francisco, CA: Institute of Language and Phonology.

Costello, J., & Ferrer, J. (1976). Punishment contingencies for the reduction of incorrect responses during articulation instruction. *Journal of Communication Disorders, 9,* 43–61.

Crary, M. (1993). *Developmental motor speech disorders*. San Diego, CA: Singular Publishing Group.

Cruttenden, A. (1986). *Intonation*. Cambridge, UK: Cambridge University Press.

Crystal, D. (1982). *Profiling linguistic disability*. London: Edward Arnold.

Cummins, J. (1984). *Bilingualism and special education: Issues in assessment and pedagogy*. Clevedon, UK: Multilingual Matters, Ltd.

Das, J-P. (2002). A better look at intelligence. *Current Directions in Psychological Science, 11,* 28–33.

Davis, B. L., Jakielski, K. J., & Marquardt, T. P. (1998). Developmental Apraxia of Speech: Determiners of differential diagnosis. *Clinical Linguistics and Phonetics, 12,* 25–45.

Davis, B., & MacNeilage, P. (1990). Acquisition of correct vowel production: A quantitative case study. *Journal of Speech and Hearing Research, 33,* 16–27.

Dawson, G. & Watling, R. (2000) Interventions to facilitate auditory, visual, and motor integration in autism: A review of the evidence. *Journal of Autism and Developmental Disorders, 30,* 415-421.

Dialect Accent Specialists, Inc. Lyndonville, VT.

Diedrich, W. (1971). Procedures for counting and charting a target phoneme. *Language, Speech, and Hearing Services in Schools,* 18–32. (Note: There is no volume number. The 1972 issues under this serial name are labeled Volume 1.)

Diedrich, W., & Bangert, J. (1980). *Articulation learning.* Houston, TX: College-Hill Press.

Dunn, L. M. (1965). *Expanded manual for the Peabody Picture Vocabulary Test* (Rev. ed.). Circle Pines, MN: American Guidance Service.

Dunn, L. M. & Dunn, L. M. (1997). *Peabody Picture Vocabulary Test, Third Edition (PPVT-III).* Circle Pines, MN: American Guidance Service.

Dyson, A. (1988). Phonetic inventories of 2- and 3-year-old children. *Journal of Speech and Hearing Disorders, 53,* 89–93.

Edwards, H. T., & Strattman, K. H. (1996). *Accent modification manual.* San Diego, CA: Singular Publishing Group.

Elbert, M., Dinnsen, D. A., Swartzlander, P., & Chin, S. B. (1990). Generalization to conversational speech. *Journal of Speech and Hearing Disorders, 55,* 694–699.

Elbert, M., & Gierut, J. (1986). *Handbook of clinical phonology: Approaches to assessment and treatment.* San Diego, CA: College-Hill Press.

Elbert, M., Shelton, R., & Arndt, W. (1967). A task for evaluation of articulation change: 1. Development of methodology. *Journal of Speech and Hearing Research, 10,* 281–288.

Ertmer, D. J., & Ertmer, P. A. (1998). Constructivist strategies in phonological intervention: Facilitating self-regulation for carryover. *Language, Speech, and Hearing Services in Schools, 29,* 67–75.

Fairbanks, G. (1960). *Voice and articulation drill book.* New York: Harper and Row.

Fenson, L., Dale, P., Reznick, J. S., Thal, D., Bates, E., Hartung, J. P., Pethick, S., & Reilly, J. S. (1993). *MacArthur Communicative Development Inventories.* San Diego, CA: Singular Publishing Group.

Fey, M. (1991). *Language intervention with young children.* Needham Heights, MA: Allyn & Bacon.

Fey, M., & Gandour, J. (1982). Rule discovery in phonological acquisition. *Journal of Child Language, 9,* 71–81.

Forrest, K. (2002). Are oral-motor exercises useful in the treatment of phonological/ articulatory disorders? *Seminars in Speech and Language, 23,* 15–25.

Fudala, J. B. (2000). *Arizona Articulation Proficiency Scale, Third Revision (Arizona-3).* Los Angeles: Western Psychological Services.

Gibbs, E., Sherman-Springer, A. & Cooley, C. (1990, November). *Total Communication for Down syndrome children? Patterns across six children.* Paper presented at the annual convention of the American Speech-Language-Hearing Association, Seattle, WA.

Gierut, J. (1989). Maximal opposition approach to phonological treatment. *Journal of Speech and Hearing Disorders, 54,* 9–19.

Gierut, J. A., Elbert, M., & Dinnsen, D. A. (1987). A functional analysis of phonological knowledge in generalization learning in misarticulating children. *Journal of Speech and Hearing Research, 30,* 462–479.

Gierut, J. A., Morrisette, M. L., Hughes, M. T., & Rowland, S. (1996). Phonological treatment efficacy and developmental norms. *Language, Speech, and Hearing Services in Schools, 27,* 215–230.

Giromaletto, L., Pearce, P. S., & Weitzman, E. (1997). Effects of lexical intervention on the phonology of late talkers. *Journal of Speech, Language, and Hearing Research, 40,* 338–348.

Goldman, R., & Fristoe, M. (2000). *Goldman-Fristoe Test of Articulation-2 (GFTA-2).* Circle Pines, MN: American Guidance Service.

Goldstein, B. (2000). *Resource guide on cultural and linguistic diversity.* San Diego, CA: Singular Publishing Group.

Gordon-Brannan, M., & Hodson, B. (2000). Intelligibility/severity measurements of prekindergarten children's speech. *American Journal of Speech-Language Pathology, 9,* 141–150.

Gresham, F., Beebe-Frankenberger, M., & MacMillan, D. (1999). A selective review of treatments for children with autism: Description and methodological considerations. *School Psychology Review, 28,* 559–575.

Gruber, F. (1999). Probability estimates and paths to consonant normalization in children with speech delay. *Journal of Speech, Language, and Hearing Research, 42,* 448-459.

Grunwell, P. (1985). *Phonological Assessment of Child Speech (PACS).* San Diego, CA: College-Hill Press.

Guitar, B. (1998). *Stuttering: An integrated approach to its nature and treatment.* Second Edition. Baltimore: Williams & Wilkins.

Hadley, P. A., & Rice, M. L. (1991). Conversational responsiveness of speech- and language-impaired preschoolers. *Journal of Speech and Hearing Research, 34,* 1308–1317.

Hall, P. K. (2000). The oral mechanism. In J. B. Tomblin, H. L. Morris, & D. C. Spriestersbach, (Eds.). *Diagnosis in speech-language pathology* (2nd Ed., pp. 91–128). San Diego, CA: Singular Publishing Group.

Hall, P. K., Hardy, J. S., & LaVelle, W. (1990). A child with signs of Developmental Apraxia of Speech with whom a palatal lift prosthesis was used to manage palatal dysfunction. *Journal of Speech and Hearing Disorders, 55,* 454–460.

Hall, P. K., Jordan, L. S., & Robin, D. A. (1993). *Developmental Apraxia of Speech.* Austin, TX: Pro-Ed.

Hammill, D. (1985). *Detroit Tests of Learning Aptitude-2.* Austin, TX: Pro-Ed.

Hayden, D., & Square, P. (1999). *The Verbal Motor Production Assessment for Children (VMPAC).* San Antonio, TX: The Psychological Corporation.

Haynes, W. O., & Pindzola, R. H. (1998). *Diagnosis and evaluation in speech-language pathology* (5th Ed.). Boston: Allyn & Bacon.

Helfrich-Miller, K. (1984). Melodic Intonation Therapy with developmentally apraxic children. *Seminars in Speech and Language, 5,* 119–125.

Helm-Estabrooks, N., Nicholas, M., & Morgan, A. R. (1989). *Melodic intonation therapy*. San Antonio, TX: Special Press, Inc.

Hickman, L. A. (1997). *The Apraxia Profile*. San Antonio, TX: Communication Skill Builders.

Hodge, M. M. (1994). Assessment of children with Developmental Apraxia of Speech: A rationale. *Clinics in Communication Disorders, 4*, 91-101.

Hodge, M. M., & Hancock, H. R. (1994). Assessment of children with Developmental Apraxia of Speech: A procedure. *Clinics in Communication Disorders, 4*, 102–118.

Hodson, B. (1986). *The Assessment of Phonological Processes*. Danville, IL: The Interstate Publishers and Printers.

Hodson, B. W. (1998). Research and practice: Applied phonology. *Topics in Language Disorders, 18*, 58–70.

Hodson, B. W., & Paden, E. (1991). *Targeting intelligible speech*. Austin, TX: Pro-Ed.

Hoffman, P. R. (1993). A whole-language treatment perspective for phonological disorder. *Seminars in Speech and Language, 14*, 142–152.

Hoffman, P. R., Schuckers, G. H., & Daniloff, R. G. (1989). *Children's phonetic disorders: Theory and treatment*. Boston: Little, Brown.

Howell, J., & Dean, E. (1994). *Treating phonological disorders in children: Metaphon-theory to practice* (2nd Ed.). London: Whurr.

Hurt, M. (1991). Changes in parent-child interactions as child's intelligibility improves. Unpublished master's thesis, Kansas State University, Manhattan, KS.

Ingram, D. (1981). *Procedures for the phonological analysis of children's language*. Baltimore: University Park Press.

Jarrold, C., Baddeley, A. D., & Phillips, C. (1999). Down Syndrome and the phonological loop: The evidence for, and importance of, a specific verbal short-term memory deficit. *Down Syndrome: Research and Practice, 6*, 61–75.

Jusczyk, P., Storkel, H.L., & Vitevitch, M. (2000). *The lexicon in development*. Paper presented at the Annual Convention of the American Speech-Language-Hearing Association, Washington, DC.

Kamhi, A., & Catts, H. (1991). *Reading disabilities: A developmental perspective*. Boston: Allyn & Bacon.

Kent, R., & Forner, L. (1980). Speech segment duration in sentence recitations by children and adults. *Journal of Phonetics, 9*, 157–168.

Kent, R., & Murray, A. (1982). Acoustic features of infant vocalic utterances at 3, 6, and 9 months. *Journal of the Acoustical Society of America, 72*, 353–365.

Kent, R., & Read, C. (1992). *The acoustic analysis of speech*. San Diego, CA: Singular Publishing Group.

Kent, R., & Shriberg, L. (1995). *Clinical phonetics* (2nd Ed.). Boston: Allyn & Bacon.

Khan, L., & Lewis, N. (1986). *The Khan-Lewis Phonological Analysis (KLPA)*. Circle Pines, MN: American Guidance Service.

Khan, L., & Lewis, N. (2002). *The Khan-Lewis Phonological Analysis, Second Edition (KLPA-2)*. Circle Pines, MN: American Guidance Service.

Klein, E. S. (1996). Phonological/traditional approaches to articulation therapy: A retrospective group comparison. *Language, Speech, and Hearing Services in Schools, 27*, 314–323.

Kwiatkowski, J., & Shriberg, L.D. (1998). The capability-focus treatment framework for child speech disorders. *American Journal of Speech-Language Pathology, 7*, 27–38.

Lehiste, I. (1970). *Suprasegmentals*. Cambridge, MA: The M.I.T. Press.

Leonard, L. (1985). Unusual and subtle behavior in the speech of phonologically disordered children. *Journal of Speech and Hearing Disorders, 50,* 4–13.

Lippke, B., Dickey, S., Selmar, J., & Soder, A. (1997). *Photo Articulation Test—Third Edition (PAT-3)*. Austin, TX: Pro-Ed.

Locke, J. L. (1980a). The inference of speech perception in the phonologically disordered child. Part I: A rationale, some criteria, the conventional tests. *Journal of Speech and Hearing Disorders, 45,* 431–434.

Locke, J. L. (1980b). The inference of speech perception in the phonologically disordered child. Part II: Some clinically novel procedures, their use, some findings. *Journal of Speech and Hearing Disorders, 45,* 435–468.

Locke, J. L. (1983). *Phonological acquisition and change*. New York: Academic Press.

Long, S., Fey, M., & Channell, R. (2000). *Computerized Profiling (CP), Version 9*. Cleveland, OH: Department of Communication Sciences, Case Western Reserve University.

Macken, M., & Ferguson, C. (1983). Cognitive aspects of phonological development: Model, evidence and issues. In K.E. Nelson (Ed.), *Children's language, 4*. Hillsdale, NJ: Lawrence Erlbaum.

MacNeilage, P., & Davis, B. (1990). Acquisition of speech production: Frames then content. In M. Jeannerod (Ed.)., *Attention and performance XIII: Motor representation and control* (pp.453–475). Hillsdale, NJ: Lawrence Erlbaum.

Madison, C. L. (1979). Articulatory stimulability reviewed. *Language, Speech, and Hearing Services in Schools, 10,* 185–190.

Marquardt, T. P., & Sussman, H. M. (1991). Developmental Apraxia of Speech: Theory and practice. In D. Vogel & M. P. Cannito (Eds.) *Treating disordered speech motor control* (pp. 341–390). Austin, TX: Pro-Ed.

Masterson, J., Long, S., & Buder, E. (1998). Instrumentation in clinical phonology. In J. Bernthal & N. Bankson (Eds.)., *Articulation and phonological disorders, Fourth Edition* (pp. 378–406). Boston: Allyn & Bacon.

Masterson, J., & Pagan, F. (1994). *The Macintosh Interactive System for Phonological Analysis*. San Antonio, TX: The Psychological Corporation.

Matheson, P. B. (1986). Evaluation of a Total Communication approach for children with Down Syndrome. (Doctoral dissertation, Hofstra University, 1986). Dissertation Abstracts International, 47-09B, 3984.

McCabe, P., Rosenthal, J., & McLeod, S. (1998). Features of developmental dyspraxia in the general speech-impaired population? *Clinical Linguistics and Phonetics, 12,* 105–126.

McDonald, E. (1964a). *Articulation testing and treatment: A sensory-motor approach*. Pittsburgh, PA: Stanwix House.

McDonald, E. (1964b). *A Deep Test of Articulation*. Pittsburgh, PA: Stanwix House.

McLean, J. E. (1970). *Extending stimulus control of phoneme articulation by operant techniques*. Rockville, MD: American Speech and Hearing Association Monographs, Number 14.

McNutt, J., & Hamayan, E. (1984). Subgroups of older children with articulation disorders. In R. Daniloff (Ed.), *Articulation assessment and treatment issues* (pp. 51–70). San Diego, CA: College-Hill Press.

McReynolds, L., & Elbert, M. (1981). Criteria for phonological process analysis. *Journal of Speech and Hearing Disorders, 46,* 197–204.

McReynolds, L., & Engmann, D. (1975). *Distinctive feature analysis of misarticulations.* Baltimore: University Park Press.

McReynolds, L., & Kearns, K. (1983). *Single-subject experimental designs in communicative disorders.* Baltimore: University Park Press.

Miccio, A. W., Elbert, M., & Forrest, K. (1999). The relationship between stimulability and phonological acquisition in children with normally developing and disordered phonologies. *American Journal of Speech-Language Pathology, 8,* 347–363.

Milisen, R. (1954). A rationale for articulation disorders. *Journal of Speech and Hearing Disorders, Monograph Supplement 4,* 5–18.

Moskowitz, A. (1973). The acquisition of phonology and syntax: A preliminary study. In K. Hintikka, J. Moravcsik, & P. Suppes (Eds.) *Approaches to natural language* (pp. 48–84). Dordrecht, The Netherlands: Reidel.

Mowrer, D. (1982). *Methods of modifying speech behaviors* (2nd Ed.). Columbus, OH: Charles E. Merrill Publishing Company.

Netsell, R. (1986). *A neurobiologic view of speech production and the dysarthrias.* San Diego, CA: College-Hill Press.

Oller, K., & Delgado, R. (2000). *Logical International Phonetic Programs.* Miami, FL: Intelligent Hearing Systems.

Olswang, L. B., Bain, B. A., & Johnson, G. A. (1992). The zone of proximal development: Dynamic assessment of language disordered children. In S. Warren & J. Reichle (Eds.), *Causes and effects in communication and language intervention* (pp. 187–216). Baltimore: Paul H. Brooks.

Paul, R. (2001). *Language disorders from infancy through adolescence: Assessment and intervention.* St. Louis, MO: Mosby, Inc.

Paul, R., & Shriberg, L. (1982). Associations between phonology and syntax in speech-delayed children. *Journal of Speech and Hearing Research, 25,* 536–547.

Perrine, S. L., Bain, B. A., & Weston, A. D. (2000, November). Dynamic assessment of phonological stimulability: Construct validation of a cueing hierarchy. Paper presented at the annual convention of the American Speech-Language–Hearing Association, Washington, DC.

Peters-Johnson, C. (1992, November). Caseloads in schools. *Asha, 34,* 12.

Pickett, J. (1999). *The acoustics of speech communication.* Boston: Allyn & Bacon.

Pindzola, R., Jenkins, M., & Lokken, K. (1989). Speaking rates of young children. *Language, Speech, and Hearing Services in Schools, 20,* 133–138.

Portwood, M. (2000). *Understanding developmental dyspraxia.* London: D. Fulton Publishers.

Powell, T. W., Elbert, M., & Dinnsen, D. A. (1991). Stimulability as a factor in the phonological generalization of misarticulating preschool children. *Journal of Speech and Hearing Research, 34,* 1318–1328.

Rice, M. L., Sell, M. A., & Hadley, P. A. (1991). Social interactions of speech- and language-impaired children. *Journal of Speech and Hearing Research, 34,* 1299–1307.

Robb, M., & Bleile, K. (1994). Consonant inventories of young children from 8 to 25 months. *Clinical Linguistics & Phonetics, 8,* 295–320.

Robertson, C., & Salter, W. (1995). *Phonological Awareness Test.* East Moline, IL: LinguiSystems, Inc.

Robin, D. (1992). Developmental Apraxia of Speech: Just another motor problem. *American Journal of Speech-Language Pathology, 1,* 19–22.

Ruscello, D. M. (1984). Motor learning as a model for articulation instruction. In J. M. Costello (Ed.), *Speech disorders in children: Recent advances* (pp. 129–156). San Diego, CA: College-Hill Press.

Rvachew, S., & Nowak, M. (2001). The effect of target-selection strategy on phonological learning. *Journal of Speech, Language, and Hearing Research, 44,* 610–623.

Sax, M. (1972). A longitudinal study of articulation change. *Language, Speech, and Hearing Services in Schools, 1,* 41–48.

Schmidt, R. A., & Lee, T. D. (1999). *Motor control and learning: A behavioral emphasis* (3rd Ed.) Champaign, IL: Human Kinematics Press.

Schwartz, R., & Leonard, L. (1982). Do children pick and choose? An examination of phonological selection and avoidance in early lexical acquisition. *Journal of Child Language, 9,* 319–336.

Secord, W. A. (1981). *Eliciting sounds: Techniques for clinicians.* San Antonio, TX: The Psychological Corporation.

Secord, W. A. (1989). The traditional approach to treatment. In N. Creaghead, P. Newman, & W. Secord (Eds.), *Assessment and remediation of articulatory and phonological disorders* (2nd Ed; pp. 129–158). New York: Macmillan.

Secord, W., & Donohue, J. (2002). *Clinical Assessment of Articulation and Phonology (CAAP).* Greenville, SC: Super Duper Publications.

Secord, W. A., & Shine, R. (1997). *Secord Contextual Articulation Tests (S-CAT).* Greenville, SC: Super Duper Publications.

Shipley, K. G., & McAfee, J. G. (1998). *Assessment in speech-language pathology: A resource manual.* San Diego, CA: Singular Publishing Group.

Shriberg, L. (1975). A response-evocation program for /ɝ/. *Journal of Speech and Hearing Disorders, 40,* 92–105.

Shriberg, L. (1986). *Programs to Examine Phonetic and Phonologic Evaluation Records: Version 4.0.* Hillsdale, NJ: Lawrence Erlbaum.

Shriberg, L. D. (1993). Four new speech and prosody-voice measures for genetics research and other studies in developmental phonological disorders. *Journal of Speech and Hearing Research, 36,* 105–140.

Shriberg, L. D. (1994). Five subtypes of developmental phonological disorders. *Clinics in Communication Disorders, 4,* 38–53.

Shriberg, L. (1997). Developmental phonological disorders: One or many? In B. Hodson & M. Edwards (Eds.), *Perspectives in applied phonology* (pp. 105–131). Gaithersburg, MD: Aspen Publishers, Inc.

Shriberg, L. D., Aram, D. M., & Kwiatkowski, J. (1997a). Developmental Apraxia of Speech II. Toward a diagnostic marker. *Journal of Speech, Language, and Hearing Research, 40,* 286–312.

Shriberg, L. D., Aram, D. M., & Kwiatkowski, J. (1997b). Developmental apraxia of speech III. A subtype marked by inappropriate stress. *Journal of Speech, Language, and Hearing Research, 40,* 313–337.

Shriberg, L., & Kent, R. (1995). *Clinical phonetics* (2nd ed.). Boston: Allyn & Bacon.

Shriberg, L., & Kwiatkowski, J. (1982a). Phonological disorders III: A procedure for assessing severity of involvement. *Journal of Speech and Hearing Disorders, 47,* 256–270.

Shriberg, L., & Kwiatkowski, J. (1982b). Phonological disorders I: A diagnostic classification system. *Journal of Speech and Hearing Disorders, 47,* 226–241.

Shriberg, L., & Kwiatkowski, J. (1988). A follow-up study of children with phonologic disorders of unknown origin. *Journal of Speech and Hearing Disorders, 53,* 144–155.

Shriberg, L., & Kwiatkowski, J. (1994). Developmental phonological disorders I: A clinical profile. *Journal of Speech and Hearing Research, 37*, 1100–1126.

Skinner, B. F. (1954). The science of learning and the art of teaching. *Harvard Educational Review, 24*, 86–97.

Slater, S. (1992 August). Portrait of the professions. *Asha, 34*, 61–65.

Sloane, H., Johnston, M., & Harris, F. (1968). Remedial procedures for teaching verbal behavior to speech-deficient or -defective young children. In H. Sloane & B. MacAulay (Eds.), *Operant procedures in remedial speech and language training* (pp. 77–101). Washington, DC: University Press of America, Inc.

Small, L. (1999). *Fundamentals of phonetics*. Boston: Allyn and Bacon.

Smit, A. B. (2000, June). *Pressure Points phonological intervention for preschoolers who are severely unintelligible*. Paper presented at the Child Phonology Conference, Cedar Falls, IA.

Smit, A. B., & Bernthal, J. E. (1983). Performance of articulation-disordered children on language and perception measures. *Journal of Speech and Hearing Research, 26*, 124–136.

Smit, A.B., & Hand, L. (1997). *Smit-Hand Articulation and Phonology Evaluation*. Los Angeles: Western Psychological Services.

Smit, A. B., Hand, L., Freilinger, J., Bernthal, J. B., & Bird, A. (1990). The Iowa Articulation Norms Project and its Nebraska replication. *Journal of Speech and Hearing Disorders, 55*, 779–798.

Square, P. (1999). Treatment of Developmental Apraxia of Speech. In A. Caruso & E. Strand (Eds.), *Clinical management of motor speech disorders in children* (pp. 149–185). New York: Thieme.

Stackhouse, J. (1997). Phonological awareness: Connecting speech and literacy problems. In B. Hodson, & M. Edwards (Eds.), *Perspectives in applied phonology* (pp. 157–196). Gaithersburg, MD: Aspen Publishers, Inc.

Stephens, I., Hoffman, P., & Daniloff, R. (1986). Phonetic characteristics of delayed /s/ development. *Journal of Phonetics, 14*, 247–256.

Stoel-Gammon, C. (1985). Phonetic inventories, 15–24 months: A longitudinal study. *Journal of Speech and Hearing Research, 28*, 505–512.

Stoel-Gammon, C., & Dunn, C. (1985). *Normal and disordered phonology in children*. Baltimore: University Park Press.

Strand, E. A., & McCauley, R. J. (1999). Assessment procedures for treatment planning in children with phonologic and motor speech disorders. In A. Caruso & E. Strand (Eds.), *Clinical management of motor speech disorders in children* (pp. 73–107). New York: Thieme.

Strand, E. A., & Skinder, A. (1999). Treatment of Developmental Apraxia of Speech: Integral stimulation methods. In A. Caruso & E. Strand (Eds.), *Clinical management of motor speech disorders in children* (pp. 109–148) New York: Thieme.

Templin, M. (1957). *Certain language skills in children*. Westport, CT: Greenwood Press, Publishers.

Templin, M., & Darley, F. (1969). *The Templin-Darley Tests of Articulation*. Iowa City, IA: University of Iowa Bureau of Educational Research and Service.

Tiffany, W. (1980). The effects of syllable structure on diadochokinetic and reading rates. *Journal of Speech and Hearing Research, 23*, 894–908.

Tingley, B. M., & Allen, G. D. (1975). Development of speech timing control in children. *Child Development, 46*, 186–194.

Tomblin, J. B., Morris, H. L., & Spriestersbach, D. C. (2000). *Diagnosis in speech-language pathology* (2nd ed.). San Diego, CA: Singular Publishing Group.

Torgeson, J., & Bryant, B. (1993). *Phonological Awareness Test*. Austin, TX: Pro-Ed.

Tyler, A., & Watterson, K. (1991). Effects of phonological versus language intervention in preschoolers with both phonological and language impairment. *Child Language Teaching and Therapy, 7*, 1–160.

Van Riper, C. (1978). *Speech correction: Principles and methods* (6th ed.). Englewood Cliffs, NJ: Prentice-Hall.

Vargas, S., & Camilli, G. (1999). A meta-analysis of research on Sensory Integration treatment. *American Journal of Occupational Therapy, 53*, 189–198.

Velleman, S., & Strand, K. (1994). Developmental verbal dyspraxia; In J. E. Bernthal & N. W. Bankson (Eds.), *Child phonology: Characteristics, assessment, and intervention with special populations* (pp. 110–139). New York: Thieme.

Vygotsky, L. (1978*). Mind in society: The development of higher psychological processes*. Cambridge, MA: Harvard University Press.

Vygotsky, L. (1986). *Thought and language*. Cambridge, MA: MIT Press.

Wade, C. (1996). *A case study: The effects of Melodic Intonation Therapy and oral-motor treatment on initial consonant production by a child with Developmental Verbal Dyspraxia*. Master's thesis, Kansas State University, Manhattan, KS.

Watling, R., Deitz, J., Kanny, E., & McLaughlan, J. (1999). Current practice of occupational therapy for children with autism. *American Journal of Occupational Therapy, 53*, 498–505.

Weiner, F. (1981). Treatment of phonological disability using the method of meaningful minimal contrast: Two case studies. *Journal of Speech and Hearing Disorders, 46*, 97–103.

Westby, C. E. (2000). A scale for assessing development of children's play. In K. Gitlin-Weiner, A. Sandgrund, & C. Schaefer (Eds.), *Play diagnosis and assessment* (2nd Ed., pp. 15–57). New York: John Wiley & Sons, Inc.

Wilcox, K., & Morris, S. (1999). *Children's Speech Intelligibility Measure*. San Antonio, TX: The Psychological Corporation.

Williams, A. L. (2000). Multiple oppositions: Theoretical foundations for an alternative contrastive intervention approach. *American Journal of Speech-Language Pathology, 9*, 282–288.

Williams, A. L. (2003). Speech Disorders: Resource Guide for Preschool Children. New York: Thomson Delmar Learning.

Williams, P., & Stackhouse, J. (2000). Rate, accuracy, and consistency: Diadochokinetic performance of young, normally developing children. *Clinical Linguistics and Phonetics, 14*, 267–293.

Winitz, H. (1969). *Articulatory acquisition and behavior*. Englewood Cliffs, NJ: Prentice-Hall.

Winitz, H. (1975). *From syllable to conversation*. Baltimore: University Park Press.

Yavas, M., & Goldstein, B. (1998). Phonological assessment and treatment of bilingual speakers. *American Journal of Speech-Language Pathology, 7*, 49–60.

Yorkston, K., Beukelman, D., & Tice, R. (2000). *Sentence Intelligibility Test (SIT)*. Communication Disorders Software, Lincoln, NE: Tice Technology Services, Inc.

Zimmerman, I. L., Steiner, V. G., & Pond, R. E. (1992). *Preschool Language Scale-3*. San Antonio, TX: The Psychological Corporation.

# INDEX

••••••••••••••••••••••••••••••••••••••••

Note: Tables are indicated with a letter *t*; figures are indicated with a letter *f*.